ONCOLOGY NURSING

ONCOLOGY NURSING

Cynthia Chance Snyder, R.N., M.N.

Executive Director
LifeCare Services

Little, Brown and Company   Boston   Toronto

Non ridere, non lugere, neque detestari, sed intelligere. (Not to laugh, not to lament, not to curse, but to understand.)

—Spinoza

Library of Congress Cataloging-in-Publication Data

Snyder, Cynthia Chance.
  Oncology nursing.

  Includes index.
  1. Cancer—Nursing. I. Title. [DNLM: 1. Oncologic
Nursing.   WY 156 S675o]
RC266.S68   1986   610.73'698   85-23097
ISBN 0-316-80234-4

Library of Congress Catalog Card No. 85-23097

ISBN 0-316-80234-4

9 8 7 6 5 4 3 2

Published simultaneously in Canada
by Little, Brown & Company (Canada) Limited

Printed in the United States of America

ALP

*The author gratefully acknowledges permission to use the following
material:* p. 275: Myra Bluebond-Langner, *The Private Worlds of Dying
Children.* Copyright © 1978 by Princeton University Press. Fig.,
p. 169, reprinted by permission of Princeton University Press.

Preface

This book is based on my experience teaching oncology nursing to hundreds of undergraduate and graduate nursing students and to professional nurses. The book may be used as a required or adjunct text in undergraduate, graduate, and in-service nursing courses in cancer nursing or in nursing courses about medical-surgical nursing, pediatric nursing, critical care nursing, nursing care of the client with multiple-system failure or care of the client with chronic disease. The text will also be valuable as a resource for hospital oncology units, physicians' offices, clinics, and home health care agencies. Professional nurses who provide continuing education in the various aspects of cancer nursing should find the text to be an invaluable tool.

Oncology Nursing is based on the Snyder Stress-Adaptation Model of Nursing Practice (see "To the Reader"). A teaching structure based on this model and incorporating the use of concepts provides organization to the material. A *concept* as defined here is a clear, singular statement regarding one aspect of a major content area in the broad yet specialized field of oncology nursing. The expression of the concept is followed by explanation or discussion of it in detail and from different perspectives. Whether dealing with content areas containing primarily objective information or with what has been described as "logical mysteries," the concepts themselves have the following points in common:

1. The concepts progress from general to specific, from easy, basic information toward complex, difficult information.
2. The concepts and ensuing discussions deal with definitions of terms, the meaning and significance of the ideas they express, the application of theoretical data to clinical situations, and the nursing implications.
3. The concepts incorporate current research data and provide discussion of conflicting research or controversial views.
4. The presence or absence of certain factors that alter the application of theoretical data to clinical situations is recognized.
5. The interrelationships of the major content areas in oncology nursing are recognized and clarified by the use of concepts.
6. Concepts in the content areas that are defined as "logical mysteries" raise questions rather than merely discuss my value judgment of what is "right." They recognize how the additional sum of involved caregivers impacts on the day-to-day clinical situation and the care received by the client.
7. The concepts show the need for clarifying one's own interpretation of the meaning and nursing implications of the ideas presented.
8. The concepts also demonstrate the learner's need for other involved caregivers to clarify their interpretations of the meaning and implications of the ideas presented.

I hope this approach to the broad but very specialized field of cancer nursing will prove valuable to students and practicing oncology nurses alike.

The author wishes to gratefully acknowledge:

JOVETA K. WESCOTT, R.N., B.S.P.A.
MARILYN SCHULZE, R.N., M.N.
ELEANOR A. SCHUSTER, R.N., D.N.Sc.
MICHAEL GOODWIN, R.N., M.S., M.N.
    who have taught me so much about the uniquely discernible profession of nursing, with its special blend of scientific knowledge and the art of responding with sensitivity and compassion to those who are broken and in need of healing.

DENNIS F. MOORE, M.D.
P. N. KIM, M.D.
JIM CONGDEN, M.D.
STEPHEN A. FIELDS, D.O.
    who consistently demonstrate the unique ability to provide excellent clinical expertise, while carefully acknowledging the intrinsic value and dignity of each ill person who seeks out their care.

CARL M. CHRISTMAN, M.D.
    who so beautifully displays the skill of healing a broken heart . . . a special thank you.

MY STUDENTS
    who consistently challenge me to grow and learn.

MY PARENTS, BILL AND JULIE
    for their consistent support, belief, and love.

MY CHILDREN, CHRISSY, KELLY, STEPHANIE, DEREK, AND JONATHAN
    the apples of my eye, who have no idea of the pleasure and joy that they have brought to the author. They are God's opinion that the world should go on.

MY HUSBAND, DANIEL SNYDER
    who is the personification of the Heavenly Room in the Parable of the Spoons. His splendid love has made the author a wealthy woman in ways not experienced by many.

And finally, I humbly and gratefully acknowledge those persons with cancer—past, present, and future—who touch my life and leave me richer, wiser, and more tender each and every time.

—CCS

To the Reader

The conceptual framework and the teaching structure for this book grew directly out of my experience as a nurse educator and researcher. Although they are closely linked, there is a distinct difference between a conceptual framework and a teaching structure, and it is important to make this distinction clear.

CONCEPTUAL FRAMEWORK

Even though many of us in nursing and the other helping professions speak of theory development, education, clinical practice, and research as though they were separate and distinct entities, they cannot in truth be separated. They blend into one another and, most importantly, are interpreted and carried out in terms of the conceptual framework upon which they rest. Every nurse bases his or her nursing practice on a conceptual framework even though that framework is not often articulated. The conceptual framework provides the theoretical base for every aspect of nursing practice. Nursing education, clinical practice, and nursing research are the visible expressions of a conceptual framework.

This book is based on the *Snyder Stress-Adaptation Model of Nursing Practice and Health Care*, which is described in detail in the first section of the text. Briefly, this theoretical model is comprised of three basic concepts: stress and the individual's response to it, holistic health care, and the concept of self-care. The synthesis of these three perspectives of nursing and the other helping professions form the Snyder Stress-Adaptation Model of Nursing Practice and Health Care, which is the theoretical foundation for the teaching structure used in this text.

TEACHING STRUCTURE

Teachers and learners both discover very quickly that *any* topic must be taught within a structured framework of some kind. If a teaching framework is not developed and consistently used, the teaching is purposeless and unmethodical. Use of a teaching framework gives shape and direction to the presentation of content that might otherwise meander indefinitely within a broad content area in a chaotic, rambling manner.

Oncology nursing covers a vast range of nursing areas: nutrition, pain, various medical treatment modalities, prevention, rehabilitation, terminal care, client teaching, and so on. Without a structured teaching framework firmly based on a sound theoretical conceptual framework, the teaching—and thus the learning— becomes chaotic and confused. All of the major content areas in oncology nursing are intricately intertwined and interdependent, and thus it is crucial that a well-developed conceptual framework and teaching structure be consistently used not only to present effectively the major content areas but also to show clearly the lines of interdependence among those content areas.

CONCEPTS

As a teacher of adult students in cancer nursing, I presented the content in a structured way by using concepts. *Concept,* as it appears in this book and in this teaching framework, is defined as *a singular, coherent element of thought—the expression of one idea about one aspect of a major content area.* The study of the specialty of oncology nursing, like any other area of study, necessitates the understanding of concepts peculiar to its content. Within the major content areas in oncology nursing, a concept is presented as a statement of a singular element or idea and then followed by in-depth explanation of that idea. The explanation that follows the statement of the concept includes exploration of current research focusing on that concept, nursing implications of the application of theoretical data to clinical situations, and discussion of conflicting and sometimes controversial views of various nurses and other health care professionals about that one idea.

The concepts within the major content areas are arranged from easy, basic material to more difficult, complex material. Thus, as the learner progresses through the content, his or her knowledge base increases both in scope and depth as one concept builds and expands on the previous ones. This method has proven to be valuable and hugely successful for hundreds of adult learners. They are able not only to deepen and broaden their knowledge about one aspect of cancer care, but also to clarify the relationships between one aspect of care and another.

It must be emphasized that *concept* as used in this learning style is a single idea that draws the learner's attention to the *meaning* of the concept, to the *implications* stemming from that singular idea, and to the *interrelationships* of that one aspect of cancer care to other aspects of oncology nursing. In this teaching framework, the use of concepts helps both the teacher and the learner to define more clearly and precisely those ideas with which we are concerned.

OBJECTIVE CONCEPTS

Some of the content areas—and thus the concepts presented—are primarily concerned with objective, empirical definitions and facts (e.g., content regarding medical treatment modalities, pathophysiology, etc.). These concepts and the ensuing exploration of the concepts' meanings and implications draw the learner's attention to the development of precise definitions and the interrelationships of specific and primarily objective facts in order to form definitive conclusions.

SUBJECTIVE CONCEPTS

Other content areas deal with subjects that are much more subjective and without exact definitions. In the broad area of chronic cancer pain or care of the dying, for example, there are no clear-cut, well-defined rules. The concepts developed in these content areas present ideas that are essentially "logical mysteries." The conceptual statements and ensuing discussion raise questions to which there are no answers that are indisputably right or wrong, and no single "right" conclusion can be drawn.

A certain amount of objective data are certainly part of these content areas. For example, definitive and objective information about analgesics and methods of pain control are important parts of any teaching about chronic pain, enabling the knowledgeable nurse to assess the client with chronic cancer pain more accurately, develop and implement an effective plan of nursing treatment, and evaluate the degree of the plan's success. These objective data are the logical portion of the "logical mystery."

However, the nurse cannot approach the problem of chronic cancer pain without simultaneously addressing the very subjective and real accompanying problem of suffering. Primarily subjective problems that require (and deserve) nursing and medical intervention—problems such as suffering, helplessness, family dysfunction, the dying process, and so on—are the mystery portion of the "logical mystery."

Concepts addressing these "logical mysteries" present singular, cohesive ideas about aspects of the content, and the ensuing discussion explores the merits of the idea from different perspectives. These particular content areas are the most difficult for both teachers and learners because the very nature of these concepts deals with discernment, clarification, and communication of such ideas as values, ethics, morals, accountability, responsibility, power, authority, etc. As was previously emphasized, no single "right" answer or conclusion can be drawn in response to the questions raised by the conceptual ideas. Instead, the learner is prodded into thinking about an aspect of a logical mystery—thinking that may clarify or reshape the way very real people are treated in very real, day-to-day clinical situations.

For example, when we, as nurses, are faced with the situation of providing care to a client who is dying, we cannot truly separate the nursing and the medical care: they are interdependent. Not only must we deal with the needs of the client, but we must also deal with the attitudes and value judgments of the family, other nurses, attending and consulting physicians, administrators, laboratory and X-ray staff, and so on. Each one of the involved individuals has an attitude not only about what is appropriate terminal care, but also about a particular dying client, and it is the sum of these attitudes that largely determines the care received by a particular dying person. We tend to judge attitudes different from our own as morally or ethically wrong but such attitudes may simply reflect differences about a particular person engaged in the process of dying. This attitudinal sum—the various meanings and clinical applications by all involved persons—becomes intricately enmeshed with and may well change the life-reality for the client.

Contents

PART I

INTRODUCTION TO
ONCOLOGY NURSING

Chapter 1

Concepts of Oncology Nursing

CONCEPT I:
The traditional health care system is based on a superior/inferior relationship between caregiver/recipient of care and is a destructive, nonhealing relationship.

Each discipline has become differentiated from its parent science by examining different phenomena or by asking different questions about the same phenomena, resulting in unique and varied bodies of knowledge [13], and it carries out its problem-solving activities by use of a conceptual model as a framework. A model has a closely linked protocol for observing and analyzing phenomena under study [26]. Much debate exists regarding the validity and viability of nursing theories and models, yet a theory or model *of* nursing is not of great value. What is of significance is a workable theory or model *in* nursing that describes, explains, and predicts client disorders and provides the rationale for effective management of these disorders.

MEDICAL MODEL

Nursing's parent discipline is medicine, which describes and explains client disorders and provides rationale for treatment by the medical model, which in turn is based upon the scientific method. The scientific method reduces the phenomena under study to the smallest possible parts (reductionism). Reductionism is considered the appropriate method of inquiry for any problem [31]. Nursing, however, must expand beyond the method used by its parent discipline since reductionism is not wholly appropriate as a model in nursing. The medical model, because of its acceptance of reductionism, reduces humankind to physiological, psychological, or sociological beings, which in turn can be further subdivided.

The medical model maintains a multitude of polarizations, for example, expert versus laity, superior versus subordinate, healthy versus ill, which legitimizes an ethic of domination that is destructive and profoundly nonhealing in nature. The present traditional health care delivery system promotes fragmentation of care, the person with cancer gives up the role of independent adult and ultimately becomes a captive in the closed world of health care practitioners. In the traditional system, nursing and medicine receive legitimacy for what they claim to do rather than for what actually is done, and thus gain a type of infallibility [4]. An ill person being admitted to a teaching hospital, for example, is often submitted to numerous procedures of questionable value, interminable interviews, mismanaged care, and a

multitude of other horrors. Caregivers speak of invasive and noninvasive procedures, for example, when actually the only difference is in visibility of the invasion.
Invasion of body, mind, and spirit are carried out with impunity and without question by those health care professionals practicing within the framework of the traditional system. Naming intricate, specific diagnoses and being able to put a label
on a chart seems to take precedence over healing, ill persons being reduced to
objects under repair rather than persons being helped to heal. The acutely-ill person most often receives priority attention, but for the individual chronically ill with
cancer, hospitalized living usually is only not dying. Just what is being taught in
teaching hospitals is seemingly never questioned. Technology is primary, and "we
can" somehow becomes "we ought."

Professionals practicing within the framework of the traditional health care delivery system become immune to the physical, psychological, and social impact and
meaning of the care that is delivered to the individual person. Repetition of horror
scenes—"having trouble getting a vein for an IV," bone marrow aspirations, long
periods of time on X-ray tables, autopsies, and so on—eventually result in the
inability to be horrified. Iatrogenic illnesses, or those physical or mental disequilib-
riums *caused* by medical and/or nursing treatments, are not uncommon complications that must be endured by persons with cancer. Sadly, a continually expanding
ethical framework commensurate with the rapidly developing health care technology has not evolved, and procedures are too often done merely because we know
how to do them. The medical model, with its emphasis on reductionism and technology, does not view humankind as physiological, psychological, *and* social
beings, and thus it cannot account for the whole person as an integrated being
who functions as a totality.

NEW PARADIGM OF HEALTH

The health care delivery system in our society has begun to experience
fundamental change, and the new paradigm of health is painfully emerging from
the old paradigm of medicine and sickness. The new paradigm incorporates the
skills and knowledge of the old one but simultaneously is validating old intuitions
and new knowledge about the interaction of mind, body, and environment. In
addition to treating disease and symptoms of disease, the new paradigm of health
seeks to heal the underlying problem causing the disease/disharmony. Aspects of
the old paradigm of medicine and sickness and the new paradigm of health have
been delineated [10], illustrating the transitions being experienced by nursing as
well as all other health professions (See Table 1.1).

CONCEPT II:
Cancer frequently elicits responses of hopelessness and helplessness among caregivers.

Anxiety about cancer is not restricted to those persons who suffer from the
disease but is also experienced by people around them. An overall review of literature reveals that health care professionals have pessimistic and fearful attitudes

Table 1.1. Old Paradigm of Sickness Versus New Paradigm of Health.

Old Paradigm of Sickness	New Paradigm of Health
Medical treatment of symptoms.	Search for patterns and causes, plus treatment of symptoms.
Specialized, with resulting fragmentation of care.	Integrated, concerned with the whole person.
Professional should be emotionally neutral.	Professional's caring and involvement is a component of healing.
Pain and disease are completely negative.	Pain and disease provide information about conflict and disharmony.
Primary intervention with drugs, surgery, radiation treatments.	Intervention with technology is complemented with full armamentarium of noninvasive techniques (psychotherapies, diet, exercise).
Body seen as machine in good or bad repair.	Body seen as dynamic system, as a field of energy within other fields of energy.
Disease or disability seen as thing or entity.	Disease or disability seen as process.
Emphasis on eliminating symptoms, disease.	Emphasis on achieving optimal wellness.
Patient is dependent.	Patient (or client) is or should be autonomous.
Professional is authority.	Professional is therapeutic partner.
Body and mind are separate. Psychosomatic illness is mental, should be referred to psychiatrist.	Bodymind perspective. Psychosomatic illness is province of all health care professionals.
Mind is secondary factor in organic illness.	Mind is primary or coequal factor in all illness. There is no such thing as "pure" organic illness.
Placebo effect shows the power of suggestion or demonstrates that patient's pain is "phony."	Placebo effect shows the mind's ability to control pain and assist in the healing process.
Primary reliance on quantitative information (charts, tests, etc.).	Primary reliance on qualitative information, including client's subjective reports and professional's intuition. Quantitative data important as adjunct information.

Source: Adapted by permission from *The Aquarian Conspiracy: Personal and Social Transformation in the 1980s* by M. Ferguson. Copyright © 1980 by Jeremy P. Tarcher Inc.

about cancer that are very similar to the attitudes of the general public, often including responses of helplessness and hopelessness [6, 9, 28]. Nurses seem to perceive cancer as a dreaded disease and a terminal event, sharing with the layperson feelings of hopelessness in the face of a diagnosis of cancer [1, 22, 23]. It also appears that hospital staff nurses fear cancer more than nurses in other positions, such as clinics or community health, and that this fear is unrelated to knowledge of the disease process or length of nursing experience [11].

These attitudes of fear, hopelessness, and helplessness are inevitably perceived by persons who receive care from nurses, and it is immensely more difficult for individuals with cancer to maintain hope when their caregivers neither share nor support realistic hope.

CONCEPT III:
Nursing management of persons with cancer is complex and multimodal, and may threaten the nurse's sense of professional competence and lead to the desire to escape stressful situations.

Management of nursing care for persons with cancer is systematic, complex, and multimodal. It must be precise in order for it to be effective. With increasing survival times, the problems to be resolved are both more numerous and more complex. As the time following diagnosis of cancer increases, ill persons sense that they have decreased control over their own health and a reduction in the change-effectiveness of their own actions [15]. Decision-making control regarding their lives and health is subtly relinquished to nurses and other health care professionals, increasing the power and concurrent responsibility held by caregivers. Persons with recurrent malignancy experience periods of increased anxiety and disrupted communication [1], depending upon nurses, physicians, and other caregivers to manage not only their physical symptoms of disease but also their emotional reactions to cancer and its treatment.

When compared with nononcology nurses, cancer nurses are more constantly exposed to the emotional turmoil and physical distresses experienced by persons with cancer and their families. Thus, making one's job in oncology nursing the sole life focus will lead to certain psychological devastation for the nurse [21]. Many common problems are intensified for oncology nurses by the very nature of the chronicity and complexity of the disease process and its treatment. Time conflicts are particularly frustrating when the nurse perceives that the ill person needs emotionally supportive, and thus time consuming, conversation. Nurses may experience intense dilemmas over participation in investigational treatment or in therapy that results in distressing and painful side effects, thus jeopardizing the open and communicative relationships necessary with caregivers and clients [21]. Depression and grieving because of disease progression and impending death is common among cancer nurses, and identification with dying persons leads to an intensely profound recognition of the nurse's own mortality. The nurse's subconscious anger at the very ill or dying person's "refusal" to respond to treatment is commonly experienced by the nurse as a sense of guilt for having failed [21]. Frustration over the inability to completely alleviate the physical and emotional pain of the ill person and the family unit may threaten the nurse's sense of competence and professional self-esteem and may lead to avoidance behavior and the desire to escape stressful situations involving the person with cancer [7].

Danger signs indicative of emotional decompensation among oncology nurses have been identified [21]. Depression may be exhibited by sleep disorders, profound malaise, or excessive irritability. The endangered nurse may have dreams filled with conflict material symbolizing conscious defenses that are being overwhelmed by cancer-generated feelings and fears. There may be an inability to emotionally detach oneself from one's job, demonstrated by excessive involvement with persons with cancer and their families, and an inability to stop thinking about the job during nonworking hours. Repetitive accidents or feeling guilty about taking vacation time are also danger signs of emotional decompensation. Strategies to minimize the psychic distress of oncology nurses, which allow the nurse to prevent or heal emotional trauma, are discussed in Chapter 15.

CONCEPT IV:
The art of oncology nursing is rooted in skillful communication, the therapeutic use of self, and a willingness to be accountable for one's nursing actions.

COMMUNICATION AND THE THERAPEUTIC USE OF SELF

The multitude of complex, acute problems encountered by the person with cancer during the chronic course of the disease process causes significant physical, personal, and social distress, and it is a difficult challenge indeed for the caregiver to reduce the ill person's distress. Difficult experiences by persons with cancer are visible, evident, and distressing not only to the ill person but also to the family and caregivers.

By definition, nurses diagnose and treat human responses to actual or potential health problems [2]. This definition implies relationships with those persons who receive nursing care that encompass physical care, emotional support, preventive counseling, and health education. Unfortunately, few nurses, particularly hospital nursing staff, satisfactorily fulfill aspects of nursing other than mere physical care. Nurses are apparently relatively confident of their skills in fulfilling the physical needs of persons with cancer but feel insecure about skills necessary to fulfill emotional, religious, and interpersonal needs [6].

Persons with cancer tend to perceive a *lack* of support from health care providers, including nurses, with even the provision of information relative to surgery and postoperative events perceived to be inadequately presented [12, 16, 23, 33]. In one study, only 25 percent of the persons with cancer identified nurses as a significant source of emotional support, and only 20 percent perceived nurses as significant sources of information [3].

Communication is reliable only if the words serve to reveal, rather than conceal, information. Often in situations of stress, nurses and other caregivers use a variety of communicative defenses in attempts to avoid further distress for the ill person and to reduce the nurses' own discomforts. There may be attempts to convey a high level of intelligence by using words with a high level of unintelligibility. Highly technical language—or the use of common abbreviations such as "N.P.O." or "P.R.N."—instills a sense of awe, ignorance, and fear in the ill person, thus reducing further questions or attempts to communicate [4].

Overintellectualization of the situation is yet another common way for care providers to escape the psychic discomfort generated within the relationship with persons having cancer. In this communication phenomenon, the ill person may say, "Tell me about my cancer," and the caregiver replies with X-ray results, laboratory levels of blood components, and so on. The ill person may actually be voicing a need to discuss the human, experiential, and thus painful meaning and implications of the disease process, yet receives instead quantitative nonanswers about things he or she does not understand. Unless the nurse takes the time to explore the nature of the actual question, nonanswers will be offered under the guise of therapeutic communciation.

Another common block to therapeutic communication is the phenomenon of labeling. This is a means of dehumanizing both the ill person and the caregiver. By labeling an ill person as "confused" or "combative," for example, caregivers are given an excuse for not explaining procedures, offering health teaching, or facilitating self-care. The ill person becomes locked into the closed world of the health care providers. Things are done *to* the ill person, rather than in collaboration, and any sense of autonomy or self is negated [4].

Words may be used to intimidate persons with cancer and their families, further deepening their sense that caregivers are infallible and godlike. Words such as *"I'll give* him 3 months to live," "physician's *orders*," and "you'll have to *ask* your doctor" intimidate many ill persons and their families. Questioning by the person with cancer is viewed as suspicious, for it implies a lack of faith in those who define what is good and bad, appropriate and inappropriate, healthy and sick. Many persons with cancer fear that their "inappropriate" behavior will jeopardize their relationships with caregivers. Caregivers are perceived to be the ill person's link with life and surcease from pain, so the relationship is jealously guarded and protected— even at the expense of the ill person's autonomy.

Both verbal and nonverbal communication may be used as swords to further wound the ill person rather than being used as modalities of healing. Nontherapeutic use of words and self may result in iatrogenic despair, as many caregivers do not have a good understanding of the role played by emotion in wellness and illness. Iarogenic despair may prevent cure and precipitate or perpetuate illness. By decreasing stereotyping of persons with cancer, nurses are more able to see each person as unique and with individual characteristics and needs that are the nurse's responsibility to recognize[6].

"Nurse," in the changing paradigm of health, is a verb as well as a noun, and it is a different verb than "doctor." The fundamental difference between the verbs "nurse" and "doctor" is that one would discover it to be virtually impossible to effectively doctor another person without tools or medicines yet one may indeed effectively nurse without such things. Peripheral definitions of the verb "nurse" include to nourish, to seek to cure, and to handle carefully or fondly [30]. "Nurse" as a verb refers to the process of facilitating wholeness in the client, thus implying relationship. One of the basic tenets of holism is that any addition to the system changes it [32]. Therefore, the nurse cannot remain neutral in the relationship but will facilitate or impede the ill person's wholeness by the process of "to nurse."

ACCOUNTABILITY

To be accountable is to be responsible and answerable. Implicit in the concept of accountability is the premise that nurses must conform to prevailing legal, ethical, and social expectations that are held for one's performance of nursing care directed toward other people. Nurses have multiple sources of accountability, including the recipient of care, peers within the profession of nursing, colleagues in related fields, the employing agency, society, and themselves. The nurse is often in the position of interface between the physician and client, or between the ill person and other health care professionals. This aspect of nursing, in addition to nurses' heavy responsibilities with little actual power for primary decision making in bureaucratic health care settings, results in confusion about the focus of primary nurs-ing accountability.

Accountable nursing care is not a linear process but rather the consideration of many aspects of the ill person's needs, strategies for need fulfillment, and any con-straints to need fulfillment. Nurses make provisional commitments to plans of care but recognize that, given more information or different circumstances, different plans of care may be indicated. Reflection on and clarification of difficult, complex, or ambiguous decisions regarding the ill person's care allow the involved caregivers to clarify and understand points of disagreement.

When care providers refuse to be accountable for the delivery of quality health care, iatrogenic disorders—any abnormal mental or physical condition induced by effects of treatment [31]—may develop. Iatrogenic distress implies a condition that may have been avoided by proper, judicious, and accountable treatment. Nurse-perpetuated iatrogenic distress stems from a variety of commonly observed behav-iors.

Nurses most often act as advocates for physicians, the hospital or clinic, and other nurses, rather than for the person with cancer. When the nurse takes offense to the ill person's rebellion against oppressive agency routines and practices, this emphasizes to the person with cancer that the "rules" of this closed world are to be followed without question, thus increasing perceptions of helplessness and futil-ity. If the caregiver justifies unnecessary or harmful procedures or treatments out of fear of legal reprisal, iatrogenic distress is perpetuated in physical, personal, and social aspects of the ill person's life. Participation in the concealment of professional errors and inadequacies further extends the ill person's perception of caregivers as infallible beings without whom the ill person cannot survive, again increasing the sense of helplessness and the inadequacy of the change-effectiveness of the client's own actions. Loyalties to physicians and health care agencies seem to take prece-dence over the nurse's basic sense of loyalty and accountability to the person with cancer and to himself or herself.

Each time nurses remain silent when they know that they should speak up and thus break the silence that induces iatrogenic distress, accountability to self and to the person with cancer is sacrificed. The personal power of the nurse is lost, rein-forcing the syndrome of polarization and iatrogenesis. The current health care de-livery system is such that it facilitates and rewards blindness, deafness, muteness, inactivity, and inertia.

The nurse who is committed to the provision of accountable nursing care to persons with cancer will formulate a plan of care and evaluate the efficacy of that plan. Nurses must collaborate with the ill person and the family to devise a plan of care that is innovative, flexible, and comprehensive, specific to the person's unique needs and resources.

Although nurses often act as physician-extenders and carry out medical regimes of treatment, they do not often question the propriety or efficacy of either medical or nursing treatment protocols. Questioning the physician seems to produce tension and suspicion between the two health care professionals rather than collaboration regarding problem management. Nurses must learn to act as advocates for the per-son with cancer despite interprofessional and bureaucratic constraints. The deci-sion-making structure within which nursing is presently practiced must be modified into one that is more conducive to accountable practice since therapeutic communication and use of self, along with the underlying accountability to persons with cancer, presupposes collegial relationships between nurses, physicians, and other caregivers.

CONCEPT V:
The science of oncology nursing is rooted in a solid knowledge base of adaptive and maladaptive human behaviors and responses to the disease process and treatment modalities.

ANALYSIS OF THE STRESS-ADAPTATION MODEL

Stress-adaptation models in nursing that have been developed by Roy [25] and Neuman [20] constitute the basis of the nursing design developed for application to client care and nursing education. In this model, the person is not fragmented but rather is visualized as a dynamic whole system with biological, personal, and social components.

Person

The Matrix of Body-Mind-Social Being. The biological component is comprised of all physiological aspects and responses of the person. The personal component is composed of all intrapersonal aspects and responses of the person: psychological, emotional, spiritual, and cognitive. The social component of the person consists of all aspects of interrelationships: sexual, familial, societal, and cultural. Precise, clear delineation of boundaries between the three components is not possible since personhood emerges from a body-mind-social being matrix, each component blending into and affecting the others. The individual is viewed as a biological-personal-social being who functions as a totality.

Core Structure. The core structure of the dynamic system is composed of those particular physiological, personal, and social moieties that must be maintained if the person is to survive, e.g., adequate oxygenation, a functional ego, a meaningful relationship with a significant other. Core structure varies in extent and complexity not only from person to person, but also may vary within the same individual depending on the situation, biological age, or developmental stage.

Lines of Defense and Resistance. Lines of defense and resistance protect the core structure from injury by environmental stimuli. For example, the physiological body will attempt to defend the core structure from inadequate oxygenation by a circulatory system shift of blood from nonvital organs to those essential for life, the personal mind will defend the core structure from the ego-threatening diagnosis of fatal illness by denial, and the social being will defend the core structure from the loss of a significant other by eliciting the comforting presence of other persons.

Lines of defense and resistance can be strengthened or weakened by a variety of influencing factors that may be biological, personal, or social in nature. For example, a person's defense against the development of a bacterial infection may be weakened by the presence of immunodeficiency, fatigue, or malnutrition. Conversely, immunocompetence, physical and mental rest, and adequate nutrition may strengthen the person's defense.

Environments

Sources of Stimuli.   The person is in constant interaction with continually changing internal and external environments that provide continuous sources of stimuli. Three types of stimuli that emanate from the internal and external environments have been identified: focal, contextual, and residual [25]. Focal stimuli refer to the degrees of change immediately confronting the person. Contextual stimuli are all other environmental stimuli that are simultaneously affecting the person, and residual stimuli consist of those beliefs and past experiences that have an effect on the person's responses.

Stressors.   Stressors are defined as tension-producing stimuli with the potential for causing disequilibrium [27]. Stressors are situations in which environmental demands tax or exceed the adaptive responses of the person [17]. An interaction is forced between the person and environment and a change occurs to maintain balance between the stressor's demand from the person and the resources to deal with it [26]. Stressors vary in quality, intensity, meaning, and effect from one person to another [20], thus differing in ability to penetrate lines of defense and resistance. Each person's interpretation of stressors as harmful or innocuous is influenced by his or her unique configuration of influencing factors, which include genetic endowment, past experiences, and current resources. More than one stressor may occur at one time, demanding response from the person, and the presence of one stressor reduces the person's ability to effectively adapt to any additional stressor [20]. A stressor is harmful when it jeopardizes the person's steady state of functioning and progression toward optimal levels of wellness.

Adaptation

Adaptive Response.   Adaptation is both a process and an end state. When stressors produce disruption in the person's steady state of functioning, adaptive mechanisms are activated to return the person to a state of equilibrium. Adaptive mechanisms are innate or acquired ways of doing or acting that mediate between the demands of environmental stressors and the person's adaptive resources. Four basic areas of need underlie adaptive mechanisms: physiological, self-concept, role function, and interdependence [25]. Each mode arises out of the biological-personal-social being matrix—the person—and influences and interacts with the others in attempts to adapt to stressors and thus enable the person to maintain or regain equilibrium. The person interacts with the internal and external environments either by adapting the self to the environments or the environments to the self [20], using those innate or acquired adaptive mechanisms that have proven successful in previous experiences. Adaptation occurs when adaptive mechanisms to maintain or regain equilibrium are successful in establishing a balance between environmental demands and the power to deal with them. Thus, stress and the person's response to it constitute the major components of the stress-adaptation model in nursing practice.

Maladaptive Responses.   If adaptive mechanisms are not successful in enabling the person to maintain or regain equilibrium, maladaptation occurs. Maladaptive responses require intervention either by the addition of resources of another person or by the individual's search for the discovery of new adaptive mechanisms that are successful in maintaining or regaining equilibrium.

Wellness-Illness Continuum

Wellness-illness is viewed as a continuum, and the person has the potential to move with or without assistance from point to point along this continuum. Wellness is a dynamic progression toward optimal levels of biological, personal, and social functioning and exists when the person is successfully adapting to stressors within the external and internal environments. Illness exists when the response to stressors is maladaptive and thus inadequate in maintaining or restoring equilibrium. Illness results in reduced ability to progress toward optimal levels of functioning.

At some point in time for each person, the ability to maintain physiological equilibrium is beyond the capacity of the person's adaptive resources. Death is a normal event in the life cycle. Although experiential, personal knowledge of death itself remains a mystery, the process of dying is one that must be experienced by each person. Dying, like birthing, is a visible process usually requiring some help. Achievement of a healthy death implies cohesion within and among the personal and social spheres. Maladaptive personal and social responses, when coupled with progressive biological deterioration, result in the phenomenon of unhealthy death. Equilibrium can exist despite the presence of pathology, so varying degrees of wellness-illness are differentiated by the focus of energy expenditure as well as the presence or absence of adaptation and equilibrium. Well individuals have varying degrees of illness, and ill individuals have varying degrees of wellness.

Nursing

Nursing is a scientific, practice-oriented discipline that is concerned with persons as total beings. Nursing functions to collaborate with the person when his or her own efforts (or the efforts of significant others) to adapt are ineffective, resulting in illness. Nursing assists the person to maintain or regain effective adaptation in order to restore or continue equilibrium and function at optimal levels. Nursing attempts to eliminate potentially harmful stressors before impact with the person; assesses influencing factors; maximizes lines of defense and resistance; and protects core structure when lines of defense and resistance are broken. Nursing supports maintenance of adaptive responses and intervenes into maladaptive responses to facilitate conversion into adaptation. Finally, nursing acts to facilitate achievement of a healthy death when return to optimal adaptive biological functioning is no longer possible.

The nursing process is a systematic, cyclic, problem-solving tool utilizing five steps: assessment, analysis, planning, implementation, and evaluation. The assessment component relies on both qualitative and quantitative data, including client history and assessment of stressors, influencing factors, strengths, and weaknesses. Analysis of assessment data yields determination of specific client problems and various factors causing or influencing the problems. Knowledge of the manifestations and precipitants of problems is crucial to effective treatment. The planning component includes determination of long-term client goals, short-term client objectives, evaluative criteria, and appropriate, specific nursing interventions. All aspects of the planning component must be mutually congruent and aimed at the achievement of optimal client functioning or healthy death. Implementation of the plan is carried out by the nurse and/or client, and evaluative criteria are used as measurement tools to determine efficacy of the plan and its implementation. Evaluations serve as data for further assessment, thus completing the cycle.

SYNTHESIS OF THE STRESS-ADAPTATION MODEL

After specific client problems and causative factors are determined, they must not remain isolated but instead must be viewed in context of the whole person. Data support a relationship between adaptation and the magnitude of the stress *response* rather than between adaptation and the number and/or magnitude of the stressors themselves [8]. Since the client's adaptive or maladaptive response to stressors cannot be separated from the client's self—which is a biological-personal-social being matrix—it is clear that the whole person's response to the stressor, rather than the stressor itself, determines equilibrium (wellness) or disequilibrium (illness).

NURSING DIAGNOSES FOR PERSONS WITH CANCER

Central to the nursing process is the nursing diagnosis, the process of inferring the nature and causative stressor of an undesirable actual or potential situation. The nursing diagnosis is based on data that are then analyzed to produce an inferential, judgmental statement. Nursing diagnoses identify those unhealthful responses actually occurring or at risk to occur [18], and specify the causal relationship between the unhealthful response and the stressor inducing it [19]. Without identification of the causative stressor, only symptomatic treatment is possible; however, identification of the causative stressor allows attempts to eliminate the cause of the symptoms rather than merely the symptoms alone. The more specific nursing diagnoses are, the more specific and effective the treatment will be.

Nursing diagnoses for persons with cancer have been divided into three groups: involuntary physical, voluntary physical, and emotional/psychological [18]. Each problem statement, or nursing diagnosis, contains both the undesired situation and the causative stressor. It must be remembered that problems experienced by persons with cancer often have a complex etiology, with several causative stressors working together to elicit the clinical symptom exhibited by the ill person. Again, the more precise the nursing diagnosis is, especially if several stressors are implicated in the development of the problem, the more precise and effective nursing management will be. For example, if nausea and vomiting are results of chemotherapy, offensive odors, and the taste of red meat, the problem will be much less severe if repugnant odors and red meat are eliminated from the ill person's environment and diet in addition to the administration of antiemetics than if the gastrointestinal distress was treated with drugs alone. Examples of nursing diagnoses may be found in Figure 1.1. It must be noted, however, that nursing diagnoses for persons with cancer are as many and varied as the ill persons themselves, with each person having a unique configuration of factors interrelating to elicit clinical symptoms of distress.

Figure 1.1. Partial List of Nursing Diagnoses for Cancer Clients.

I. INVOLUNTARY PHYSICAL
1. **Pain** secondary to stretching of organ capsule by growing tumor or edema, tumor pressure on nerves, tumor pressure causing ischemic pain, obstructed lumen, nerve compression by edema, pathological fractures, inflammation, infection, stress, medical/nursing procedures.
2. **Upper Gastrointestinal Dysfunction (Nausea, Vomiting)** secondary to chemotherapy, external or internal beam radiotherapy, constipation, paralytic ileus, reduced peristalsis, increased intracranial pressure, possible metabolic by-product of tumor, offensive odors, dysgeusia (altered sensation of taste), poor oral hygiene.
3. **Lower Gastrointestinal Dysfunction (Diarrhea)** secondary to chemotherapy, external or internal beam radiotherapy, intestinal inflammation or infection, oral antibiotics, inadequate diet, improper use of tube feeding formulas.
4. **Lower Gastrointestinal Dysfunction (Constipation)** secondary to immobility, routine use of narcotic analgesics, inadequate diet, chemotherapy with vinca alkaloids.
5. **Malnutrition and Negative Nitrogen Balance** secondary to nausea, vomiting, dysgeusia, anorexia, decreased nutritional intake, intravenous "feedings" without adequate protein and fatty acids, "regular diet" without supplementation, protein-losing enteropathy, stomatitis/esophagitis.
6. **Skin Breakdown** secondary to negative nitrogen balance and malnutrition, edema, immobility, weight loss, circulatory impairment, reduced capacity of the blood to adequately oxygenate body tissues, dehydration.
7. **Increased Vulnerability to Infection** secondary to chemotherapy-induced leukopenia, negative nitrogen balance and subsequent impaired cellular immunity, tissue necrosis, increased exposure to pathogens in the hospital setting.
8. **Increased Vulnerability to Bleeding and Hemorrhage** secondary to chemotherapy-induced thrombocytopenia, clotting factor dysfunctions, loss of ability to synthesize Vitamin K after certain intestinal surgeries, increased weakness and resultant increased risk of injury.
9. **Fatigue and Weakness** secondary to impaired oxygen-carrying capacity of erythrocytes, circulatory dysfunctions, malnutrition, muscle wasting, immobility, general feelings of unwellness and malaise.
10. **Disrupted Bone Integrity and Resultant Increased Vulnerability to Pathologic Fractures** secondary to osteolytic lesions (bone metastases).
11. **Hypercalcemia** secondary to osteolytic lesions and some hormonal chemotherapy.
12. **Hyperuricemia** (especially in leukemia and lymphoma clients undergoing chemotherapy) due to massive cell lysis as a result of antineoplastic treatment.

Figure 1.1 Continued.

13. **Hyperkalemia** (especially in leukemia and lymphoma clients undergoing chemotherapy) secondary to massive cell lysis as a result of antineoplastic treatment.

II. VOLUNTARY PHYSICAL
  1. **Deficits in Performance of Activities of Daily Living** secondary to mobility dysfunctions, pain, fatigue, premature dependence on others.
  2. **Noncompliance with Nursing/Medical Therapy** secondary to lack of knowledge, denial of diagnosis, psychic distress.
  3. **Refusal to Eat** secondary to pain, stomatitis, depression, anger.

III. PERSONAL
  1. **Prolonged or Unchanging Denial** secondary to lack of effective adaptive coping mechanisms.
  2. **Severe, Crippling Anxiety** secondary to uncertain outcomes of treatment, inadequate pain control.
  3. **Isolation, Loneliness, Despair** secondary to unresolved depression, helplessness, hopelessness, unremitting pain.
  4. **Hostility** secondary to unresovled anger, sense of helplessness.
  5. **Loss of Self-Esteem** secondary to feelings of hopelessness, meaninglessness, uselessness, being burdensome to significant others, altered body image.
  6. **Fear** secondary to pain, perceived or threatened abandonment by significant others and/or caregivers, loss of dignity, loss of control over life situation, anticipated death.

IV. SOCIAL
  1. **Social Isolation** secondary to stigma of cancer, extensive or frequent hospitalization, possible loss of job or career, decreased ability to perform family or career roles.
  2. **Undue Reliance on Caregivers (Professionals or Family)** secondary to lack of knowledge about the possibility and efficacy of self-care, inducement of the phenomenon of "premortem dying" induced by professionals or family.

Source: Adapted from Mundinger, M.O., Nursing Diagnoses for Cancer Patients. *Cancer Nurs* 1:221, 1978.

CONCEPT VI:
Nursing assessments, diagnoses, and treatments must be ongoing and holistic in order to provide a high quality of care for persons with cancer.

The profession of nursing, which has the knowledge to make the diagnosis, must also have the skills to successfully resolve the unwanted condition [18]. After the diagnosis has been made and causative stressors identified as much as possible, skills unique to nursing are utilized to assist the person to attain, maintain, or regain optimal health.

Cancer nursing activities that are perceived by oncology nurses to be important have been partially identified [5]. Resolving physiological distress, such as treatment side effects, pain, and special physical needs, is perceived as an important cancer nursing activity. Educational activities are also regarded as of great significance in cancer nursing, such as teaching early detection and prevention of cancer. Of highest priority, however, are those nursing activities encompassing psychosocial aspects, such as helping the ill person to deal with an uncertain future and changes in body image, assisting the person to accept the reality of a diagnosis of cancer, and helping the ill person manage enforced dependency. Also identified as highly important are communicative aspects of cancer nursing, such as therapeutic communication with the ill person, family, and physician; making referrals; and being able to talk openly about death and dying. Dealing with the nurse's own feelings about cancer is also perceived to be of importance.

Cancer nursing is now a distinct specialty and must take into account all related physiological, personal, and social problems resulting from or affecting the ill person's response to the disease process. Cancer is increasingly a chronic illness with longer survival times and intermittent acute crises, rather than always an acute disease rapidly culminating in death. Using an intensive nursing approach that gives ill persons the opportunity to understand their disease and treatment, and to verbalize and work through their feelings, may actually significantly reduce the physical, personal, and social distress experienced by the person with cancer [29]. In addition, making the attempt to deal with *nurses'* feelings about cancer may result in a radical alteration of the emotional climate of a hospital unit or clinic, with less depression and increased physical activity exhibited by the persons receiving care [14]. The use of the stress-adaptation model in nursing practice will facilitate provision of high-quality care, the kind of care that makes cancer nursing discernibly unique and of crucial importance to the ill persons who need that care.

REFERENCES

1. Abrams, R. D. The Patient with Cancer—His Changing Patterns of Communication. *N Engl J Med* 214:317, 1966.
2. American Nurses' Association. *Nursing: A Social Policy Statement.* Kansas City, MO: American Nurses' Association, 1980. P. 9.
3. Bullough, B. Nurses as Teachers and Support Persons for Breast Cancer Patients. *Cancer Nurs* 4:221, 1981.
4. Connors, D. D. Sickness Unto Death: Medicine as Mythic, Necrophilic, and Iatrogenic. *ANS* 2(3):39, 1980.
5. Craytor, J. K., Brown, J. K., and Morrows, G. R. Assessing Learning Needs of Nurses Who Care for Persons with Cancer. *Cancer Nurs* 1:211, 1978.
6. Craytor, J. K. and Fasse, M. L. Changing Nurses' Perception of Cancer and Cancer Care. *Cancer Nurs* 5:43, 1982.
7. Davitz, L. J. and Davitz, L. R. How Do Nurses Feel When Patients Suffer? *Am J Nurs* 75:1505, 1975.
8. Donovan, M. I. Study of the Impact of Relaxation with Guided Imagery on Stress Among Cancer Nurses. *Cancer Nurs* 5:43, 1982.
9. Easson, E. C. Cancer and the Problem of Pessimism. *Cancer* 17:7, 1967.
10. Ferguson, M. *The Aquarian Conspiracy: Personal and Social Transformation in the 1980s.* Los Angeles: J. P. Tarcher, 1980. Pp. 246–248.
11. Gillmer, R. and Hassels, A. Nurses' Practices and Attitudes Toward Cancer. *Am J Nurs* 64:84, 1964.
12. Jamison, K. R., Wellisch, D. K., and Pasnau, R. O. Psychosocial Aspects of Mastectomy: I. The Woman's Perspective. *Am J Psychiatry* 135:432, 1978.

13. Johnson, D. E. State of the Art of Theory Development in Nursing. In National League for Nursing. *Theory Development: What, Why, How?* New York: National League for Nursing, 1978. Pp. 1–10.

14. Klagsbrun, S. C. Cancer, Emotion, and Nurses. *Am J Psychiatry* 126:1237, 1970

15. Lewis, F. M. Experienced Personal Control and Quality of Life in Late-Stage Cancer Patients. *Nurs Res* 31:113, 1982.

16. Lindsey, A. M., Norbeck, J. S., Carrieri, V. L., and Perry, E. Social Support and Health Outcomes in Post-Mastectomy Women: A Review. *Cancer Nurs* 4:377, 1981.

17. Monat, A. and Lazarus, R. S. (Eds.). *Stress and Coping.* New York: Columbia University Press, 1977.

18. Mundinger, M. O. Nursing Diagnoses for Cancer Patients. *Cancer Nurs* 1:221, 1978.

19. Mundinger, M. O. and Jaurun, G. D. Developing a Nursing Diagnosis. *Nurs Outlook* 23(2):94, 1975.

20. Neuman, B. The Betty Neuman Health Care Systems Model: A Total Person Approach to Patient Problems. In J. P. Riehl and C. Roy. *Conceptual Models for Nursing Practice* (2nd Ed.). New York: Appleton-Century-Crofts, 1980. Pp. 119–134.

21. Newlin, J. J. and Wellish, D. K. The Oncology Nurse: Life on an Emotional Roller Coaster. *Cancer Nurs* 1:477, 1978.

22. Olson, K. B. Cancer and the Patient. *Ann Intern Med* 81:696, 1974.

23. Quint, J. C. The Impact of Mastectomy. *Am J Nurs* 63(11):88, 1963.

24. Quint, J. C. Institutionalized Practices of Information Control. *Psychiatry* 28:119, 1965.

25. Roy, C. The Roy Adaptation Model. In J. P. Riehl and C. Roy. *Conceptual Models for Nursing Practice* (2nd Ed.). New York: Appleton-Century-Crofts, 1980. Pp. 179–188.

26. Scott, D. W., Oberst, M. T., and Dropkin, M. J. A Stress-Coping Model. *ANS* 3(1):9, 1980.

27. Selye, H. *The Stress of Life.* New York: McGraw-Hill, 1956.

28. Sherman, C. D. Jr., and Williams, C. M. A Survey of the Attitudes of Second, Third, and Fourth Year Medical Students Toward the "Curability" of Breast Cancer. *CA* 20:365, 1970.

29. Sonstegaard, L., Hansen, N., Johnston, M. J., and Zillman, L. A Way to Minimize Side Effects from Radiation Therapy. *Am J Maternal Child Nurs* 1:27, 1976.

30. Stein, J. (Ed. in Chief). *The Random House College Dictionary* (Rev. Ed.). New York: Random House, 1980. P. 913.

31. Thomas, C. L. (Ed.). *Taber's Cyclopedic Medical Dictionary.* Philadelphia: F. A. Davis, 1973. Pp. I–1.

32. Winstead-Fry, P. The Scientific Method and Its Impact on Holistic Health. *ANS* 2(4):1, 1980.

33. Woods, N. F. and Earp, J. Women with Cured Breast Cancer: A Study of Mastectomy Patients in North Carolina. *Nurs Res* 27:279, 1978.

CHAPTER 2

Holistic Care of the Person With Cancer

CONCEPT I:
Cancer is a severe insult to the physiological, personal, and social aspects of a human being.

The disease process known as cancer is greatly feared in our society, with one study revealing that the public fears cancer more than any other world danger, even more than violent crimes and atomic war [11]. Cancer remains a stigmatizing illness, viewed as repugnant and dreadful, and persons with even early cancerous processes may be viewed as different from other people and even as dying [89].

Malignant diseases may be considered to be chronic illnesses, since they are usually permanent, leave residual disability, are caused by nonreversible pathological dysfunction and may be expected to require long-term observation and/or care [65]. Yet, cancer as a chronic illness has a clinically abrupt onset and specific protocols of medical treatment. There are profound deleterious effects on personal and family adaptation to the enforced new life situation, and cancer and its treatment threaten the physical and personal resources of both the ill person and the family unit [49], requiring additional or new coping behaviors.

The person with cancer is plunged into the new, sometimes bizarre, often frightening world of long-term specialized health care. Contact with a trusted family physician is often lost as care is turned over to oncologists and oncology nurses. The ill person often has difficulties establishing an open, communicative relationship with the new physicians and nurses, perhaps feeling constrained by the caregivers' time limits or feeling in awe of the specialized professionals and not wanting to appear stupid by asking naive questions. The ill person may also exhibit reluctance to ask questions because of fear of the answers [46], and thus the person with cancer further withdraws into himself, intensifying feelings of loneliness, helplessness, and despair.

CONCEPT II:
Persons with cancer often experience common fears and psychic distresses secondary to the diagnosis of cancer, responses from others, and perceived threats to survival.

Generalized categories of fears or burdens common to persons with cancer include fear of disfigurement or mutilation, fear of antineoplastic treatments, loss of work role in job or career, enforced dependency on others, alienation from significant others, and concern about the future [30]. Persons with cancer commonly experience ambiguity about treatment outcomes, and they often perceive loss of control and mastery over their own life situations. Fear of disruption of positive relationships with their caregivers is often observed, as is the nightmare fear that the cancer will be invulnerable to treatment.

Learning how to live with the uncertainties of the disease is a difficult challenge, since the ill person does not know if or when symptoms will recur or if exacerbation of the disease will take place. This unpredictable outcome increases the person's stress level [27] and contributes to the sense of loss of mastery over life events.

It is not surprising, therefore, that persons with cancer experience more anxiety than do persons with nonmalignant disease conditions [58], and that as time following diagnosis increases, levels of self-reported anxiety increase [54].

Changes in perceptions of body image also contribute to the ill person's psychic distress and anxiety. There is a close relationship between a person's body image and the resulting organization and functioning of the personality, so perceptions of negative alterations in body image have profound effects on the ill person's intra- and interpersonal aspects of being.

All fears experienced by the person with cancer, whether generalized or specific, are of concern and importance to caregivers, but the greatest fear of all is not one of death but rather fear of abandonment [101]. Persons with cancer often have deep, troublesome anxieties about the possibilities that significant others will abandon them because of fear and repugnance or that caregivers will abandon them as "dying failures." If the ill person acknowledges his or her possible growing dependence upon significant others and caregivers as essential to physical and psychic survival or for relief of distressing symptoms, fear of abandonment becomes even deeper, resulting in a variety of unhealthful behavioral responses.

CONCEPT III:
Instead of demanding compliant patients, caregivers must enable persons with cancer to retain the role of independent adult capable of making informed decisions and must nonjudgmentally accept the ill person's decisions even if contrary to the caregivers' opinions.

The definition of the word "patient" includes such adjectives as long-suffering, victimized, bearing pain without complaint or anger, and untiring [91]. "Patient" implies compliance, passivity, submission, and relinquishment of life control to powerful others. Much professional literature speaks to the "problem of noncompliance" among ill persons. If the ill person exhibits noncompliance with treatment protocols because of lack of knowledge, depression, or a sense of helplessness, then noncompliance is indeed a valid nursing diagnosis worthy of intervention. In this case, if compliance with treatment protocols would increase the ill person's chance of survival or enhance quality of life, the deleterious effects of noncompliance could be avoided through appropriate education and counseling. If, however, the ill person is fully informed of all consequences and implications of both compliance and noncompliance with medical or nursing treatment and still chooses to refuse the proposed treatment, noncompliance is *not* an appropriate nor valid nursing diagnosis. Caregivers must learn to nonjudgmentally accept informed refusals of proposed treatment, even if the refusal will result in the ill person's death, since the client is exercising his or her right to participate in decisions concerning his or her own care. Nurses can minimize noncompliance secondary to knowledge deficits, depression, and perceived helplessness by establishing a trusting, openly communicative, caring relationship with the client during the initial hospitalization.

Client management problems may be viewed as stemming from three areas: reluctance, reactance, and recidivism [1]. Reluctant clients are the "no-shows," those persons who choose not to avail themselves of health services even when medical or nursing treatments are crucial to the maintenance of life. This group of clients is not as amenable to intervention by health professionals as clients in the other two problem areas.

Reactance refers to a variety of behaviors exhibited by clients in response to necessary treatment or changes in life style necessary to improve or ensure health. Reactance may be expressed by outright refusal to comply with treatment protocols but more often is observed in a variety of covert reactions. For some clients, the restraints of hospitalization and/or therapy impose heavy burdens that conflict with their needs to independently direct their own lives. For more passive persons, compliance may be a depleting experience and may result in lowered self-esteem and feelings of helplessness because of the continuous direction and supervision provided by health professionals.

Recidivism refers to backsliding by clients who may have initially exhibited willingness and ability to comply with treatment protocols and changes in life style but are unable to sustain successful compliance over prolonged periods of time. Recidivism requires further intervention by health professionals in order to maintain therapy, promote health, and prevent feelings of helplessness and loss of control within the client.

CONCEPT IV:
Insights into the psychic and social distress experienced by persons with cancer can be obtained through examination of the concepts of locus of control, learned helplessness, and stress-adaptation.

The derivation of the word "cancer" is "pernicious, spreading evil" and invokes the immediate thought of the possibility that nothing can be done. Common initial responses to unacceptable news are either attacking the problem or running away from the situation. If such activities are not effective, feelings of helplessness may ensue and all externally directed activity may be discontinued [82]. This reaction of quiescence and helplessness has been commonly observed in cancer clients with life expectancies of less than six months [48, 94].

Few health professionals would discount the importance of the will to live, especially in life-threatening situations. The secure possession of an individual's own body as a safe entity under his or her control empowers that person to overcome a sense of vulnerability to powerful external forces [7]. Negative effects of stress are especially potent when feelings of lack of control are present [84]. Yet, institutional systems are often insensitive to clients' needs to control important life events.

INTERNAL-EXTERNAL LOCUS OF CONTROL

Internal-external locus of control refers to the degree to which one perceives that environmental control is contingent upon his or her own actions. The theory implies that persons have a choice in how they will behave; before choosing a particular action, they must first determine the value of the outcome (reinforcement value) and their estimation or expectance of the probability that the desired outcome will occur [79, 80]. Persons judge their chances for success by assessing the immediate situation (situational expectancy), as well as by considering what they have learned from past experiences that were similar to the present event (generalized expectancy). Because generalized expectancies influence perceptions and meanings ascribed to present situations [1], the importance of the role of generalized expectations in determining behavior is clear.

Individuals with an internal locus of control perceive environmental changes as a direct consequence of their responses. Individuals with external locus of control perceive that environmental changes are independent of their behavior and are instead related to luck, chance, fate, or powerful others [80].

Learned helplessness and the internal-external locus of control construct both view the individual's perceived control of external events as a crucial variable [32, 53, 86]. The more control one perceives oneself to have, the less threatening situations will seem. Conversely, the less control one perceives oneself to have—or the more helpless the individual perceives himself or herself to be—the more threatening situations will appear to be.

Persons with an internal locus of control believe that what happens to them is primarily the result of their own actions [1, 80]. These individuals appear to be more motivated and better able to extract relevant situational data and use these data in effective problem solving [1, 19, 70, 103]. Persons with an internal locus of control seem to value health more highly than do people with an external locus of control, thus enhancing health-related learning [97, 98] and achieving greater success in the initial mastery of health information [40, 45, 57, 85]. Individuals with an internal locus of control exhibit denial when confronted by a threat [56, 73, 77], but this denial does not stop them from attempting to change the threatening situation [73]. Individuals with an internal locus of control exhibit greater trust in strangers [20] and are more willing to approach, use, and benefit from assistance from authority figures, e.g., health professionals [23].

Persons with an external locus of control believe that what happens to them is primarily the result of fate, luck, chance, or powerful others, or is unpredictable because of the complexity of the situation [1, 80, 81]. These individuals view events as being independent of their own actions. People with an external locus of control exhibit less denial and less assumption of responsibility for outcomes in threatening situations [1, 17], and they prefer situations that enable them to rationalize failures [72]. If these individuals cannot reach their goals, they may display aggression [8] or simply devalue the goal [71].

The secure possession of one's body as a safe entity under one's own control empowers a person to overcome a sense of vulnerability to external forces [7]. Illness, however, is an externalizing event. Internal-external locus of control studies comparing sick and well people show increased externality among the ill [25, 38,

100], with even greater externality exhibited by people with chronic, nonacute disease [9]. Cancer, in particular, is an externalizing disease, invoking the strong idea that one's body is no longer safely under one's control. The diagnosis of cancer usually elicits responses of fear, which initially is an adaptive mechanism. It is postulated that fear is an adaptive motivator to control unwanted events [86]. As long as the individual is uncertain whether or not trauma can be controlled, fear is adaptive because it maintains a search for responses that will control the unwanted situation. Once the trauma is under the person's control, fear has little use and normally will then decrease. However, when the person is convinced that the trauma is uncontrollable, several phenomena may occur: fear decreases, feelings of helplessness and depression may occur, and all externally directed activity may cease [82, 86]. Cancer, with its problems and chronicity, results in a greater possibility that clients will perceive that what happens to them is the result of fate or powerful others (such as health professionals) rather than their own actions.

LEARNED HELPLESSNESS

Helplessness is defined as the feeling or belief that important life events are beyond one's control [86]. If one believes that internally initiated actions will not influence or control the environment, helplessness ensues.

The defining characteristic of helplessness is the failure to escape from an unwanted situation [32]. When exposed to uncontrollable events, both animals and humans learn that responding is futile [86], and, if aversive events are perceived to be inescapable, organisms learn that responding and reinforcement (e.g., the termination of unwanted events) are independent [33]. The aversive, unwanted situation is then seen as being beyond the individual's control.

Animal Studies

Animal studies have supported the proposition that helplessness is a causal factor in unexpected physiological dysfunction and death [34, 75, 86]. Common physiological findings in all animal studies point to a parasympathetic death with bradycardia, arrhythmias, and engorgement of the heart with blood. One researcher suggested that death was directly due to "giving up the struggle" [75].

Human Studies

Helplessness can be experimentally induced in human beings wholly parallel to animal manifestations of helplessness, with humans showing more failures to escape a threatening situation after they have failed to escape previous threatening situations than following escapable undesirable events [32, 39, 86]. It has been proposed that when animals and humans learn that their actions are futile, they become more vulnerable to death. It is also thought that belief in environmental control can prolong life [10, 24, 60, 75, 86, 102].

Human subjects transfer learned helplessness to a second task that, in fact, may offer control. The subjects seem to give up the pursuit of goals since this has proven to be useless in the past [63, 95]. This finding is congruent with the proposal that generalized expectancies influence a person's perception of current situations as being either controllable or uncontrollable by the person's own actions.

Implications for Persons with Cancer

Cancer is one of the most devastating events that can occur in a human being's life. The nature of the disease process, as well as its treatment, imposes tremendous biological, personal, and social disruptions in the ill person's life and the family unit. The problems associated with cancer are magnified by the chronicity of the disease, demanding additional or new coping behaviors.

Experienced personal control over life events, rather than state of health, appears to be a most meaningful and statistically significant correlate of psychological well-being in late-stage cancer clients [54]. As the time following diagnosis increases, subjects appear to express increased externality in regard to health status and increased levels of self-reported anxiety, both of which are consistent with Seligman's hypothesis on uncontrollable trauma and learned helplessness. This external locus of control orientation and perception of helplessness may predispose the individual to failure in coping; a generalized emotional pattern of helplessness, depression, and anxiety; and a diminished ability to express anger [4, 16, 29]. Loss of personal control is also associated with unresolved grief and feelings of despair [62]. Self-devaluation, psychomotor retardation, feelings of sadness, and the expectancy that further responding would be futile are associated with perceived helplessness [33], and clients often exhibit disengagement from the external environment [82]. Additionally, the negative effects of stress are especially potent when feelings of lack of control and helplessness are present [84], and losing personal control over life events may even lead to physical aberrations and/or unexpected death [21, 24, 29, 68, 82, 84, 86]. The perception of helplessness magnifies reactions of anxiety [39], seems to decrease pain tolerance [90], and may result in anorexia plus decreased absorption and metabolism of ingested nutrients [82]. Thus, learned helplessness and external locus of control appear to result in biological, personal, and social disturbances by undermining the motivation to respond and by retarding the ability to learn that responding is effective.

STRESS-ADAPTATION

An organism's physiological/psychological stress reaction in response to internal or external stimuli is exhibited in four general ways [53]. First, the ill person may report or exhibit a disturbed affect, such as fear, anxiety, or depression. The second general group of stress reactions involve motor-behavioral responses, such as increased muscle tension, tremors, or speech disturbances. Third, there may be changes in the person's cognitive ability, with decreased learning potential resulting from high stress levels. Finally, physiological changes are characterized by overstimulation of the sympathetic nervous system and adrenal glands.

It has been postulated that control or progression of malignant processes is a result of the interplay of the adaptive resources of the biological, personal, and social aspects of the individual. Evidence is stronger in support of the theory that excessive stress is a factor in the *progression* of established disease rather than in the precipitation of the malignancy [13]. The General Alarm System results in thymi-colymphatic involution [87], resulting in immunosuppression and possible facili-tation of tumor growth.

The excessive stress that may be imposed by cancer and its treatment also has tremendous ramifications in the personal sphere of being. Resulting lowered self-esteem, external locus of control, and feelings of despair, depression, and helpless-ness have already been addressed. In addition, when a person is locked into a demeaning life situation that is inconsistent with his or her self-concept as a worth-while human being, one way of reducing this psychic dissonance is to change one's perceptions of the situation being faced, thus enabling adaptation to occur. By changing perceptions of the demeaning situation, the ill persons' perceived impo-tence to extricate themselves from it is decreased [12]. The person with cancer may also demonstrate a lack of interest in the cancer and treatment experience, which may be attributed to defensive psychological reactions. If the ill person is fearful of the possible negative reactions of caregivers if criticisms are made, then the person is likely to retreat into an apparent lack of interest that further increases perceptions of helplessness and great stress [6].

Additionally, the individual with cancer may experience temporary alterations in cognitive abilities resulting from the conflict between old patterns of behavior and the pull to fit the person's cognitive world to new situations [76].

The social aspect of being is also profoundly affected by cancer and its treatment, and the client may even be at greater risk than persons without cancer for disrup-tions in social relationships. The most consistent finding in life event research with respect to cancer clients has been the loss of a major love relationship within months or years prior to the onset of disease symptoms [42], and one study indi-cated a marked lack of closeness to parents in people with cancer [93]. Increased life changes and high stress levels seem to increase the likelihood of major health changes [36, 37, 41, 52, 74, 96]. Development of a personality characterized by inhibition, rigidity, repression, and regression is theorized to precede cancer devel-opment [2], which is, in fact, *cellular* regression. Research seems to support a rela-tionship between a high hopelessness potential, or recent profound feelings of hopelessness, and the development of malignant processes [83]. These findings may indicate weaknesses in family support systems for persons with cancer, thus increasing the possibility of maladaptive social responses.

The stress of loss and depression, when combined with certain personality and ego-defensive characteristics, seems to increase vulnerability to clinical cancer through neurological, endocrine, and immunological dysfunction [3]. However, re-gardless of whether one sees the role played by excessive stress, learned helpless-ness, and external locus of control as directly precipitating the development of ma-lignancy or as a part of a more complex syndrome that weakens the cancer client's adaptive resources, the clinical significance of these phenomena is clear. Excessive stress, learned helplessness, and external locus of control weave a complex web of negativity within the biological-personal-social being matrix that is the person, de-creasing the likelihood of adaptive responses and increasing the probability of mal-adaptation and worsening of the pathological condition.

Perception of participation in the turn of events, with the hope of mastery, is less anxiety-arousing than no activity at all or activity that leaves individuals feeling helpless victims of inevitable events [69]. The traditional health care delivery system, however, is often insensitive to clients' needs to control important life events. Health professionals are commonly perceived by clients to know all and tell little, whereas clients are expected to sit back "patiently" and rely on professional treatment. There has been little for individuals with cancer to do to directly participate in their treatment in order to control the disease process and assure recovery, or to ensure quality of life until death. This is in contrast to many other chronic diseases in which individuals have an important, active role in carrying out treatment regimes. Feelings of helplessness and external locus of control orientation may be precipitated when health professionals' demands for passivity and compliance are perceived by clients as a loss of their ability to control the environment.

DANGER OF MODELS

Using conceptual models to attempt to better understand the behavior patterns of ill persons and their families carries a danger for the caregiver. It is possible that the model can be misused to stereotype persons with cancer and reduce the complexity of human behavior to simplistic patterns locked into predetermined modes. This results in the evolution of emotional distance between health professionals and their clients and diminishes the caregiver's awareness of the uniqueness of each person. Models for understanding the behavior of persons with cancer and their families must be used only as a framework for the analysis and interpretation of those behaviors.

CONCEPT V:
Most persons with cancer exhibit common major defense mechanisms in attempts to cope with the impact of the disease process and its treatment.

Coping mechanisms are cognitive and motor activities that the ill person uses to preserve his or her physical and psychic integrity. Other uses for coping mechanisms include recovery of reversible dysfunction and compensation for limits imposed by irreversible impairment. Prior personality factors and life experiences profoundly affect the type and degree of usage of coping mechanisms used by the person with cancer. Denial, withdrawal, rationalizations, intellectualization, suppression, repression, compensation, and regression are all general types of coping mechanisms commonly used by persons with cancer [78], but each person will use the type and degree of coping mechanisms that have been characterstic of the preillness life style.

TIME PERSPECTIVE OF PERSONS WITH CANCER

Persons with cancer report a shorter future time perspective than do healthy persons or people ill with nonmalignant diseases, and people with cancer report more time pressure even though they have more free time [26]. For persons without cancer, death is not usually perceived to be even a remote possibility. However, since our cultural meaning ascribed to cancer includes concepts of suffering and death, even persons with early cancer may perceive death as a concrete, very real possibility within the foreseeable future. This may explain the individual's perception of a more limited future and more time pressure.

MAJOR COPING STRATEGIES

Those who cope best seem to be those individuals who are optimistic, openly confront even unpleasant realities, ask for and accept support from significant others, and deal with singular problems as they arise without being overwhelmed by the entire problem burden as a totality [31, 99]. Those individuals who have the most difficult time in coping with their disease are those who suppress, avoid, and deny reality, and those who are by nature domineering and controlling people [14]. Common negative defense mechanisms include repression, filtering of information so that only manageable data is "heard," regression to a childlike state of dependency on others, transference of decision-making power to caregivers, and denial of the reality of their cancer [6]. The major coping strategies (which may be either positive or negative), commonly observed in persons with cancer, have been identified as coping as in past crises, seeking information, compliance with medical treatment, denial or escape, searching for meaning in the disease, returning to one's job, tension-reducing strategies, blaming others or external situations, preparing for death, and seeking support [28].

Utilization of Past Coping Mechanisms

Unless proven to be inadequate or ineffective in coping with the crisis of cancer, the ill person will first attempt to utilize coping strategies that were successful in dealing with past crises. By assisting the person with cancer to explore old coping mechanisms, nurses can help the ill individual to discover skills already possessed to effectively cope with this new crisis.

Seeking Information

Appropriate information can allay anxiety and fear. The seeking of information about cancer, its treatment, and its effect on the person's life, therefore, is a positive coping strategy to be encouraged. If ill persons hold large amounts of appropriate information, their sense of control over life events will increase. However, a negative twist to this coping strategy is the filtering of information. The ill person "hears" only what is desired to be heard. This is an example of the use of a cognitive defense mechanism, stemming from repression, to minimize the intake of painful or unacceptable information [64].

Compliance with Medical Treatment

Many persons with cancer believe that the meticulous following of medical treatment protocols is their best defense against the disease. Although the ill person's active participation in his or her health care is certainly positive, the danger exists that the person will develop an overly submissive dependency on caregivers, resulting in lowered self-esteem and increased perceptions of personal helplessness. Nurses can minimize these negative effects by facilitating self-care and encouraging the client to collaborate in planning and implementation of health care.

Denial and Escape

The defense mechanisms of denial and escape can benefit or impede adaptive coping by either protecting the ill person from news as yet unbearable or by inducing isolation and withdrawal. Nurses must take care not to forcefully break through the denial, and nurses must facilitate sharing between the person with cancer and the family unit. Denial is indeed a crutch, yet nurses should not forcefully remove that crutch any more than they would remove canes or walkers from persons with orthopedic dysfunctions.

Finding Meaning in the Disease

Many persons with cancer attempt to cope with their disease by searching for humanistic meaning in the disease. In other words, they attempt to answer the question, "Why me?" Common activities utilized to search for meaning in the disease include helping others and involvement in work, activity, and other aspects of living.

Returning to Employment

Reinvolvement in job activities is considered to be a sign of positive, healthy coping. Persons who return to their jobs exhibit better self-esteem, increased morale, reduced anxiety and depression, and are less threatened by the implications of their disease. Nurses may facilitate a return to employment by securing the services of occupational or physical therapy to help clients obtain prostheses or transportation, and by education of employers and peers within the work setting to reduce the stigma of cancer.

Tension-reducing Strategies

Again, tension-reducing strategies may be positive or negative in nature. Healthy means of reducing tension may include physical activity, arts and crafts, music, meditation, relaxation exercises, or expression of feelings. However, tension-reducing strategies such as smoking, drinking, overeating, and focusing on symptoms are frequently maladaptive and unhealthy. Nurses can enhance the ability of the ill person to transform maladaptive responses into adaptive ones, thus enhancing quality of life.

Blaming Others

The person with cancer may use the coping strategy of blaming others, God, or situations external to themselves for their disease. They may question religious or spiritual attitudes. Allowing the ill person to vent hostile and negative feelings is sometimes effective, and provision of professioanl religious or spiritual counseling may help. A serious pitfall to avoid, however, is the verbal or nonverbal message to the ill person of "It's God's will." No one knows what "causes" cancer, and attitudes such as these will only exacerbate the blaming process.

Preparing for Death

This coping strategy may also be either adaptive or maladaptive. Preparing for death, finishing one's unfinished business, and setting things in order may signify acceptance of the reality of impending death. If, however, death is not soon expected, preparation for death is premature and unhealthy, indicative of "giving up."

Turning to Others for Support

This coping strategy is usually healthy and adaptive if the interpersonal relationships are interdependent. Maladaptive social support is characterized by the ill person's inappropriate and total dependence on others for physical and personal need fulfillment. Social support systems are comprised of networks of relationships emerging from the family, social and role relationships (job peers, friends), health care professionals, and the community[55].

Social support is defined as that situation in which ill persons believe that they are loved, that they are an important part of a network of communication, that they are esteemed and valued, and that there exists a network of mutual obligations exclusive of tangible or material aid [15]. Positive, strong social support seems to buffer or mediate the threat of fearful situations [55, 92], and persons who are part of a strong social network are better able to cope with crises and adapt to changes [55]. People who are exposed to fearful or threatening experiences often increase their quantity of interpersonal relationships in order to maximize their social support as they face the threat. Indeed, persons with cancer appear to value interpersonal relationships more highly and to express desires for increased physical closeness with others [35]. Persons with cancer who have few significant others seem to experience increased fears of disease recurrence [67] and have more difficulty coping with the cancer situation [99], so maximizing social support systems is a crucial nursing activity. Turning to others for support may take many forms, including one-to-one relationships, support groups, and healthy reliance on caregivers, family, friends, and/or clergy. If, however, the nurses assess the ill person to be inappropriately dependent upon others for need fulfillment, then strong encouragement of self-care—physical and personal—is indicated. As ill persons begin to acknowledge their own capabilties for self-fulfillment of needs, maladaptive dependency will decrease and healthy interpersonal relationships will emerge.

One of the most significant interpersonal relationships is between ill persons and their spouse or primary significant other. Stable marital relationships enhance adaptive coping to the crisis of cancer [30], and a basic way of maintaining that stability and intimacy is through sexual activity with the loved one. Human sexuality is a complex aspect of life that is both influenced by and influences a wide range of biological and sociocultural aspects of being. Sexuality pervades our biological existence, our sense of self, and the ways in which we relate and respond to others [50]. Femininity and masculinity are not merely physiological phenomena but are biopsychosocial in nature and reflect a wide range of human behaviors and attitudes. Sexual health is defined as the integration of physical, emotional, intellectual, and interpersonal aspects of sexual being in a manner that is personally enriching and enhances one's personality, communication, and expression and acceptance of love.

Persons with cancer may actually find that their sexuality is enhanced because of reevaluation of self-concept and the relationship with the spouse. Sexual activity may reinforce the human experience of being alive, and this may have a special meaning for those ill persons whose cancer experience has caused them to question their own humanness and the value of life. Physical, intimate closeness with one's mate may allay fears, give encouragement to continue to endure distressing treatments, and may even enable the ill person to transcend some of the dehumanizing aspects of the cancer experience. Sexual activity may validate acceptance from one's mate, which is particularly important for those experiencing physical disfigurement. For those persons who are fatally ill, sexual activity is a way of enriching that cherished relationship and validating that they are still alive. Conversely, cessation of active sexual expression may indicate that the dying person is "letting go," relinquishing his or her hold on this life and preparing for death.

The cancer experience, however, often impedes sexual expression in ways that decrease quality of life. Fatigue, malaise, or a generalized sense of feeling unwell often interferes with desire or ability for sex. Physiological malignant processes that lower serum androgen levels will reduce libido in both men and women and will also decrease male erectile ability. This phenomenon may also be observed in estrogen chemotherapy and some testicular tumors. Disruption of central nervous system pathways by tumor growth or surgery may have deleterious effects on both desire and tactile sensation. Similarly, intracranial tumors in the frontal or temporal lobes may alter libido, and disruption of the spinal cord may reduce sexual sensations or interfere with the reflex mechanisms necessary for erection or ejaculation. Pain is a significant stressor upon the ill person's sexuality, since competition will exist between painful and pleasurable stimuli. Changes in body image and self-esteem commonly observed in persons who have undergone a colostomy, pelvic exenteration, or mastectomy may radically alter sexual expression in a negative way. Limitations of mobility may result in physically uncomfortable sexual expression, thus reducing both the quantity and quality of sexual activity.

The stress of the cancer experience may precipitate performance anxiety and faulty communication between partners, negatively affecting sexual expression. Many persons also have fears that the malignancy is contagious or that sexual intercourse will cause spread or recurrence of the cancer [44]. The "well" partner may view the ill spouse as fragile and may thus hesitate to initiate sexual activity, perhaps feeling guilty about "making demands" upon the person with cancer [50].

Nurses can assist cancer clients and their spouses to reestablish a satisfactory sexual relationship by offering information that will minimize stressors impeding sexual expression. Nurses must recognize the legitimacy and importance of sexual needs and establish an open, nonthreatening, nonjudgmental relationship with the client so as to more effectively deal with this often emotionally charged, very private issue.

The stressor of pain can be minimized by analgesic medication before intercourse, although an excessive amount of medication will decrease libido and erectile ability. Relaxation exercises before and after intercourse will often reduce any accompanying discomfort, and experimentation with pillows and comfortable positions will decrease pain during sexual activity. Dyspareunia, or painful sexual intercourse, may be minimized by avoidance of deep vaginal penetration.

Fatigue may be minimized if the ill person rests before and after intercourse and if heavy meals and liquor are avoided before sexual activity. Choosing comfortable positions, such as sidelying or the well person astride, will decrease the ill person's exertion and resultant fatigue.

Comfortable positions and the use of pillows to support body weight may compensate for limitations in mobility. Relaxation exercises before and after sexual activity and a warm bath before intercourse will reduce the muscle tension, fatigue, and discomfort often accompanying range of motion difficulties.

Alternative methods of expressing physical love are possibilities that may satisfy sexual needs even if genital intercourse is not possible. Simple touching is important, as it satisfies skin hunger and enhances intimacy and closeness. Manual, digital or oral stimulation, or intrathigh or intramammary intercourse may be satisfactory expressions of physical love if vaginal penetration is not possible.

In summary, turning to others for support is a way for the ill person to compensate for the psychosocial deteriorations induced and perpetuated by the cancer experience. The social costs of cancer, which extend to the family, imply negative alterations in family roles, career, sexuality, social relationships, and ultimately the quality of life [5]. Extending and strengthening the ill person's network of social support is an important nursing activity that will minimize the trauma inflicted by the disease process and treatment.

CONCEPT VI:
Each person with cancer has unique needs for information about the disease process, its treatment, and its implications.

Most people receive information about cancer and cancer treatment from mass media sources [59], information that is often incomplete or inaccurate. Persons with cancer, or their families, often cling to unrealistic hopes generated by inaccurate media information. Gentle teaching about accurate information must be carefully and judiciously carried out in a manner that will correct misinformation without extinguishing hope.

There appears to be a significant difference between nurses' perceptions of learning needs and the perceptions of the clients themselves [51]. Individuals with cancer have unique learning needs, different with each person, and the nurse must assess what the ill person perceives as important information before initiating teaching. Persons with cancer seem especially concerned about receiving information that will facilitate realistic planning for immediate as well as long-range needs.

There seems to be little concern with information that would not significantly contribute to the person's understanding of the disease process or its implications for necessary changes in life style [18].

CONCEPT VII:
Cancer is a disease process that has tremendous economic costs for the affected family unit.

The direct economic costs of cancer are all related to the prevention, diagnosis, and treatment of the disease, whereas indirect costs refer to idle resources and lost personal productivity. Time off work necessary for medical treatment is an example of an indirect economic cost, as is the situation of a cancer client dying at age forty and thus losing twenty-five years of occupational productivity [5, 61]. Psychosocial costs refer to the personal effects of spending for medical and nursing care, such as the loss of savings, forced sale of a home, family disintegration, or the cost related to additional family members who move into the home to assist with care [61].

Hospital care is the single most important direct economic cost of cancer [5], and annual costs to the family often exceed its annual income [61]. For example, a 1976 study (see Table 2.1) revealed a direct cost of treatment for a person with acute leukemia over a period of less than one year to be $40,022 [22]. Economic costs are related to the extent of disease and to the type and duration of the treatment, and many persons with cancer do not have coverage by health insurance and are personally responsible for their own bills.

By being cognizant of the enormous financial burden accompanying the cancer experience, nurses can assist the family to cope with the stressor of high economic costs. Prudent and judicious use of supplies, equipment, and medications will minimize hospital charges. Teaching skills necessary for adequate and effective home care will enable the family to reduce the number and duration of hospitalizations, and referral to a home health care agency or community health nursing service may allow home care despite special physical needs of the ill person.

Table 2.1.   Cost of Leukemia Treatment for All Problems for 11.5 Months [22].

Time Intervals	Charge per day	Days	Cost
Admission to remission	$376*	30	$11,280
Remission to relapse	32	180	5,760
Relapse to remission	376	30	11,280
Remission to relapse	32	90	2,880
Relapse to death	401	22	8,822
			$40,022

*Mean

Source: R. J. Esterhay, Jr., et al., Cost Analysis of Leukemia Treatment: A Problem-Oriented Approach, *Cancer* 37 (1976): 650. Reprinted by permission of J. B. Lippincott and the author.

CONCEPT VIII:
Nurses can facilitate holistic care of the person with cancer by instituting and maintaining a healing milieu and by minimizing stressors that decrease quality of life.

RELATIONSHIP BETWEEN THE NURSES AND PERSON WITH CANCER

A positive relationship between the nurse and the person with cancer is based upon the ill person being treated as a unique individual with assets and strengths as well as needs. Overt acceptance of the ill person's behavior, purposeful and attentive listening, and teaching by the nurse will enhance development of a healing relationship.

Acknowledgement of the appropriateness of the ill person's feelings will increase a sense of being understood and cared about, and recognition of the client's unique strengths will enhance a sense of security and trust between the person with cancer and the nurse. Reinforcing the ill person's sense of personal control will reduce anxiety and positively affect self-esteem and the sense of meaningfulness in life.

THE HEALING MILIEU

Caregivers often overestimate the psychological pain experienced by persons with cancer, resulting in protective communication by the nurse and heightened feelings of isolation and loss of identity by the ill person [43]. Accurate assessment of the biological, personal, and social status of the ill individual is necessary before a healing milieu can be established. Simply knowing that a person is anxious or sad does not give information about the specific stressors precipitating the negative situation. Use of the stress-adaptation model in nursing practice will enable caregivers to provide specific treatment for specific problems rather than merely giving symptomatic treatment for stressors that may or may not exist in reality.

STRESS-INOCULATION TECHNIQUES

Stress-inoculation techniques have proven to be effective in altering anxiety-related behaviors and is a process inclusive of both cognitive and behavioral interventions. Cognitive coping skills are threefold: (1) identification and monitoring of maladaptive anxiety-arousing thoughts about one's response to a stressful situation, (2) generation of adaptive anxiety-reducing thoughts about the situation, and (3) conscious substitution of the latter for the former. Behavioral coping skills used in stress-inoculation training include deep muscle relaxation, imagery, and deep breathing.

There are three phases in stress-inoculation training. The first, or educational, phase has as its purpose to assist the ill person to understand the nature of his

Figure 2.1. Relaxation Technique [88]

1. Use a quiet room with soft lighting. Sit in a comfortable chair with eyes closed and feet flat on the floor.
2. Concentrate on and become aware of your own breathing.
3. Take in a few deep breaths and think "relax" as you exhale.
4. Concentrate on feeling and becoming aware of the tension in your face. Make a mental picture of the tension in your face, then imagine your facial muscles relaxing and becoming limp.
5. As your face relaxes, feel that wave of relaxation spreading throughout your body.
6. Physically tense and then relax your other body parts, moving downward from your face: jaw, neck, shoulders, and so on to your feet and toes.
7. After your entire body is relaxed, simply rest quietly for two or three minutes in this state of deep relaxation.
8. Let your eyelid muscles become lighter and become aware of the room and your external environment.
9. Open your eyes, get up from your chair, and resume your normal activities feeling refreshed and relaxed.

Figure 2.2. Imagery Process [88].

1. Attain a deep state of relaxation by using the Relaxation Technique.
2. Mentally picture your cancer in realistic or symbolic terms. Think of the cancer as a group of very weak, confused cells. Remember that our bodies destroy cancerous cells thousands of times during a normal lifetime. Think about returning your body's defenses to their natural, healthy state.
3. If you are currently receiving treatment, mentally picture the treatment entering your body. For example, you may choose to think of radiotherapy as a beam of millions of bullets of energy hitting your body's cells. Your normal cells are able to repair the damage; but the cancer cells cannot repair themselves because they are so weak, and thus they die. Another example is to visualize chemotherapy as poison in your bloodstream. Your normal cells are intelligent and strong and so don't take up the poison. Cancer cells, however, are weak and it takes very little to kill them. The cancer cells absorb the poison, die, and are flushed out of the body.
4. Mentally picture the white blood cells in your circulation. They recognize the cancer cells as abnormal and destroy them. Vast armies of white blood cells are there in your bloodstream, and they are very aggressive, strong, and smart. Cancer cells just can't win against the strong white blood cells.
5. Mentally picture the cancerous tumor shrinking or the number of leukemic cells getting smaller and smaller. The dead cancer cells are carried away by the white blood cells and flushed out of the body through urine and stool.
6. Picture yourself with increased energy, increased appetite, and feeling better.
7. If you have pain, mentally picture an army of white blood cells flowing into the painful area and soothing the pain. Visualize your body getting well.
8. Mentally picture yourself well, free from disease, full of energy, reaching your goals, and fulfilling your life's purpose. Picture your relationships with significant others taking on new meaning and beauty. Focus clearly on your priorities in life, realizing that having strong reasons for being well will *help* you to be well.
9. Congratulate yourself for participating in your own recovery.
10. Let your eyelid muscles become lighter, and become aware of the room and your external environment.
11. Open your eyes, get up from your chair, and resume your normal activities feeling refreshed and relaxed.

or her response to stressful situations. The second phase is rehearsal, in which the individual learns an array of new and adaptive coping skills. The third phase, application, occurs when the person tests the new skills in actual stressful situations [66].

RELAXATION WITH GUIDED IMAGERY

Relaxation techniques accompanied by guided imagery are not intended to replace but rather to support traditional antineoplastic treatment. Implicit in the concept of relaxation with guided imagery is the tenet of holism—that mind, body, and environment are inextricably interrelated and that what affects one aspect inevitably affects the others. The purpose of the technique is to stimulate the immune system by an unknown action to destroy malignant cells and to increase the cancer cells' vulnerability to traditional treatment [47]. Figures 2.1 and 2.2 summarize the technique of relaxation with guided imagery.

REFERENCES

1. Arakalien, M. An Assessment and Nursing Application of the Concept of Locus of Control. *ANS* 3(1): 25, 1980.
2. Bahnson, C. B. Stress and Cancer: The State of the Art, Part 1. *Psychosom* 21:1975, 1980.
3. Bahnson, C. B. Stress and Cancer: The State of the Art, Part 2. *Psychosom* 22:207, 1981.
4. Bahnson, M. and Bahnson, C. Development of Psychosocial Screening Questionnaire for Cancer. *Cancer Detect Prev* 2:295, 1979.
5. Baird, S. B. Economic Realities in the Treatment and Care of the Cancer Patient. *Topics Clin Nurs* 2(4):67, 1981.
6. Bean, G., Cooper, S., Alpert, R., and Kipnis, D. Coping Mechanisms of Cancer Patients: A Study of 33 Patients Receiving Chemotherapy. *CA* 30:256, 1980.
7. Becker, E. *The Denial of Death.* New York: Free Press, 1973.
8. Bhatia, K. and Golin, S. Role of Locus of Control in Frustration-Produced Aggression. *J Consult Clin Psychol* 46:364, 1978.
9. Bruhn, R. J., Hampton, J. W., and Chandler, B. C. Clinical Marginality and Psychological Adjustment in Hemophilia. *J Psychosom Res* 15:207, 1971.
10. Burrell, R. J. W. The Possibility Bearing of Curse Death and Other Factors in Bantu Culture on the Etiology of Myocardial Infarction. In T. N. James and J. W. Keyes (Eds.). *The Etiology of Myocardial Infarction.* Boston: Little, Brown and Co., 1963. Pp. 95–97.
11. Cantor, R. C. *And a Time to Live.* New York: Harper and Row, 1978.
12. Carp, F. M. Ego-Defense or Cognitive Consistency Effects on Environment Evaluations. *J Gerontol* 30:707, 1975.
13. Carroll, R. M. Stress and Cancer: Etiological Significance and Implications. *Cancer Nurs* 4:467, 1981.
14. Chaney, P. Surviving. *Nurs 76* 6:42, 1976.
15. Cobb, S. Social Support as a Moderator of Life Stress. *Psychosom Med* 38:300, 1976.
16. Cohen, F. Personality, Stress, and the Development of Physical Illness. In G. Stone, F. Cohen, and N. Adler (Eds.). *Health Psychology.* San Francisco: Jossey-Bass, 1979. Pp. 77–111.
17. Davis, W. L. and Davis, D. E. Internal-External Control and the Attribution of Responsibility for Success and Failure. *J Pers* 40:123, 1972.

18. Dodge, J. S. Factors Related to Patients' Perceptions of Their Cognitive Needs. *Nurs Res* 18:502, 1969.

19. DuCette, J. and Wolk, S. Cognitive and Motivational Correlates of Generalized Expectancies for Control. *J Pers Soc Psychol* 26:420, 1973.

20. Duke, M. P. and Nowicki, S. Personality Correlates of the Nowicki-Strickland Locus of Control Scales for Adults (ANSIE). *Psychol Rep* 33:267, 1967.

21. Engel, G. L. Sudden and Rapid Death During Psychological Stress: Folklore or Folkwisdom? *Ann Intern Med* 74:771, 1974.

22. Esterhay, R. I. Jr., Vogel, V. G., Fortner, C. L., Shapiro, H. M., and Wiernik, P. H. Cost Analysis of Leukemia Treatment: A Problem-Oriented Approach. *Cancer* 37:646, 1976.

23. Ferguson, B. and Kennelly, K. Internal-External Locus of Control and Perception of Authority Figures. *Psychol Rep* 34:1119, 1974.

24. Ferrari, N. A. *Institutionalization and Attitude Change in an Aged Population: A Field Study in Dissonance Theory.* Unpublished doctoral dissertation, Western Reserve University, 1962.

25. Finlayson, M., Aoan, J., and Rourke, B. P. Locus of Control as a Predicator Variable in Rehabilitative Medicine. *J Clin Psychol* 34:367, 1978.

26. Fitzpatrick, J. J., Donovan, M. J., and Johnston, R. L. Experience of Time During the Crisis of Cancer. *Cancer Nurs* 3:191, 1980.

27. Friedenbergs, I., Gordon, W., Hibbard, M., and Diller, L. Assessment and Treatment of Psychosocial Problems of the Cancer Patient: A Case Study. *Cancer Nurs* 3:111, 1980.

28. Friedman, B. D. Coping with Cancer: A Guide for Health Care Professionals. *Cancer Nurs* 3:105, 1980.

29. Greer, S., Morris, T., and Pettingale, K. W. Psychological Response to Breast Cancer: Effect on Outcome. *Lancet* 2(8146):785, 1979.

30. Hinton, J. Bearing Cancer. *Br J Med Psychol* 46:105, 1973.

31. Hinton, J. The Influence of Previous Personality on Reactions to Having Terminal Cancer. *Omega* 6:95, 1975.

32. Hiroto, D. S. Locus of Control and Learned Helplessness. *J Exp Psychol* 102(2):187, 1974.

33. Hiroto, D. S. and Seligman, M. E. P. Generality of Learned Helplessness in Man. *J Pers Soc Psychol* 3:311, 1975.

34. Hofer, M. A. Cardiac and Respiratory Function During Sudden Prolonged Immobility in Wild Rodents. *Psychosom Med* 32:633, 1970.

35. Holland, J. Psychologic Aspects of Oncology. *Med Clin North Am* 61:737, 1977.

36. Holmes, T. H. and Rahe, D. H. The Social Readjustment Rating Scale. *J Psychosom Res* 11:213, 1967.

37. Holmes, T. S. and Holmes, T. H. Short-term Intrusions Into the Life Style Routine. *J Psychosom Res* 14:121, 1970.

38. Houpt, J. L., Goudl, B. S., and Morris, F. H. Psychological Characteristics of Patients with Amyotrophic Lateral Sclerosis. *Psychosom Med* 39:299, 1979.

39. Houston, B. K. Control over Stress, Locus of Control, and Response to Stress. *J Pers Soc Psychol* 21:249, 1971.

40. Ireland, R. E. Locus of Control Among Hospitalized Emphysema Patients. *Diss Abstr Internat* 33:6091-A, 1973.

41. Jeffers, J. M. *Life Experiences as a Variable in Carcinogenesis.* Unpublished master's thesis, Wichita State University, 1977.

42. Jenkins, D. Psychosocial Modifiers of Response to Stress. *J Hum Stress* 5:3, 1979.

43. Jennings, B. M. and Muhlenkamp, A. F. Systematic Misperception: Oncology Patients' Self-Reported Affective States and Their Care-Givers' Perceptions. *Cancer Nurs* 4:485, 1981.

44. Jusenius, K. Sexuality and Gynecologic Cancer. *Cancer Nurs* 4:479, 1981.

45. Kirscht, J. P. Perceptions of Control and Health Behavior. *Can J Behav Sci* 4:225, 1972.

46. Klagsbrun, S. S. Communication in the Treatment of Cancer. *Am J Nurs* 71:944, 1971.

47. Klisch, M. L. The Simonton Method of Visualization: Nursing Implications and a Patient's Perspective. *Cancer Nurs* 3:295, 1980.

48. Krant, M. J. and Johnston, L. Family Members' Perceptions of Communications in Late Stage Cancer. *Int J Psychiatry Med* 8:203, 1977.

49. Krouse, H. J. and Krouse, J. H. Cancer as Crisis: The Critical Elements of Adjustment. *Nurs Res* 31:96, 1982.

50. Lamb, M. A. and Woods, N. F. Sexuality and the Cancer Patient. *Cancer Nurs* 4:137, 1981.

51. Lauer, P., Murphy, S. P., and Powers, M. J. Learning Needs of Cancer Patients: A Comparison of Nurse and Patient Perceptions. *Nurs Res* 31:11, 1982.

52. Lauer, R. H. Rate of Change and Stress: A Test of the "Future Shock" Thesis. *Social Forces* 52:510, 1974.

53. Lazarus, R. S. *Psychological Stress and the Coping Process.* New York: McGraw-Hill, 1966.

54. Lewis, F. M. Experienced Personal Control and Quality of Life in Late-Stage Cancer Patients. *Nurs Res* 31:113, 1982.

55. Lindsey, A. M., Norbeck, J. S., Carrieri, V. L., and Perry, E. Social Support and Health Outcomes in Postmastectomy Women: A Review. *Cancer Nurs* 4:377, 1981.

56. Lipp, L., Kolstoe, R., James, W., and Randall, M. Denial of Disability and Internal Control of Reinforcements: A Study Using a Perceptual Defense Paradigm. *J Cons Clin Psychol* 32:73, 1968.

57. Lowery, B. and DuCette, J. Disease-Related Learning and Disease Control in Diabetics as a Function of Locus of Control. *Nurs Res* 25:358, 1976.

58. Lucente, F. E. and Fleck, S. A. A Study of Hospitalization Anxiety in 408 Medical and Surgical Patients. *Psychosom Med* 34:304, 1972.

59. Luther, S. L., Price, J. H., and Rose, C. A. The Public's Knowledge About Cancer. *Cancer Nurs* 5;109, 1982.

60. Mathis, J. L. A Sophisticated Version of Voodoo Death: Report of a Case. *Psychosom Med* 26:104, 1964.

61. McNaull, F. W. The Costs of Cancer: A Challenge to Health Care Providers. *Cancer Nurs* 4:207, 1981.

62. Mechanic, D. Stress, Illness, and Illness Behavior. *J Hum Stress* 2:2, 1976.

63. Melges, F. T. and Bowlby, J. Types of Hopelessness in Psychopathological Processes. *Arch Gen Psychiatry* 20:690, 1969.

64. Miller, C. L., Denner, P. R., and Richardson, V. E. Assisting the Psychosocial Problems of Cancer Patients: A Review of Current Research. *Int J Nurs Stud* 13:161, 1976.

65. Miller, M. W. and Nygren, C. Living with Cancer-Coping Behaviors. *Cancer Nurs* 1:297, 1978.

66. Moore, K. and Altmaier, E. M. Stress Inoculation Training with Cancer Patients. *Cancer Nurs* 4:389, 1981.

67. Northouse, L. L. Mastectomy Patients and the Fear of Cancer Recurrence. *Cancer Nurs* 4:213, 1981.

68. Parkes, C. M., Benjamin, B., and Fitzgerald, R. G. Broken Heart: A Statistical Study of Increased Mortality of Widowers. *Br Med J* 1:740, 1949.

69. Pervin, L. A. The Need to Predict and Control Under Conditions of Threat. *J Pers* 31:570, 1963.

70. Phares, E. J. Differential Utilization of Information as a Function of Internal-External Control. *J Pers* 36:649, 1968.

71. Phares, E. J. Internal-External Control and the Reduction of Reinforcement Value after Failure. *J Cons Clin Psychol* 37:386, 1971.

72. Phares, E. J. and Lamiell, J. T. Internal-External Control and Defensive Preferences. *J Cons Clin Psychol* 42:872, 1974.

73. Phares, E. J., Ritchie, D. E., and Davis, W. J. Internal-External Control and Reaction to Threat. *J Pers Soci Psychol* 10:402, 1968.

74. Rahe, R. H., McKean, J. D., and Arthur, R. J. A Longitudinal Study of Life-Change and Illness Patterns. *J Psychosom Res* 10:355, 1967.

75. Richter, C. P. On the Phenomenon of Sudden Death in Animals and Man. *Psychosom Med* 19:191, 1957.

76. Roberts, S. L. Piaget's Theory Reapplied to the Critically Ill. *ANS* 2(2):61, 1980.

77. Rosenbaum, M. and Raz, D. Denial, Locus of Control, and Depression Among Physically-Disabled and Nondisabled Men. *J Clin Psychol* 33:672, 1977.

78. Rosillo, R. H., Welty, M. J., and Graham, W. B. The Patient with Maxillofacial Cancer: II. Psychological Aspects. *Nurs Clin North Am* 8:153, 1973.

79. Rotter, J. B. *Social Learning Theory and Clinical Psychology.* Englewood Cliffs, NJ: Prentice-Hall, 1954.

80. Rotter, J. B. Generalized Expectancies for Internal Versus External Control of Reinforcement. *Psych Monogr* 80:1, 1966.

81. Rotter, J. B. and Mulry, R. C. Internal Versus External Control of Reinforcement and Decision Time. *J Pers Soc Psychol* 2:598, 1965.

82. Schmale, A. H. Jr. Psychological Aspects of Anorexia. *Cancer* 43:2087, 1979.

83. Schmale, A. H. Jr. and Iker, H. P. The Effect of Hopelessness in the Development of Cancer: Part I. Identification of Uterine Cervical Cancer in Women with Atypical Cytology. *Psychosom Med* 26:714, 1964.

84. Schulz, R. and Aderman, D. Effect of Residential Change on the Temporal Distance to Death of Terminal Cancer Patients. *Omega* 4:157, 1973.

85. Seeman, M. E. and Evans, J. W. Alienation and Learning in a Hospital Setting. *Am Sociol Rev* 27:72, 1962.

86. Seligman, M. E. P. *Helplessness on Depression, Development, and Death.* San Francisco: W. H. Freeman and Co., 1975.

87. Selye, H. A Code for Coping with Stress. *AORN J* 25:35, 1977.

88. Simonton, O. C., Matthews-Simonton, S., and Creighton, J. *Getting Well Again.* Los Angeles: J. P. Tarcher, 1978. Chapter II.

89. Sonstegard, L., Hansen, N., Johnston, M. J., and Zillman, L. A Way to Minimize Side Effects from Radiation Therapy. *Am J Maternal Child Nurs* 1:27, 1976.

90. Staub, E., Tursky, B., and Schwartz, G. E. Self-Control and Predictability: Their Effects on Reactions to Aversive Stimulation. *J Pers Soc Psychol* 18:157, 1970.

91. Stein, J. (Ed. in Chief). *The Random House College Dictionary* (Rev. Ed.). New York: Random House, 1980. P. 974.

92. Sullivan, H. S. *Clinical Studies in Psychiatry.* New York: W. W. Norton Co., 1956.

93. Thomas, C. and Duszynski, D. Closeness to Parents and the Family Constellation in a Prospective Study of Five Disease States: Suicide, Mental Illness, Malignant Tumor, Hypertension, and Coronary Heart Disease. *Johns Hopkins Med J* 134:251, 1974.

94. Thomas, S. G. Breast Cancer: The Psychosocial Issues. *Cancer Nurs* 1:53, 1978.

95. Thornton, J. W. and Jacobs, P. P. Learned Helplessness in Human Subjects. *J Exp Psychol* 87:367, 1971.

96. Vinokur, A. and Selzer, M. L. Desirable Versus Undesirable Life Events: Their Relationship to Stress and Mental Distress. *J Pers Soc Psychol* 32:329, 1975.

97. Wallston, B., Wallston, K. A., Kaplan, G. D., and Maides, S. Development and Validation of the Health Locus of Control Scale. *J Cons Clin Psychol* 44:580, 1976.

98. Wallston, K. A., Wallston, B., and DeVellis, R. Development of the Multidimensional Health Locus of Control Scales (MHLC). *Health Educ Monogr* 6:160, 1978.

99. Weisman, A. and Worden, W. The Existential Plight in Cancer: Significance of the First 100 Days. *Int J Psychiatry Med* 7:1, 1976–1977.

100. Wendland, C. J. Internal-External Expectancies of Institutionalized Physically-Disabled. *Rehabil Psychol* 20:180, 1973.

101. Williams, J. Understanding the Feelings of the Dying. *Nurs 76* 6:53, 1976.
102. Wintrob, R. M. Hexes, Roots, Snake Eggs? M. D. Versus Occult. *Med Opinion* 1(7):54, 1972.
103. Wolk, S. and DuCette, J. Intentional Performance and Incidental Learning as a Function of Personality and Task Dimensions. *J Pers Soc Psychol* 29:90, 1974.

CHAPTER 3

Family in Crisis

CONCEPT I:
The family of a person with cancer is a unit in crisis and thus the target of nursing care.

It is estimated that 855,000 Americans were newly diagnosed with cancer in 1983 and 440,000 Americans died from a malignancy during that same time period [1]. Frequently overlooked is the fact that each of these persons with cancer has a family, including spouse, parents, children, and extended family members. The family unit, which had formerly served as the first line of defense to support a member in crisis, is suddenly plunged into the alien world of hospitals, chemotherapy, radiation treatments, difficult decisions, and other aspects of cancer care that often seem bizarre and frightening when first encountered. One of its significant members is threatened by disease, mutilation, and death; yet instead of being able to successfully defend that member, the family may perceive that the disease itself renders the family impotent and vulnerable and that the care team relegates them to a position of passive observers without the ability or knowledge to assist the person with cancer in any significant way.

The catastrophic event of cancer disrupts family structure and function, resulting in disequilibrium and alteration of the entire system. The ill member may not be able to fulfill former role functions and may be simultaneously creating new demands upon existent family resources. Other family members may have to assume additional or new roles and obligations, demanding coping skills not normally used. Role reversals, relinquishment of roles, and acquisition of new roles and obligations—all imposed by the cancer experience—may cause tremendous disruption in the family's dynamic equilibrium. Fear of the unknown, perceptions of helplessness and vulnerability, and watching the loved one experience treatment side-effects, pain, and disease progression all add immense burdens to the family's attempts to cope.

Spouses of persons with cancer face different problems than do spouses of persons ill with nonmalignant disease. Perceptions of helplessness and anger with the medical system are more common among spouses of persons with cancer, and spouses may feel abandoned by physicians and nurses as their mates become sicker. Thus, these spouses experience greater difficulties during both illness and bereavement [15].

When the person with cancer dies, survivors may be at high risk for physical and emotional illnesses and even death. Physical health seems to deteriorate during bereavement, with an increased probability that the bereaved will receive medical care [12, 20]. The hypothesis that the death of a spouse results in increased risk of death for the surviving mate is gaining credence. Surviving spouses seem to be mortally endangered for at least the first six months of bereavement [13, 17]. White widowers aged 25 to 34 exhibit a death rate more than four times greater than their married counterparts [14], and the mortality rate among widowers aged 55 or older is 40 percent higher than the population of married men in the same age group [21].

Families of persons with cancer thus seem more vulnerable to physical, personal, and social disequilibrium because of the catastrophic, chronic nature of the disease itself as well as the depletion of family resources and the perception of loss of mastery over the family unit. When a person within a family system has cancer, the entire family may be in a crisis and thus the target of nursing care.

CONCEPT II:
The diagnosis of cancer is an assault on the integrity of the family system, and many families fail to successfully adapt to and cope with the threat to family stability.

Families tend to proceed through four stages during their experience with cancer, each stage having characteristic events and hurdles. The four stages are living with cancer, restructuring during the living-dying interval, bereavement, and reestablishment [6].

LIVING WITH CANCER

During this first stage, the family is informed that one of its members has been diagnosed with cancer. Within the stage of living with cancer, the typical family proceeds through five phases: impact, functional disruption, search for meaning, informing others, and engaging emotions.

Impact

A family enters the first phase, impact, when it learns that one of its members has been diagnosed with cancer. The other family members typically exhibit shock and strain, and the entire family unit often becomes disorganized. Key members of the family may emerge to help the others cope with the impact of the diagnosis of cancer. The hurdle for the family to overcome is despair. Nurses can assist the family by fostering hope, by assuring distressed family members that medical and nursing treatment is available and may help the ill member, and by communicating with the family clearly and with confidence and candor. Since the family can perceive caregivers' attitudes of hopefulness or hopelessness, the caregivers tremendously influence the family's ability to overcome despair.

Functional Disruption

The substage of functional disruption occurs as family members weaken their commitment to former role obligations. Time spent at the hospital interferes with usual responsibilities and family activities; and job responsibilities, household activities, and child care are adjusted to adapt to the new situation. The family may exhibit reduced initiative, and role dilemmas are common. The hurdle for the family to overcome during this time is a sense of vulnerability as each member becomes aware of his or her own mortality. If nurses provide emotional support to family members at this time, then a sense of security under the pressures of rapidly changing life situations is enhanced and strengthened.

Informing Others

The next substage might occur before the family has successfully overcome the hurdles of despair, isolation, and vulnerability. Informing others of their new catastrophic situation may be necessary before family members have fully dissipated the impact of diagnosis or assimilated information concerning prognosis, course of treatment, and expected outcomes. In our culture, cancer is still a stigmatizing condition, so the response of others to the family's news may be horror, pity, or dismay. The hurdle for the family to overcome is retreat from others because of real or imagined negative reactions. Assisting the family to clarify and share their feelings within the immediate family unit will foster courage. Search for outside sources of primary support will be lessened if family communication and cohesion is strengthened.

Engaging Emotions

The last substage commonly observed during this adaptive period is characterized by the surfacing of volatile emotions as family values, goals, and security undergo change. Engaging emotions is the result of challenge, clarification, and alteration of these values and positions of security, and the hurdle for the family to overcome is perceived helplessness in the face of the catastrophic illness of a valued member. If the ill person progresses toward recovery, the sense of helplessness and experiences of volatile emotions diminish. If, however, the ill person's condition worsens and death seems inevitable, the family begins to recognize its defeat and acknowledge its loss, and they may begin to grieve for the anticipated loss of their loved one. Anticipatory grieving enables the family to work through a portion of the psychic trauma associated with the expected loss of their family member. The beginning of mourning, the strain of fulfilling additional roles within the family structure, and the experience of intense emotion and perceived helplessness cumulatively result in an emotionally fatigued family. Some family members struggle to suppress volatile emotions, fearing that outbursts of strong feelings imply loss of self-control. Nurses can help the family during this time by facilitating emotional expression and helping the family to effectively solve the daily problems that arise. Loss of control does not occur when family members acknowledge and express intense feelings. Loss of control does occur, however, if emotions are suppressed and family members lose touch with themselves and each other. Successful daily problem solving and the opportunity to express emotions will reduce perceptions of helplessness and will help the family realize that life will continue even should their loved one die.

RESTRUCTURING DURING THE LIVING-DYING INTERVAL

In the mid-stage of the cancer experience, the ill person characteristically develops progressive, symptomatic disease with patterns of improvement and decline, remissions and exacerbations, over a period of time [4]. Indeed, the time when medical treatment begins for disease recurrence may be more disruptive for the family than the periods of initial diagnosis and treatment [9]. The ill person becomes increasingly dependent upon other family members for assistance in carrying out activities of daily living and experiences frequent acute disease-related problems requiring hospitalizaiton. These episodes of acute medical crisis may occur in rapid succession, allowing little time for either the ill person or the family to successfully adapt and cope. With longer survival times among persons with cancer, the mid-stage has also lengthened. Since the family has primary responsibility for the physical and emotional care of their chronically ill member during the patterns of improvement and decline over this lengthy period of time, the mid-stage has a high stress-producing potential. The hurdle for the family to overcome during the mid-stage is frustration. Our societal expectations of medicine include immediate, or at least rapid, cure of ailments, but the chronic nature of cancer and its accompanying complex problems are not amenable to simple, quick resolution. Thus, the family may experience mounting frustration and tension over recurrent medical crises. Nurses can assist families to clarify their perceptions of the situation and to deal with each problem as it arises. In cancer treatment, battles are usually won by inches, and assisting the family to gain this perspective will reduce frustration.

Stressors emanating from the internal and external environments have a tremendous negative impact on the family. Already burdened by the situation of serious, chronic disease in one of its members, recurrent and frequent hospitalizations of that valued member for acute crises, anticipatory grieving and the tendency for social isolation, the family must additionally attempt to cope with a wide array of other stressors. Since the presence of even one stressor will weaken the family's defenses against other stressors, the family unit is extremely vulnerable to biological, personal, and social disequilibrium as negative events and additional demands occur (see Table 3.1).

Table 3.1. Family Stressors and Nursing Interventions in the Mid-Stage of the Cancer Experience

STRESSOR	BIOLOGICAL DISEQUILIBRIUM	NURSING INTERVENTIONS
Lack of help with physical care of ill person. Lack of help with care of children. Long distance from hospital or clinic. Necessity of preparing different meals. Necessity of rearranging living quarters. Working at outside jobs.	Physical fatigue and exhaustion.	Assist family to utilize community resources and extended family for help. Help to devise simple, nutritious meals. Schedule hospital and clinic visits to produce minimal disruption of family routines. Encourage adequate rest and sleep.

Table 3.1.   Family Stressors and Nursing Interventions in the Mid-Stage of the Cancer Experience
(Cont.)

STRESSOR	BIOLOGICAL DISEQUILIBRIUM	NURSING INTERVENTIONS
Fatigue Depression	Anorexia, decreased nutritional intake	Encourage adequate nutritional intake, rest, and sleep.
Inadequate time for personal self-care. Reluctance to leave ill person alone.	Weight loss. Malnourishment.	Encourage expression of feelings. Facilitate realistic hope.
Fatigue. Malnourishment leading to immunoincompetence. Exposure to pathogens in hospital environment.	Increased vulnerability to infection.	Encourage adequate nutritional intake, rest, sleep. Encourage prompt treatment of infections.
Prolonged, persistent stress levels. Fatigue. Malnutrition. Possible infection.	Stress-related diseases.	Encourage adequate nutritional intake, rest, and sleep. Encourage expression of feelings. Assist in developing strategies to reduce stress. Encourage prompt treatment of symptomatic disease.
STRESSOR	PERSONAL DISEQUILIBRIUM	NURSING INTERVENTIONS
Fear of leaving ill person alone. Lack of help with ill person's physical and emotional needs. Difficulty in dealing with ill person's behavior.	Increased psychic pain. Isolation from external support and outside world. Sense of loneliness.	Assist family to arrange for intermittent private duty nursing help. Encourage family to spend regularly scheduled hours away. Encourage expression of feelings. Assure family that negative feelings are normal. Assist family to devise strategies to modify ill person's disruptive behavior.
Knowledge deficits regarding care of ill person. Communciation deficits with health professionals.	Increased sense of helplessness. Frustration. Inaccurate or incomplete information. Possibility of turning to "quack" treatments.	Collaborate with family to assess learning needs. Devise clear, easily understood teaching plans. Encourage family to ask questions. Avoid technical jargon.
STRESSOR	SOCIAL DISEQUILIBRIUM	NURSING INTERVENTIONS
Reluctance to repeatedly ask for help. Social isolation.	Paucity of external support. Family conflict. Behavioral problems among children.	Advise family of community groups and services. Referral to professional counseling.

Stressors Leading to Biological Disequilibrium in Family Members

Demands placed upon family members escalate during the mid-stage of the cancer experience. Lack of help with the ill person's physical care and with care of children living at home [19] impose excessive physical demands on immediate family members, often resulting in significant physical fatigue and exhaustion. Many families live a long distance from the hospital or outpatient clinic, necessitating lengthy, time-consuming drives for hospital visits or scheduled treatments. The necessity of preparing different meals for the ill person and for the rest of the family, and rearrangement of household living quarters to accommodate the needs of the ill person, add to the complexity of and time invested in necessary household duties. In addition, a large percentage of family members must continue to work in their outside jobs while concurrently attempting to manage the home care of the ill person or to make regular visits to their hospitalized family member. These stressors, occurring individually or in combination, impose tremendous physical burdens and commonly result in excessive physical fatigue.

Fatigue, depression, and inadequate time for personal self-care commonly lead to anorexia, decreased ingestion of a nutritionally adequate diet, weight loss, and malnourishment. While the ill person is hospitalized, it is a common occurrence for family members to exhibit reluctance about leaving their loved one and so often skip meals or eat skimpy meals brought to them. Within the home setting, the family member responsible for meal preparation is often so fatigued by the extent of preparation of different foods that he or she may tend to prepare quick, easy meals for himself or herself, sometimes not bothering to eat at all. Depression and fatigue occurring simultaneously will often greatly reduce the person's desire for food, and this inadequate intake of a nutritious diet results in weight loss and malnutrition and further weakens the person's defense against worsening fatigue.

The fatigue and malnourishment so often encountered in family members lead to a greatly increased susceptibility to infectious disease. Malnutrition has been assoicated with both cellular and humoral immunoincompetence [19], rendering the person vulnerable to bacterial and viral infection. Additionally, if the person with cancer is hospitalized, the vulnerable family member is exposed to a variety of pathogens not usually encountered in the nonhospital environment.

Stress-related diseases may be biological manifestations of the escalation of stressors to intolerable levels. Prolonged and persistent high stress levels produce alteration in neurophysiological functioning, eventually producing clinical symptoms of disease and requiring medical and/or nursing treatment. The concurrent conditions of fatigue, malnourishment, and possible infection even further weaken the family member's defense against development of stress-related disease, and the disease condition may be worsened by the person's reluctance to seek medical treatment for a seemingly trivial physical problem.

Biological disequilibrium can be minimized by preventive or curative nursing measures. Assisting the family to utilize community resources and extended family members may lessen the burden imposed by home care of the ill person and care of small children. Helping the home caregiver to devise simple, nutritious meals for both the ill person and for well family members will simplify and reduce time expenditure in meal preparation.

Ensuring that hospital and outpatient clinic visits are scheduled with as little disruption as possible to the entire family's time availability will reduce unnecessary driving and time expenditure. Encouraging family members to obtain adequate nutritional intake, rest, and sleep will be more effective if the family is reminded that they will be more helpful to their ill member if they are as well as possible. Treatment of infections or stress-related disease symptoms must be strongly encouraged; the family member should be reminded that prevention, or at least prompt treatment, of these conditions will better enable them to minister to the needs of their loved one.

Stressors Leading to Personal Disequilibrium of Family Members

Personal demands placed upon the immediate family also mount during the mid-stage of the cancer experience. When the ill person is being cared for at home, a primary stressor for the immediate family is the fear of leaving their sick member alone [19]. When coupled with the stressor of lack of sufficient help with the ill person's emoitonal needs, this fear of leaving home and the resulting isolation from physical contact with external support persons and the outside world may intensify the family's psychic pain, causing psychological disequilibrium.

Caregivers at home may find it difficult to constantly deal with the ill person's behavior in a patient, nonjudgmental, caring manner. Being the primary caregivers in the home often means being the *only* caregivers, and the inability to remove oneself from a distressing situation even for short periods of time results in a constantly escalating stress level. The family must continually deal with the ill person's anorexia, intolerance of certain foods, inability to mechanically manage oral nutrients, nausea, and vomiting. Sleep patterns in the chronically ill are often altered, adding to the caregivers' fatigue and frustration. Management of pain may require specialized assessment and intervention skills beyond the normal abilities of the family, and watching a loved one suffer chronic, unrelieved pain adds tremendously to the family's feelings of helplessness and guilt. Continuously trying to deal with the ill person's emotional lability, especially deep depression, drains the family's psychic resources. These stressors, plus others unique to each family situation, may result in maladaptive family responses and psychological disequilibrium.

Knowledge deficits regarding appropriate physical and psychological care of the ill member heightens the family's sense of helplessness and frustration. Skills and information necessary for adequate home care of persons with cancer are not often easily attainable by families, leaving them to manage the care on a trial-and-error basis or by garnering what information they can from professional literature that they may not understand, frequently inaccurate or sensationalized media offerings, or advice form well-meaning acquaintances. Skills and information needed by families providing home care for persons with cancer are summarized in Table 3.2.

Communication deficits between family and health professionals may preclude effective teaching and learning. Families often are in awe of health professionals and are reluctant to ask questions for fear of seeming stupid. To complicate the communication problem, health professionals all too often hide their discomfort with unpleasant questions by using highly technical language that the family cannot understand or by evading discussions with the family concerning the ill per-

Table 3.2. Skills and Information Needed by Families Providing Home Care for Persons with Cancer [4, 7]

Skills and Information Related to Biological Needs	1. What observations to make in assessing the ill person's condition. 2. Strategies to manage activities of daily living. 3. Comfort care. 4. Bed bath. 5. Changing an occupied bed. 6. Wound and skin care. 7. Ambulation skills. 8. Transferring from bed to chair. 9. Bedpan and urinal. 10. Bladder and bowel management. 11. Ostomy care. 12. Management of anorexia and nausea. 13. Nutrition and feeding. 14. Tube feedings. 15. Pain management and injections. 16. Oxygen administration. 17. Oropharyngeal suctioning.
Skills and Information Related to Personal Needs	1. Information about cost of home care. 2. Coping with financial stressors. 3. Using support systems.
Skills and Information Related to Social Needs	1. Information about community resources and services. 2. Dealing with children's questions. 3. Involving children in care of the ill person.

son's condition, treatment protocols, expected outcomes, or prognosis. These knowledge and communication deficits inevitably result in cognitive disequilibrium for the family, increasing their sense of helplessness and frustration and resulting in inaccurate or incomplete information and a greater possibility of turning to "quack" treatment.

Personal disequilibrium can be minimized by preventive or curative nursing interventions. Simply listening to family members and allowing them to express their frustrations, fears, and feelings of helplessness and anger will enable them to dissipate much of the energy invested in these negative emotions, freeing that energy to accomplish more positive tasks. Assuring the family that their feelings are normal and are shared by others in similar situations usually affords a great sense of relief and lessens perceptions of "being the only ones in the world who feel this way."

Behavior modification plans to decrease disruptive behavior by the ill person may be successful in reducing family tension. Nurses may help the family to devise such plans specifically tailored to their unique problems.

Assisting the family to arrange for a private duty nurse to care for the ill person on an intermittent basis will enable the family to get away from the continuous tension of the home care situation. Encouraging the family to spend regularly scheduled hours away from home will help to replenish their physical and emotional energy and enable them to better cope with home demands.

Collaboration with the family to assess learning needs will pinpoint specific skills or information necessary for the family to increase quality of care for the ill person at home. Devising a clear, easily understood teaching plan with return demonstrations or other evaluations of learning will effectively increase the abilities of the family caregivers to meet the needs of their ill members. Encouraging the family to ask questions and answering those questions clearly and in language easily understood by the family will reduce the communication deficit so commonly observed between families and health professionals. Additionally, nurses can act as translators of highly technical language and information, making sure that family members clearly understand the data being communicated.

Stressors Leading to Social Disequilibrium in Family Members

In our society, cancer remains a stigmatizing condition and, as previously mentioned, the initial reactions from others may be shock, horror, and dismay. The family may receive support from the extended family or close friends at first, but as time goes on, external support begins to wane and the family may be reluctant to repeatedly ask for assistance. As tension begins to mount within the immediate family circle, family conflict and behavioral problems among children at home may surface [11]. Personality changes, delinquency, and disrupted development may occur in the children [5], further adding to the family's stress. Social isolation increases as the family becomes more and more absorbed in the care of their ill member, and a paucity of consistent external support seems to exist. These factors may eventually result in social disequilibrium for the family.

Nursing measures may minimize social disequilibrium by intervening into the social isolation and family conflicts so commonly observed during the mid-stage of the cancer experience. Advising the family of community resources and services available to assist them may enable the family to derive support from external sources. These community resources have the added advantage of knowledge of similar family situations and have developed the skills necessary to overcome some of the obstacles of the mid-stage. Family conflict or problems with children may be eased or resolved by referral to professional counseling. Counseling services are available in most large hospitals and community mental health agencies, and payment of fees are often flexible to accommodate the needs of families who may be financially depleted.

LIVING-DYING INTERVAL

The living-dying interval is characterized by extensive disease and imminent death of the person with cancer. The ill person is cared for at home or in the hospital and ceases to fulfill roles and obligations within the family structure, necessitating redistribution of role obligations to reduce strain or overcompensation by some family members [6]. Family members must explore current needs, compromise among themselves, and consolidate new obligations and responsibilities. There may be misguided attempts to make the ill person overly dependent upon the family as a result of family members trying to compensate for their own feelings of helplessness. Unfortunately, this situation removes any control that the ill person may retain over his or her own life experiences, increasing psychic pain and perceived helplessness. Nurses can assist the family by fostering interpersonal cooperation and enhancing the ill person's personal mastery over life experiences in order to more effectively meet family goals. Cooperation and cohesion among family members—including the ill person—will facilitate a greater sense of family wholeness during this crucial time. By virtue of close and continual contact with the hospitalized person and the family, nurses are in an advantageous positon to facilitate supportive relationships among family members, to ensure maximum mastery over life events by the ill person, and to enhance the family's relationship with the member with cancer. These nursing interventions will support the family's progressive acceptance of eventual death and will foster normal grief work.

One substage in the living-dying interval is *framing of memories* [6], a time for the family to remember their dying member's life history. The hurdle for the family to overcome is the threat of anonymity for their loved one. Everyone needs to leave a shadow; and by listening to families tell their stories, nurses can assist them to solidify and clarify their perceptions of the ill person's identity as a valued family member worthy of being remembered. As the families tell their stories, their abstract image of the ill member strengthens and relinquishment of his or her physical existence becomes easier.

BEREAVEMENT

The stage of bereavement coincides with the ill member's imminent death and continues through the actual death event and the period of time immediately following. Bereavement is the objective state of deprivation secondary to the loss of the loved one, whereas grief is the subjective psychological state of intense emotional pain in response to the loss. Grieving is characterized by mental anguish and an intense focus on the deceased, and it is a process necessary to experience and complete if the survivors are to become whole persons again. Since the majority of deaths in the United States occur in institutions such as hospitals [2], nurses are in a position to facilitate the family's healthy progression through the grieving process.

The first substage in bereavement is *separation,* occurring when the ill person's level of consciousness and awareness of the external environment diminish [6]. It is at this time that the family fully experiences their loss and the loneliness of imminent separation. The hurdle for the family to overcome is self-absorption. By promoting continued verbal and tactile communication with the dying person and by fostering intimacy among family members, nurses can facilitate the family's ability to grieve within the family network and thus derive support from one another.

The period of separation is a highly stressful, emotionally charged time for family members. Withdrawal, denial of the dying person's critical condition, anger or guilt, and/or an inappropriate affect are commonly observed maladaptive responses. Depression among family members is nearly universal, usually secondary to guilt, premature resolution of the outcome, disbelief, perceptions of helplessness and the inability to change the course of events, loneliness, or overintellectualization of the situation. Unfortunately, many families perceive that nurses neglect family needs and concerns during this time, nurses being seen as "too busy" and with a tendency to avoid the family and evade their questions. In one study [8], less than 75% of families interviewed reported satisfactory fulfillment of several family needs deemed as critically important (Figure 3.1).

The most effective nursing intervention to help families cope during this crucial time of separation is not one primarily aimed at the family itself but rather nursing measures focused intensely on the dying person. If the family is assured that their loved one is receiving meticulous, quality nursing care, their feelings of apprehension and anxiety diminish [20]. It is important that nurses realize that it is the family's *perception* of support or nonsupport by health professionals that is important. Nonsupportive behaviors by caregivers include not permitting the family to talk about the past or to express feelings. Equally nonsupportive is the caregiver's expectation that the family should "control themselves" and exhibit a calm demeanor during a time of severe psychic crisis.

The second substage, *mourning*, begins with the death of the ill family member and is completed only when the memory of the dead person becomes internalized and a source of enrichment for the family's continued life [6]. Even when death is expected, the family will usually respond to the actual death event with shock, numbness, and dismay, and family members may not be able to believe that death has finally occurred. The shock and numbness result from the individual not yet admitting overwhelming emotions into conscious awareness, which is why many survivors seem to "do well" at their family member's funeral. Unfortunately, many nurses impatiently withdraw from the family's shock and disbelief since "the family knew that death was inevitable," resulting in inadequate and superficial nursing care toward survivors at this critical time. The hurdle for the family to overcome is guilt over the severed relationship. Bereaved family members commonly verbalize their feelings repeatedly at this time in an attempt to make sense of their loss and to ask the unanswerable question of "why?" This repetition is necessary before acceptance and mastery of the loss can be achieved [17]. In other words, they must tell their story again and again until it has become internalized and there is subsequently no longer a reason to tell the story. Thus, the most important nursing intervention at this time is simply to listen.

Figure 3.1. Needs of the Grieving Spouse in a Hospital Setting. [8] (Less than 75% of spouses interviewed identified needs as being met.)

To be with their dying spouses.
To be helpful to their dying spouses.
To be assured of the physical comfort of their spouses.
To be assured of the emotional comfort of their spouses.
To be informed of their spouse's condition.
To be informed privately of their spouse's impending death.
To ventilate emotions.
To receive comfort and support from family members.
To receive acceptance, support, and help from
health professions.

Good Grief

Since the bereaved are a high-risk population for physical and emotional illness and even premature death, particularly if pathological grief reactions develop, it is of great importance for caregivers to facilitate healthy and normal grieving. Unfortunately, because of their own feelings of helplessness and inadequacy in the face of intense psychic suffering and pain, nurses and other caregivers often do not respond therapeutically to family needs at this time.

Giving advice instead of simply listening in a nonjudgmental, accepting manner is a reflection of the nurse's own feelings of powerlessness, and "rushing in" to help and solve problems may prevent nurses from really hearing the needs being expressed. Additionally, our cultural emphasis on self-control, competence, strength, and adequacy as valued personal attributes may block the family's resolution of normal grieving.

Therapeutic interventions are so simple as to be often discounted as simply trivial. The mere physical presence of a trusted nurse during the immediate postdeath period usually brings immense comfort to the family, and ensuring privacy just before and after the death event enables the family to express their grieving without the feeling of being "on display." In one study, 85 percent of spouses were informed of their mate's impending death in busy, impersonal hospital corridors [8], hardly conducive to the expression of emotion. Nurses can assist the family by assuring them clearly and repeatedly that everything possible was done for their dead family member, that family members had significantly helped their loved one in his or her suffering, and that they had loved their dead member well.

After shock and numbness begin to fade, acute grief commences, a definite syndrome with both somatic and intense psychological symptomatology (see Figure 3.2). Acute grief is not related to the degree of love felt for the dead person but rather to the degree of both positive and negative feelings the individual held toward the deceased [3]. Commonly experienced somatic expressions of grief are shortness of breath, tightness in the throat, a sensation of choking, muscle weakness, a sensation of emptiness in the abdomen, anorexia and subsequent weight loss, sighing, and respiratory disturbances [10].

Psychic symptomatology of normal grieving emanates from an intense preoccupation with the image of the dead loved one [10]. The bereaved may experience a slight sense of unreality, and both visual and auditory hallucinations of the deceased are common [3]. Emotional distancing from others is common, and the bereaved may question his or her own sanity since the psychic phenomena associated with normal grieving is not congruent with the intellectual acknowledgement of the loved one's death.

Guilt, or anger turned inward, is a common experience for the bereaved. The survivor searches for evidence of his or her own failure in preventing the death, accusing himself or herself of negligence and exaggerating minor omissions. Anger may also be expressed toward others—God, the care team, other family members, and even the deceased. Feelings of hostility, irritability, and bitterness result in even further emotional estrangement from others.

Former patterns of interaction with others become disorganized, and the bereaved may exhibit apathy and despair. Behavior becomes aimless, restless, and

Figure 3.2. Symptomatology of Normal Grief [3, 10].

SOMATIC EXPRESSIONS OF GRIEF
Shortness of breath
Tightness in the throat
Sensation of choking
Muscle weakness
Sensation of emptiness in abdomen
Anorexia and weight loss
Sighing
Respiratory disturbances

PSYCHIC EXPRESSIONS OF GRIEF
Intense preoccupation with image of deceased
Slight sense of unreality
Visual and auditory hallucinations of the deceased
Emotional distancing from others
Questioning of own sanity
Guilt (anger turned inward)
    Searching for evidence of failure in preventing the death of the loved one
Hostility (anger turned outward)
    Expressions of hostility toward God, the care team, other people, deceased person
    Irritability, bitterness
    Loss of interest and warmth toward others
Altered patterns of behavior
    Disorganized patterns of interaction with others
    Apathy
    Despair
    Aimless, restless, purposeless behavior
    Sense of futility and emptiness
    Inability to initiate and maintain organized activity
    Sadness, crying
    Insomnia
    Difficulty in concentration

without purpose as a result of a sense of futility and emptiness, and there may be an inability to initiate and maintain organized activity. The bereaved may exhibit sadness, insomnia, crying, and difficulty in concentration.

REESTABLISHMENT

Reestablishment occurs as the family completes the grieving process and reexpands its social network [6]. The symptomatology of grieving may come and go as family members gradually put closure on mourning and begin to reestablish their lives without the physical presence of the dead family member. A sense of the continuity of life is reaffirmed, and the important aspects of the relationship with the deceased is integrated into the family's corporate life, enriching and deepening family relationships. The hurdle for the family to overcome is social alienation [6] after the extended time of relative social isolation during the deceased's illness and death, and the family's period of mourning. Nurses can assist the family by fostering relatedness and social interaction, thus reducing feelings of estrangement (see Table 3.3).

CONCEPT III:
Successful reestablishment of normal family life after the death of a member is thwarted by unhealthy grief reactions that impede resolution of mourning and often necessitate professional intervention.

PATHOLOGICAL GRIEF REACTIONS

It is important to remember that we as human beings do not have the choice of *whether* we will grieve; it is rather a question of *how* we will grieve. Pathological grief reactions are exaggerations of normal grieving, differing not in kind but rather in duration and intensity from normal grief [2]. Exaggerations of normal grief symptomatology may include development of symptoms characteristic of the deceased's last illness, extreme hostility with an altered affect and patterns of conduct, chronic indecisiveness, and a lack of initiative. The bereaved may exhibit abnormal behavior that is detrimental to his or her own socioeconomic survival. Agitated depression and even suicidal ideation may occur in pathological grief reactions [10].

Delayed Grief

If the bereaved seems to feel little sorrow over the loved one's death and continues on with life as though nothing of significance has occurred, the phenomenon of delayed grief may be present. The bereaved usually acts very busy and calm, and this behavior may continue for weeks. Usually, however, acute grief is suddenly triggered by another, sometimes minor, loss, such as a ring or book, or by suddenly remembering with new clarity the circumstances surrounding the loved one's death [2].

Inhibited Grief

In the phenomenon of inhibited grief, the bereaved seemingly never feels the psychic pain of mourning. However, a person cannot choose whether or not to grieve: grieving will occur either psychically or somatically. In inhibited grief, the bereaved often develops physical illnesses, such as colitis, arthritis, or asthma [2]. Since the person does not grieve psychically, the body expresses the grief with very real physical illnesses.

Chronic Grief

Normal grieving is a process with a beginning and an end, but in chronic grief, the process continues indefinitely without healthy resolution [2]. Reestablishment of normal life, expansion of the social network, and integration of memories

Table 3.3.   Family's Response to the Experience of Cancer [6]

MAIN STAGES	FAMILY EXPERIENCES	NURSE CAN FOSTER
Living with cancer: Client learns of diagnosis, tries to carry on as usual, undergoes medical/nursing treatment.	1. *Impact*—Emotional shock, despair, disorganized behavior.	*Hope* as different treatment measures are used, communication, helpful resources.
	2. *Functional disruption*— Much time spent at hospital, ignoring of home tasks and emotional needs, weakening of family structure, emotional isolation.	*Family cohesiveness*
	3. *Search for meaning*— Questioning why this happened; casting blame on various persons, deity, habits, institutions; realization that "someday I too will die."	*Security*
	4. *Informing others*—Ascent from isolation, possible need to retreat again into emotional isolation.	*Courage,* reliable help, understanding why some people can't help.
	5. *Engaging emotions*— Beginning of grieving, fear loss of self-control, assumption of roles once carried out by ill person.	*Problem-solving,* strategies will be dynamic and ongoing.
Living-Dying Interval: Client ceases to perform family roles, is cared for either at home or hospital.	6. *Reorganization*—Firmer division of family tasks.	*Cooperation* instead of competition, analysis of success of new role distribution.
	7. *Framing of memories*— Reviewing of life experiences of dying person; what he has meant and accomplished, new sense of family history, relinquishment of dependency on dying member.	*Identity,* ability of family to focus on life review rather than only on what ill person is or appears to be now.
Bereavement: Client death.	8. *Separation*—absorption in the loneliness of separation.	*Intimacy* among family members.
	9. *Mourning*—resolution of guilt.	*Relief,* release of guilt.
Reestablishment	10. *Expansion of the social network*—overcoming feelings of alienation and guilt.	*Relatedness,* looking back with acceptance and forward to new growth and socialization with a reunited, normally functioning family.

Source: From B. Giacquinta, Helping Families Face the Crisis of Cancer, *American Journal of Nursing* 77 (October 1977): 1585. Copyright © 1977, American Journal of Nursing Company. Reprinted by permission.

of the dead loved one are not accomplished, and the bereaved exists in a world of social isolation, guilt, anger, and intense psychic pain.

INTERVENTION INTO ABNORMAL GRIEVING

Patterns of abnormal grieving (see Table 3.4) usually require professional intervention through counseling, group therapy, support groups, or other measures in order to facilitate transformation of these maladaptive responses into the adaptive response of normal grief work. It must be remembered that mourning is a process that requires energy and time, and it may be as long as eighteen to twenty-four months after the death before successful resolution of normal grief has occurred. It is important, therefore, for health professionals to realize that even normal grief work is just that: *work*. It is lengthy and sometimes characterized by seemingly bizarre symptoms. Determination of the existence of abnormal grieving requires careful assessment of the bereaved as well as of all environmental factors influencing the situation.

SUMMARY

Families of persons with cancer are units in crisis and thus the target of nursing care. Significant risks of physical or emotional illness or even death are experienced by bereaved family members, rendering nursing facilitation of family progression through the stages of living with cancer and of normal grieving an important preventive aspect of nursing care. Identification of family stressors and therapeutic intervention will minimize maladaptive responses and enhance effective and successful family coping.

Table 3.4. Unhealthy Grief Reactions [3, 10]

ABNORMAL GRIEF REACTION	SYMPTOMATOLOGY
Pathological Grief Reaction	Development of symptoms characteristic of the deceased's last illness. Extreme hostility toward others. Social isolation. Repressed hostility with altered affect and patterns of conduct. Chronic indecisiveness. Lack of initiative. Abnormal behavior detrimental to socioeconomic survival. Agitated depression. Suicidal ideation.
Delayed Grief	Seems to feel little sorrow. Acts busy and calm. Acute grief triggered by minor loss or recollection of death event.
Inhibited Grief	Little or no psychic pain. Grieves somatically with physical illness.
Chronic Grief	Grief work unresolved and continues indefinitely.

REFERENCES

1. American Cancer Society. *1983 Cancer Facts and Figures*. New York: American Cancer Society, 1982.
2. Backer, B. A., Hannon, N., and Russell, N. A. *Death and Dying: Individuals and Institutions*. New York: John Wiley and Sons, 1982. Chapter 9.
3. Bowlby, J. Process of Mourning. *Int J Psychoanal* 42:317, 1961.
4. Edstrom, S. and Miller, M. W. Preparing the Family to Care for the Cancer Patient at Home: A Home Care Course. *Cancer Nurs* 4:49, 1981.
5. Evans, A. E., Combrinck-Graham, L., and Ross, J. W. Meeting the Problems of Siblings of a Child with Cancer. In American Cancer Society. *Proceedings of the American Cancer Society Second National Conference on Human Values and Cancer*. New York: American Cancer Society, 1978. Pp. 73–77.
6. Giacquinta, B. Helping Families Face the Crisis of Cancer. *Am J Nurs* 77:1585, 1977.
7. Grobe, M. E., Ilstrup, D. M., and Ahmann, D. L. Skills Needed by Family Members to Maintain the Care of an Advanced Cancer Patient. *Cancer Nurs* 4:371, 1981.
8. Hampe, S. O. Needs of the Grieving Spouse in a Hospital Setting. *Nurs Res* 24:113, 1975.
9. Holland, J., Rowland, R., and Plumb, M. Psychological Aspects of Anorexia in Cancer Patients. *Cancer Res* 37:2425, 1977.
10. Lindemann, E. Symptomatology and Management of Acute Grief. *Am J Psychiatry* 101:141, 1944.
11. Mellette, S. J. The Patient, The Family, and the Disease. In American Cancer Society. *Proceedings of the American Cancer Society Second National Conference on Human Values and Cancer*. New York: American Cancer Society, 1978. Pp. 103–108.
12. Parkes, C. M. The Effects of Bereavement of Physical and Mental Health: A Study of the Case Records of Widows. *Br Med J* 2:274, 1964.
13. Parkes, C. M., Benjamin, B., and Fitzgerald, F. G. Broken Heart: A Statistical Study of Increased Mortality Among Widowers. *Br Med J* 7:740, 1969.
14. Rees, W. and Lutkins, S. Mortality of Bereavement. *Br Med J* 4:13, 1967.
15. Shudin, S. Cancer Widows. *Nurs 78* 8:56, 1978.
16. Simos, B. Grief Therapy to Facilitate Healthy Restitution. *Soc Casework* 58(6):337, 1977.
17. Stroebe, M. S., Stroebe, W., Gergen, K. J., and Gergen, M. The Broken Heart: Reality or Myth? *Omega* 12(2):87, 1981.
18. Vredevoe, D. L. Physiological Variables Related to Cancer. In D. L. Vredevoe, A. Derdiarian, L. P. Sarna, M. Friel, and J. A. G. Shiplacoff (Eds.). *Concepts of Oncology Nursing*. Englewood Cliffs, NJ: Prentice-Hall, 1981. Chapter 2.
19. Welch, D. Planning Nursing Interventions for Family Members of Adult Cancer Patients. *Cancer Nurs* 4:365, 1981.
20. Wiener, A., Gerberg, I., Battin, D., and Arkin, A. The Process and Phenomenology of Bereavement. In B. Schoenberg, I. Gerber, A. Wiener, A. Kutscher, D. Peretz, and A. Carr (Eds.). *Bereavement: Its Psychosocial Aspects*. New York: Columbia University Press, 1975.
21. Young, M., Benjamin, B., and Wallis, C. The Mortality of Widowers. *Lancet* 2:454, 1963.

Chapter 4

Basic Concepts of Cancer

CONCEPT I:
Cancer is a group of disease processes characterized by uncontrolled growth and spread, eventually interfering with one or more vital functions of the host and leading to death.

During the last half-century, significant progress has been made in effecting cures and long-term remissions and in lengthening the survival time of persons with cancer. During the 1930s, less than one person in five was alive five years after treatment. During the 1970s, approximately one in three were alive five years after treatment [28].

Although death rates from some malignancies have decreased since 1930 (e.g., uterus, stomach), many malignancies have exhibited constant mortality rates, and the death rate from lung cancer has dramatically increased (see Figures 4.1 and 4.2 and Table 4.1). Despite advances in knowledge, treatment protocols, and technology, cancer remains the second leading cause of death in the United States, with approximately one person in five dying from a malignant process [37] (see Table 4.2).

Lung cancer is the leading cause of malignancy-related deaths in American men. For women in the United States, the leading cause of cancer death is breast malignancy [37] (see Tables 4.3 and 4.4 and Figures 4.3 and 4.4).

Cancerous processes are the second leading cause of death in American children aged one to fourteen [37]. Leukemia and central nervous system tumors are the most frequently occurring tumors in this age group (see Table 4.5).

Cancer is the leading disease killer in young adults between the ages of fifteen and thirty-four. Although mortality rates have been steadily decreasing in recent years [36], malignant disease remains a significant cause of death in this age group (see Figure 4.5).

CONCEPT II:
Cancer is not a singular, specific disease but rather a variable group of tissue responses.

Malignant tissue responses are governed by normal laws of growth, although cancerous growth is imperfectly controlled [40]. Normally, body demands for a quantitative increase in the number of cells and for cell replacement are initiated by cell loss or by extra demands for tissue function. All elements of malignant cellular growth and proliferation are found in normal tissue growth mechanisms. Cancer seems to result from progressive failure of these intrinsic normal growth

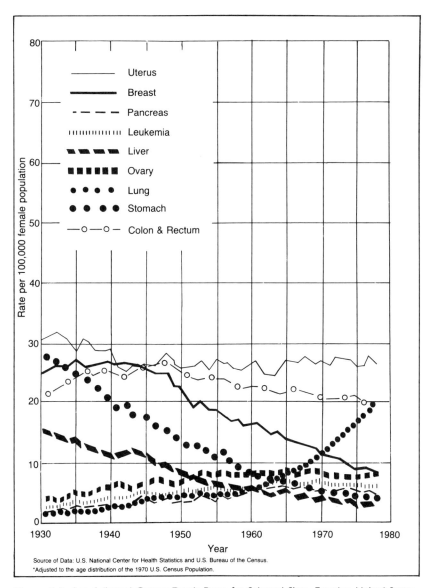

Figure 4.1. Age-Adjusted Cancer Death Rates for Selected Sites, Females, United States, 1930–1978 (From E. Silverberg, Cancer Statistics, 1982, *CA—A Cancer Journal for Clinicians* 32 (1982): 20. Reprinted by permission.)

mechanisms, and differences between malignant and normal cellular growth and proliferation are matters of degree, not kind.

Hyperplasia refers to any abnormal increase in the number of cells in a tissue or part of a tissue, resulting in increased tissue mass. Physiological hyperplasia results from the presence of an external stimulus and subsides when the stimulus is re-

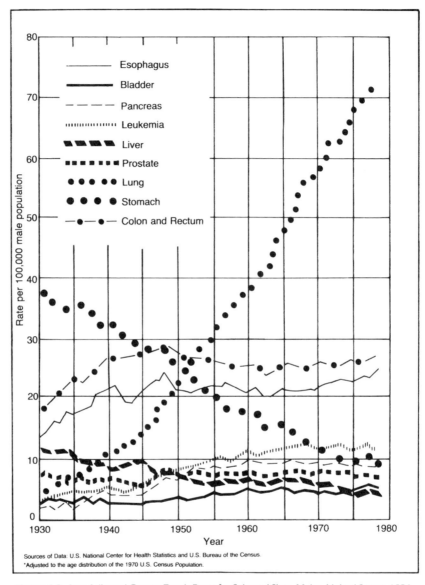

Figure 4.2. Age-Adjusted Cancer Death Rates for Selected Sites, Males, United States, 1930–1978 (From E. Silverberg, Cancer Statistics, 1982, *CA—A Cancer Journal for Clinicians* 32 (1982): 21. Reprinted by permission.)

moved (e.g., pregnancy and the subsequent hyperplasia of the uterus). Neoplastic hyperplasia is due to abnormalities within the involved cells themselves. Both types of hyperplasia may be present in a tissue simultaneously.

Metaplasia is a reversible, benign change in which an adult cell changes from one type to another. *Dysplasia* is a benign change in which an adult cell varies from its

Table 4.1. 25-Year Trends in Age-Adjusted Cancer Death Rates Per 100,000 Population 1951–52 to 1976–78

Sex	Sites	1951–53	1976–78	Percent Changes		Comments
Male	All Sites	171.9	215.7	+	25	Steady increase mainly due to lung cancer.
Female	All Sites	146.4	136.1	–	7	Slight decrease.
Male	Bladder	7.2	7.2		*	Slight fluctuations; overall no change.
Female	Bladder	3.1	2.1	–	32	Some fluctuations; noticeable decrease.
Male	Breast	0.3	0.3		*	Constant rate.
Female	Breast	26.0	27.1	+	4	Slight fluctuations; overall no change.
Male	Colon & Rectum	25.8	26.4		*	Slight fluctuations; overall no change.
Female	Colon & Rectum	24.8	20.0	–	19	Slight fluctuations; noticeable decrease.
Male	Esophagus	4.7	5.4	+	15	Some fluctuations; slight increase.
Female	Esophagus	1.2	1.5		*	Slight fluctuations; overall no change in females.
Male	Kidney	3.4	4.7	+	38	Steady slight increase.
Female	Kidney	2.1	2.2		*	Slight fluctuations; overall no change.
Male	Leukemia	7.9	8.8	+	11	Early increase, later leveling off.
Female	Leukemia	5.4	5.2		*	Slight early increase, later leveling off.
Male	Liver	6.7	4.8	–	28	Some fluctuations. Steady decrease in both sexes.
Female	Liver	7.6	3.6	–	53	
Male	Lung	25.5	69.3	+	172	Steady increase in both sexes due to cigarette smoking.
Female	Lung	5.0	17.8	+	256	
Male	Oral	5.9	5.8		*	Slight fluctuations; overall no change in both sexes.
Female	Oral	1.5	2.0		*	
Female	Ovary	8.1	8.6	+	8	Steady increase, later leveling off.
Male	Pancreas	8.6	11.2	+	30	Steady increase in both sexes, then leveling off.
Female	Pancreas	5.5	7.1	+	29	Reasons unknown.
Male	Prostate	21.0	22.6	+	8	Fluctuations all through period; overall no change.
Male	Skin	3.1	3.4		*	Slight fluctuations; overall no change in both sexes.
Female	Skin	1.9	1.9		*	
Male	Stomach	22.8	9.3	–	59	Steady decrease in both sexes; reasons unknown
Female	Stomach	12.3	4.3	–	65	
Female	Uterus	20.0	8.7	–	57	Steady decrease.

*Percent changes not listed because they are not meaningful.

Source: Reprinted from American Cancer Society 1983 Cancer Facts and Figures, Page 11. Copyright © 1982, American Cancer Society. Used with permission.

Table 4.2. Mortality for Leading Causes of Death—1978

Rank	Cause of Death	Number of Deaths	Death Rate Per 100,000 Population	Percent of Total Deaths
	All Causes	1,927,788	809.9	100.0
1.	Heart Diseases	729,510	300.4	37.8
2.	Cancer	396,992	169.9	20.6
3.	Cerebrovascular Diseases	175,629	70.8	9.1
4.	Accidents	105,561	45.8	5.5
5.	Pneumonia & Influenza	58,319	23.6	3.0
6.	Chronic Obstructive Lung Disease	50,488	12.2	2.6
7.	Diabetes Mellitus	33,841	14.2	1.8
8.	Cirrhosis of Liver	30,066	13.4	1.6
9.	Arteriosclerosis	28,940	11.1	1.5
10.	Suicide	27,294	11.6	1.4
11.	Diseases of Infancy	22,033	12.1	1.1
12.	Homicide	20,432	8.7	1.1
13.	Aortic Aneurysm	14,028	5.8	0.8
14.	Congenital Anomalies	12,968	6.8	0.7
15.	Pulmonary Infarction	10,941	4.6	0.6
	Other & Ill-defined	210,606	89.9	10.8

Source: E. Silverberg, Cancer Statistics, 1982, *CA—A Cancer Journal for Clinicians* 32 (1982): 16. Reprinted by permission.

Table 4.3. Mortality for Five Leading Cancer Sites, Males by Age Group, United States—1978

All Ages	Under 15	15–34	35–54	55–74	75 +
Lung 71,006	Leukemia 550	Leukemia 827	Lung 10,124	Lung 46,049	Lung 14,646
Colon & Rectum 25,696	Brain & Central Nervous System 344	Brain & Central Nervous System 467	Colon & Rectum 2,462	Colon & Rectum 13,717	Prostate 12,298
Prostate 21,674	Bone 47	Hodgkin's Disease 335	Pancreas 1,262	Prostate 9,047	Colon & Rectum 9,325
Pancreas 11,010	Connective Tissues 43	Testis 329	Brain & Central Nervous System 1,282	Pancreas 6,490	Pancreas 3,208
Stomach 8,529	Kidney 39	Melanoma of Skin 261	Leukemia 1,065	Stomach 4,558	Bladder 3,172

Source: E. Silverberg, Cancer Statistics, 1982, *CA—A Cancer Journal for Clinicians* 32 (1982): 17. Reprinted by permission.

Table 4.4.   Mortality for the Five Leading Cancer Sites, Women by Age Group, United States–1978

All Ages	Under 15	15–34	35–54	55–74	75 +
Breast 34,329	Leukemia 411	Breast 585	Breast 8,205	Breast 17,403	Colon & Rectum 12,626
Colon & Rectum 27,573	Brain & Central Nervous System 275	Leukemia 493	Lung 4,679	Lung 14,463	Breast 8,129
Lung 24,080	Bone 45	Brain & Central Nervous System 347	Colon & Rectum 2,210	Colon & Rectum 12,551	Lung 4,819
Uterus 10,842	Kidney 44	Uterus 295	Uterus 2,111	Ovary 5,992	Pancreas 3,939
Ovary 10,651	Connective Tissues 43	Hodgkin's Disease 223	Ovary 2,029	Uterus 5,480	Uterus 2,954

Source: E. Silverberg, Cancer Statistics, 1982, *CA—A Cancer Journal for Clinicians* 32 (1982): 17. Reprinted by permission.

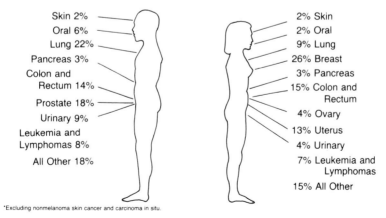

*Excluding nonmelanoma skin cancer and carcinoma in situ.

Figure 4.3. 1982 Estimated Cancer Incidence by Site and Sex (From E. Silverberg, Cancer Statistics, 1982, *CA—A Cancer Journal for Clinicians* 32 (1982): 15. Reprinted by permission.)

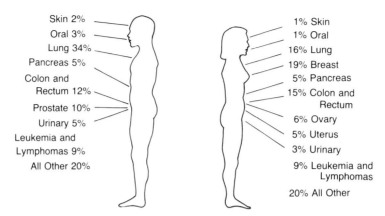

Figure 4.4. 1982 Estimated Cancer Deaths by Site and Sex (From E. Silverberg, Cancer Statistics, 1982, *CA—A Cancer Journal for Clinicians* 32 (1982): 15. Reprinted by permission.)

normal size, shape, or organization and is often due to chronic irritation. Dysplasia may reverse itself or may progress to cancer. *Anaplasia* is a malignant, irreversible alteration in which the structural patterns of adult cells regress to a more primitive level. *Differentiated* cells are those with recognizable specialized structures and functions, whereas *undifferentiated* cells are those that have lost the capacity for specialized functions. Generally speaking, the more undifferentiated a malignant cell, the more virulent it is considered to be.

Neoplasms are "new growths" and may be benign or malignant. An example of a benign neoplasm is the common wart. A cancerous solid tumor is the classic example of a malignant neoplasm.

Table 4.5.   Cancer Incidence by Site for Children Under 15, SEER PROGRAM, 1973–1976

Rank	Site	Number of Cases	Percent of Total	Rate Per 1,000,000 Children
1.	Leukemia	664	30.2	33.6
2.	Central Nervous System	409	18.6	20.7
3.	Lymphomas	298	13.6	15.1
4.	Sympathetic Nervous System	170	7.7	8.6
5.	Soft Tissue	141	6.5	7.1
6.	Kidney	135	6.1	6.8
7.	Bone	101	4.6	5.1
8.	Retinoblastoma	58	2.6	3.0
9.	Liver	26	1.2	1.3
	All Others	195	8.9	9.9
	All Sites	2,197	100.0	111.1

Source: E. Silverberg, Cancer Statistics, 1982, *CA—A Cancer Journal for Clinicians* 32 (1982): 30. Reprinted by permission.

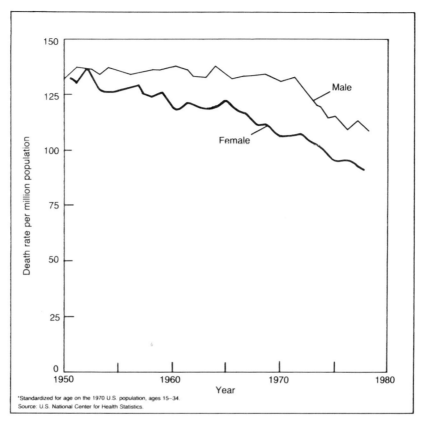

150

125

100

Death rate per million population

75

50

25

0

1950   1960   1970   1980

Male

Female

Year

*Standardized for age on the 1970 U.S. population, ages 15–34.
Source: U.S. National Center for Health Statistics.

Figure 4.5. Cancer Death Rates by Sex for Young Adults Ages 15–34, in the United States, 1950–1978 (From E. Silverberg, Cancer Statistics, 1982, *CA—A Cancer Journal for Clinicians* 32 (1982): 15. Reprinted by permission.)

CONCEPT III:
The two-stage theory of carcinogenesis [15] describes the complete process by which a normal cell is thought to become a cancer cell (see Figure 4.6).

Cancer probably begins from a single mutant cell capable of maintaining virtually uncontrolled cell division until a lethal total body burden has been reached. The two-stage theory postulates that the process of transforming a normal cell into a cancerous cell consists of two different phases (initiation and promotion) with several substages, all of which take place in the cell's DNA. *Pre-initiation* is a period in which the genome of the cell (the total gene complement of the chromosomes) is either sensitized to or protected from the effects of carcinogens. *Initiation*, or Stage 1, occurs when carcinogens contact the cell. The process responsible for initiation is thought to be mutagenic, involving permanent DNA alterations from either direct damage to DNA molecules or inhibition of DNA repair systems.

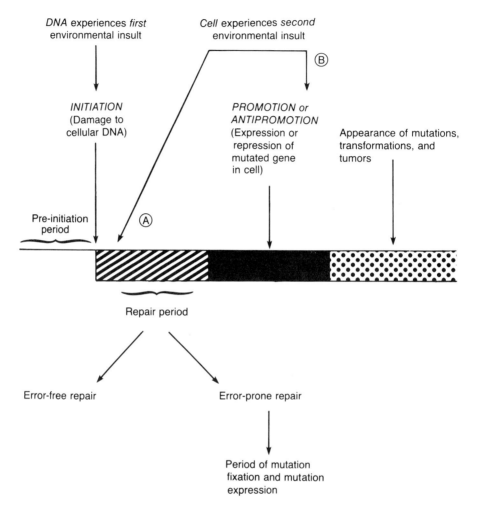

Figure 4.6. Two-Stage Theory of Carcinogenesis

At least one cell division seems to be necessary during the initiation phase in order for the neoplastic transformation to stabilize. Normal cell function is apparently not altered by initiation. *Repair* is a transitional period in which one of two repair processes take place. Error-free repair occurs if the section of damaged DNA is successfully excised and repaired by normal cellular functions. Error-prone repair occurs if DNA repair is unsuccessful. If error-prone repair occurs, the DNA lesion becomes fixed and permanent mutation results. At this point, the cell still appears to be normal and functions in a normal way because the DNA mutation has not been expressed; expression of the DNA mutation requires that the cell divide. *Promotion*, or Stage 2, occurs when a mutated gene is expressed in the cell, resulting in uncontrolled cell division and tumor promotion. The process responsible for promotion is epigenetic, involving expression or repression of genetic information. *Antipromotion* occurs when the mutated gene is repressed in the daughter cells. The affected cell is capable of normal function, but the latent mutation could be expressed at any time since the DNA lesion is still present. Host and/or environmental factors may influence the expression or repression of mutated neoplastic cells.

The two-stage theory provides sound rationale for the efforts by health professionals to prevent cancer. Cancer could theoretically be prevented if contact between cells and carcinogens is eliminated before promotion. Since both promotion and antipromotion may be influenced by host and/or environmental factors, manipulation of those factors may prevent or delay the onset of cancer.

CONCEPT IV:
Malignant cells have certain characteristics that distinguish them from nonmalignant cells.

CELL CYCLE

All cells, malignant and nonmalignant, progress through five phases of the cell cycle (see Figure 4.7). In the G_0 phase, a cell performs all cellular functions except those related to proliferation. The G_0 phase is also known as the "resting phase." Normal cells in the G_0 phase are activated to enter the reproductive cycle only by specific stimuli, e.g., death of a cell of the same type. In the G_1 phase,

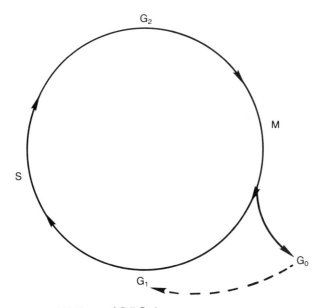

Figure 4.7. Phases of Cell Cycle

protein and RNA synthesis occur. In the S phase, synthesis of DNA takes place. In the G_2 phase, there is additional synthesis of protein and RNA. Finally, in the M phase, mitosis and cell division take place. After this, the daughter cells either return to the G_0 phase and stop dividing or, if there is continued stimulus for cell division, enter the G_1 phase again to begin the cell reproductive cycle all over again.

FACTORS CONTRIBUTING TO THE CONTINUOUS GROWTH PATTERNS OF MALIGNANT CELLS

Cancer cells apparently are unable to remain in the G_0 (resting, nondividing) phase for prolonged periods of time; thus they replicate continuously. Another factor suspected of contributing to the proclivity of cancer cells to reproduce are chalones that are thought to be glycoproteins inhibiting growth of normal cells [28]. Another substance apparently necessary for normal growth patterns is fibronectin. Fibronectin occurs in greatly reduced amounts on the membranes of both rapidly dividing normal cells and cancer cells. When fibronectin is added to cultures of some tumor cells, growth patterns temporarily normalize.

Additionally, cancer cells in culture have been observed to take up nutrients at a much greater rate than do nonmalignant cells [19, 28]. This increased transportation of nutrients may result from alterations of transport sites on the surface membrances of cancer cells. This continuous supply of nutrients may also contribute to the lack of growth control characteristic of cancer cells.

UNIQUE CHARACTERISTICS OF MALIGNANT CELLS

Cancer cells tend to be larger and more pleomorphic with specific intracellular characteristics [31]. The nuclear: cytoplasmic ratio is higher than in nonmalignant cells. Clumping of chromatin commonly occurs, and multiple and prominent nucleoli are often seen. Also, abnormal mitoses may be observed. Another characteristic of malignant cells is the frequently increased level of proteolytic enzymes, which may be involved in tumor cells' ability to invade through the basement membranes of nearby normal tissues [28].

Cancer cells also have a greater tendency to grow in a disorderly, chaotic manner that may be a reflection of their decreased adhesion to substrate tissue [31]. Malignant cells also usually display a reduced ability to adhere to one another. Reduced adhesiveness among cancer cells may be due to a lower than normal amount of calcium bound to the cell surfaces, thus forming a decreased number of calcium bridges between the cells and weakening their ability to cling to one another [9]. Alterations in the malignant cells' adhesive capacity may also involve changes in cell surface lectins [28]. Lectins, or agglutinins, are multivalent carbohydrate-binding proteins that attach to certain cell-surface receptor sites that contain sugars. In animals, lectins are thought to control the adhesion of one cell to another. Another factor in the phenomenon of decreased adhesiveness characteristic of malignant cells may be the failure of the cancer cell to recognize growth and movement inhibitory influences that are normally produced by contact with adjacent cells [45].

CONCEPT V:
The proliferative behavior of malignant cells that comprise a tumor mass may be described by tumor cell kinetics, viewing tumors as consisting of three compartments [39].

Compartment A consists of proliferating clonogenic cells undergoing active anabolism. Cells in this compartment contribute to the increase in total tumor cell population. Tumor growth occurs when proliferating cells in Compartment A exceed cell loss. *Compartment B* consists of nonproliferating nondividing cells that are not actively engaged in anabolism. Although cells in Compartment B retain a potential for proliferation and cellular division, they do not contribute to increases in total tumor cell population. *Compartment C* is comprised of permanently nonproliferating, nonclonogenic cells. These cells do not contribute to tumor growth but rather only to tumor volume (see Figure 4.8).

The *growth-fraction* of a tumor is the ratio of proliferating to nonproliferating cells (A/B + C). As tumor volume increases, growth fraction progressively decreases. As tumor volume increases, tumor doubling time also increases.

CONCEPT VI:
Malignancies must be evaluated before appropriate medical treatment can be determined.

The two methods of evaluating malignancies are based on different parameters. Grading refers to the microscopic appearance of tumor cells, specifically their degree of anaplasia. Staging refers to the extent of malignant spread within the body.

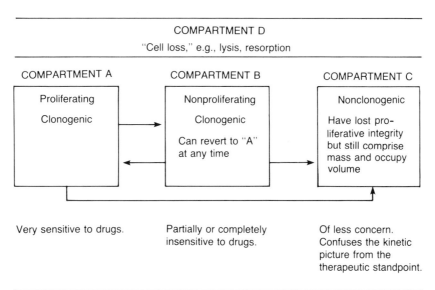

Figure 4.8. Proliferative Behavior of Subpopulations of Tumor Cells (From H. E. Skipper, Kinetics of Mammary Tumor Cell Growth and Implications for Therapy, *Cancer* 28 (1971): 1479. Reprinted by permission of J. B. Lippincott and the author.)

GRADING

Grading is a method of classifying neoplasms on a scale of I to IV and is based upon the degree of cellular anaplasia observed under the microscope. Grade I neoplasms are so well differentiated that the cells closley resemble normal parent cells. Grades II and III cells are moderately differentiated and poorly differentiated, respectively. Grade IV neoplasms are composed of undifferentiated cells that are so anaplastic that even recognition of the tissue of origin becomes difficult. If different areas of the tumor show different grades of malignancy, the tumor will be graded according to the least differentiated area.

It is the general assumption that the less differentiated the tumor cells are, the more virulent and "more malignant" the cancer is. However, grading has little or no overall prognostic value in most types of cancer. Grading has significant prognostic value in only a few cancerous tumors, such as transitional cell carcinoma of the urinary bladder, astrocytomas, and chondrosarcomas. A lower grade in these particular malignancies indicates a better prognosis.

Neoplastic progression is an unpredictable phenomenon in which the lesion progresses from a low grade to a higher one, thus becoming more malignant. The biological basis for neoplastic progression is apparently simple Darwinian selection rather than changes in the host or tumor [31]. Those cells best able to reproduce and least able to differentiate tend to "outgrow" other, less malignant cells. Thus, the nature of the tumor tends with time to become more virulent.

STAGING

Clinical staging establishes the presence and extent of a tumor within the body. Staging requires systemic evaluation of the client to determine the extent of disease and is usually based on the TNM system. "T" (tumor) indicates the degree of local extension of the primary tumor. "N" (nodes) describes clinical findings in regional lymph nodes. "M" (metastasis) indicates the presence or absence of distant metastatic disease.

A one-centimeter tumor, which is currently the usual size capable of physical diagnosis, has already progressed through thirty doublings. Forty doublings is considered to constitute a lethal body burden of tumor. Considering that few tumors are diagnosed when less than one centimeter in diameter, it is appropriate to consider most malignancies advanced at the time of diagnosis. Most cancers are treated at least one stage beyond their clinically defined stage.

Staging of Solid Tumors Other Than Large Bowel Tumors [34]

Solid tumors are described in terms of four stages. In *Stage I,* the clinical examination reveals a mass limited to the organ of origin. Because there is only local involvement, the lesion is resectable. There is no evidence of nodal or vascular spread, and the client has a 70 percent to 90 percent chance of survival.

In *Stage II,* clinical examination shows evidence of local spread into surrounding tissue and first-station lymph nodes. Although the lesion is resectable, there is uncertainty about the completeness of surgical removal. The client has a 45 percent to 55 percent chance of survival.

In *Stage III* tumors, clinical examination shows an extensive primary lesion with fixation to deeper structures, and lymph nodes exhibit evidence of malignant invasion. The tumor is operable but not resectable, and gross disease is left behind. Surgery for Stage III tumors is primarily a debulking procedure. The client has a 15 percent to 25 percent chance of survival.

In *Stage IV,* clinical examination reveals evidence of distant metastases beyond the local site of the primary tumor. The lesion is inoperable, and the client has less than a 5 percent chance of survival.

Staging of Large Bowel Solid Malignant Tumors [7]

Large bowel cancers are staged according to Dukes' Criteria. In *Stage A,* the primary tumor is restricted to the bowel wall, and the five-year survival rate is 90 percent. In *Stage B,* the tumor has invaded through the bowel wall and into the peritoneum or perirectal fat. The five-year survival rate for Stage B tumors is 65 percent. In *Stage C,* metastatic disease is observed in regional lymph nodes, and the five-year survival rate falls to 20 percent.

CONCEPT VII:
The particular types and forms of cancer are related to the tissue of origin and the degree of differentiation.

SOLID TUMORS

Solid tumors are basically divided into two types. Carcinomas are malignant neoplasms of epithelial tissues, those tissues derived from the primitive ectoderm or endoderm. Classifications of carcinomas are usually site-specific. Sarcomas are cancers of tissues of mesodermal origins. Classifications of sarcomas are generic and can usually be applied regardless of the anatomical site of origin (see Table 4.6).

Carcinomas [2]

Lung Carcinomas.   Carcinomas of the lung are divided into four types, each with definite biological characteristics. The four types are epidermoid, adenocarcinoma, oat cell (small cell), and large cell anaplastic carcinoma.

Epidermoid carcinoma of the lung is assoicated with smoking, and the largest proportion of cases is observed in males. Epidermoid lung carcinomas usually display a proximal location, can grow to large sizes, and often show central cavitation. Five-year survival rate is about 22 percent.

Adenomacarcinoma of the lung shows no association with smoking, and the largest proportion of cases is seen in females. These tumors usually display a peripheral location. They are most often small and show no central cavitation. Five-year survival rate is about 9 percent.

Table 4.6.   Types of Sarcomas [2]

TYPE OF SARCOMA	CELL OF ORIGIN
Chondrosarcoma	Chondroblast
Fibrosarcoma	Fibroblast
Fibroxanthosarcoma	Histiocyte
Hemangiosarcoma	Blood vessel endothelium
Leiomyosarcoma	Smooth muscle
Liposarcoma	Fat cell
Lymphangiosarcoma	Lymph vessel endothelium
Malignant mesenchymoma	Pluriopotential mesenchyme
Osteosarcoma	Osteoblast
Rhabdomyosarcoma	Striated muscle
Synovial sarcoma	Synovial cells
Alveolar soft part sarcoma	Uncertain cell of origin
Malignant granular cell tumor	
Kaposi's sarcoma	
Epitheloid sarcoma	
Clear-cell sarcoma of tendon sheath and aponeuroses	

Oat cell, or small cell, lung carcinoma is associated with smoking and usually displays a central location. These tumors are often associated with a large mediastinal mass. Oat cell carcinoma of the lung is extremely virulent, with a five-year survival rate approaching zero. Large cell anaplastic carcinomas of the lung include bronchioalveolar cell carcinoma.

Ovarian Carcinomas [2]. Ovarian carcinomas are divided into three large groups, depending on the cell of origin. Ovarian carcinomas may arise from surface epithelium, germ cells, or stromal cells.

Breast Carcinomas [2]. Carcinomas of the breast are classified according to local invasiveness and the tendency for axillary lymph node metastasis. Type I includes intraductal carcinoma, lobular carcinoma in situ, and papillary carcinoma confined to the ducts. Type I tumors are rarely invasive and exhibit no lymph node disease. Type II tumors include pure mucinous carcinoma, medullary carcinoma with lymphocytic infiltration, well-differentiated or "tubular" adenocarcinoma, and papillary carcinoma with stromal invasion. These tumors may be invasive but exhibit a low incidence of nodal metastasis. Type III tumors include the large majority of infiltrating ductal carcinomas whether or not they exhibit an intraductal component. Type III tumors are highly invasive and exhibit a moderate incidence of nodal metastasis. Type IV tumors consist of undifferentiated varieties and all types of tumors that have been observed to be invasive into blood vessels. Type IV tumors have the largest incidence of both regional lymph node and distant metastases.

Epidermoid Carcinomas of the Skin [2].   Epidermoid carcinomas of the skin are divided into two groups. One type arises from an active keratosis. These tumors follow an indolent course and rarely metastasize. The second group arise from normal skin tissue and are much more highly virulent cancers.

Malignant Melanoma of the Skin [2]

Malignant melanoma of the skin is divided into three distinct groups. Lentigo maligna-melanoma has the best prognosis of the three types of melanoma. Superficial spreading melanoma has a moderately good prognosis, whereas nodular melanoma is highly malignant and has a poor prognosis.

Carcinoma in Situ [2]

Carcinoma in situ is a lesion with all the histological characteristics of malignancy except invasion. The microscopic appearance of carcinoma in situ is identical to that tissue which is often seen adjacent to already-invasive carcinomas. If left untreated, these lesions will eventually become invasive cancers in a large proportion of cases.

Sarcomas

Sarcomas occur less often than carcinomas and are more frequently seen in younger age groups. Most soft-tissue sarcomas arise from normal tissue rather than from preexisting benign lesions.

DIFFUSE TUMORS

Leukemias

The classification of leukemias is based upon the predominant cell type and whether the disease process is considered to be acute or chronic (see Table 4.7). Leukemia is a disease characterized by the abnormal proliferation and release of leukocyte (white blood cell) precursors. The disease process originates during leukocyte development in the bone marrow (myeloid tissue) or lymphoid tissues.

Table 4.7. Four Main Classifications of Leukemia

Classification of Leukemia	Predominant Cell Type	Level of Cellular Maturity
Acute lymphoblastic leukemia (ALL)	Lymphoblast	Immature
Acute nonlymphoblastic leukemia (ANLL)	Varies	Immature
Chronic lymphocytic leukemia (CLL)	Lymphocyte	Mature
Chronic myelogenous leukemia (CML)	Granulocyte	Mature

Table 4.8. Summary of Differences Between Leukemic Cells and Normal Leukocytes

	Normal Leukocytes	Leukemic Cells
Appearance	Mature	Immature
	Invisible nucleolus	Nucleolus visible
	Coarse dispersement of chromosomes	Fine dispersement of chromosomes
Function	Multiply in response to body demand	Multiply continuously
	Defend the body against pathogens	Unable to defend the body against pathogens
Number	Less than 5% blasts in bone marrow	More than 5% blasts in bone marrow
	No blasts in peripheral blood	Blasts often observed in peripheral blood

Leukemic cells are abnormal, immature white blood cells, differing in appearance, function, and number from normal leukocytes (see Table 4.8). Blasts are another name for primitive white blood cells.

The leukemic process results in an alteration of homeostasis within the client's internal environment [20]. With rapid proliferation of leukemic cells, the bone marrow becomes overcrowded with immature leukocytes, which then spill over into the peripheral circulation. Crowding of the bone marrow by leukemic cells inhibits normal blood cell production. Decreased erythrocyte production results in anemia and reduced tissue oxygenation. Decreased platelet production results in thrombocytopenia and risk of hemorrhage. Decreased production of normal white blood cells results in increased vulnerability to infection, especially since leukemic cells are functionally unable to defend the body against pathogens. Leukemic cells may invade and infiltrate vital organs, such as liver, kidneys, lungs, heart, or brain, resulting in multisystem dysfunction.

Rapid destruction of circulating blood cells results in a dangerous accumulation of serum uric acid, the end-product of cell catabolism. If the uric acid crystals precipitate in and obstruct renal tubules, renal failure may occur.

Leukemia Classification.   Leukemia is classified as lymphoid or myeloid according to the predominant cell type. Leukemia originating from lymphoid tissue (lymphatic system) has "lympho" in its name. Leukemia originating in myeloid tissue (bone marrow) has "myelo" in its name. The suffix "blastic" denotes the presence of immature blast cells, whereas the suffix "cytic" refers to the presence of more mature cells.

Leukemia is classified as acute or chronic according to the level of maturity exhibited by the predominant cell type. Acute leukemia is characterized by the proliferation of blast cells, whereas chronic leukemia is characterized by the proliferation of more mature cells.

Each classification of leukemia differs according to incidence, clinical manifestation, and prognosis (see Table 4.9).

Malignant Lymphomas

Malignant lymphomas, both non-Hodgkin's lymphomas and Hodgkin's disease, are classified according to four main features: cell type, degree of differentiation, type of reaction elicited by the tumor cells, and patterns of growth [2] (see Table 4.10).

If a nodular pattern of growth is observed, the word "nodular" is used after the cell type. A better prognosis is associated with a nodular pattern. If no reference to growth pattern is made, the lymphoma is of a diffuse type.

Non-Hodgkin's lymphomas.   Non-Hodgkin's lymphomas include lymphocytic, histiocytic, and undifferentiated types [6]. Approximately 25 percent of cases develop between ages fifty and fifty-nine, with maximum risk between ages sixty and sixty-nine. A herpes-like virus is suspected in the etiology of lymphocytic and histiocytic lymphomas.

Anatomical staging of non-Hodgkin's lymphoma classifies the disease process into four stages. Stage I lymphomas display involvement of only a single extralymphatic organ or site. Stage II lymphomas exhibit involvement of two or more lymph node regions on the same side of the diaphragm, or localized involvement of an extralymphatic organ or site plus at least one lymph node region on the same side of the diaphragm. In Stage III lymphoma, there is involvement of lymph node regions on both sides of the diaphragm or involvement of the spleen, or both. Stage IV lymphomas exhibit disseminated or diffuse involvement of at least one extralymphatic organ or tissue (e.g., liver, lung, bone marrow, pleura, bone, skin) with or without associated lymph node enlargement.

Complete remission of non-Hodgkin's lymphoma has been reported as ranging between 20 percent and 60 percent. "Leukemic transformation" with high peripheral lymphocyte counts is observed in about 13 percent of the cases of lymphocytic lymphoma.

Hodgkin's disease.   Hodgkin's disease is a specific type of lymphoma, differing from all other lymphomas in its predictability of spread, microscopic characteristics, and occurrence of primary extranodal tumors [2, 6]. Hodgkin's disease accounts for about 40 percent of all cases of malignant lymphomas. Approximately 50 percent of cases occur between the ages of twenty and forty, with less than 10 percent occurring after age sixty or before age ten. The incidence of Hodgkin's disease is greater in males, and males have a poorer prognosis.

The pathway of spread in Hodgkin's disease is highly predictable. If a lymph node group is affected, the next group of lymph nodes to show evidence of disease

Table 4.9. Incidence, Manifestations, and Prognosis of Leukemias [20,23,38]

Classification of Leukemia	Incidence	Manifestations	Prognosis
Acute lymphoblastic leukemia (ALL)	85% of all childhood leukemias; 10%–20% of all adult leukemias	HEMATOPOIETIC DYSFUNCTION 1. Anemia (fatigue, pallor)-Hg ranging 2–15 mg/dl, average 7 mg/dl 2. Thrombocytopenia (bleeding)-platelets usually less than 50,000/mm^3 3. Abnormal WBC count, ranging from less than 1,000/mm^3 to more than 1 million/mm^3 LYMPHATIC DYSFUNCTION 1. Lymphadenopathy 2. Splenomegaly BONE PAIN NEUROLOGICAL DYSFUNCTION if CNS infiltration has occurred	CHILDREN: 1. Remisison achieved in 90% of cases 2. Average duration of remission 4.5 years 3. 5-year survival approching 50% ADULTS: 1. Average duration of remission 2 years 2. Average survival 33 months
Acute nonlymphoblastic leukemia (ANLL)	18% of all childhood leukemias; 80%–90% of all adult leukemias	Same as ALL	1. If left untreated, average survival 2 months 2. With intensive treatment, average survival 13 months 3. Remission achieved in 30% of cases 4. Average duration of remission 6–9 months 5. 3-year survival 30%

74

Table 4.9. Incidence, Manifestations, and Prognosis of Leukemias [20,23,38] (Continued)

Classification of Leukemia	Incidence	Manifestations	Prognosis
Chronic lymphocytic leukemia (CLL)	Uncommon before age 20	HEMATOPOIETIC DYSFUNCTION 1. Anemia 2. Neutropenia 3. Lymphocytosis 4. Thrombocytopenia LYMPHATIC DYSFUNCTION 1. Hepatosplenomegaly	1. Average survival 5–6 years
Chronic myelogenous leukemia (CML)	2% of all childhood leukemias; 15%–20% of all adult leukemias; rare before age 35	HEMATOPOIETIC DYSFUNCTION 1. Leukocytosis 2. Anemia 3. Thrombocytopenia LYMPHATIC DYSFUNCTION 1. Hepatosplenomegaly BLAST CRISIS USUALLY SIGNALS TERMINAL PHASE	1. Average survival 3 years

Table 4.10.   Classification of Lymphomas [2]

Type of Malignant Lymphoma	Component Cell
Undifferentiated lymphoma	Primitive reticular cell
Histiocytic lymphoma	Histiocyte
Hodgkin's disease	
Mixed cell type lymphoma	Histiocyte and lymphocyte
Poorly differentiated lymphocytic lymphoma	Lymphocyte
Well differentiated lymphocytic lymphoma	

is almost always immediately above or below the first group. Conversely, lymph node group involvement in non-Hodgkin's lymphomas is more unpredictable. Hodgkin's disease is microscopically characterized by a polymorphic cell infiltration comprised of lymphocytes, plasma cells, eosinophils, histiocytes, and Reed-Sternberg cells.

Hodgkin's disease may exhibit primary extranodal tumors in the lung, stomach, bowel, skin, oral cavity, and/or soft tissue. Extranodal tumors generally behave in a less malignant manner than does disease presenting in the lymph nodes. Four varieties of Hodgkin's disease have been identified: lymphocyte predominance, nodular sclerosis, mixed cellularity, and lymphocyte depletion.

There is the possibility of definitive cure in 60 percent to 90 percent of clients with localized disease and early treatment. However, the appearance of systemic symptoms and hepatic or bone involvement signifies a poor prognosis.

Multiple Myeloma

Multiple myeloma is a proliferative disease arising from plasma cells, which are normally responsible for the synthesis of immunoglobulins [25]. The annual incidence of multiple myeloma in the United States is 1 to 4 per 100,000 people. The peak incidence occurs between ages fifty and sixty-five, and less than 2 percent of cases are under age forty. Sex preference is equal.

Multiple myeloma is characterized by lytic bone lesions with bone pain, hypercalcemia, anemia, and homogenous serum and/or urinary globulin elevations. Prior to the advent of chemotherapy, the median survival time was seventeen months. Currently, however, median survival time ranges from twenty-four to fifty months.

CONCEPT VIII:
Many malignancies are associated with specific cancer markers that seem to indicate tumor progression or regression.

The most commonly known tumor marker is carcinoembryonic antigen (CEA) which is associated with tumors of the gastrointestinal tract. Another more recently discovered tumor marker is colon mucoprotein antigen (CMA), which is apparently a colon-specific substance currently under investigation. Also associated with gastrointestinal tumors, especially colorectal cancer, is the Tennessee antigen (TennaGen) which is a glycoprotein. Zinc glycinate marker (ZGM) is a tissue-associated antigen thought to have a correlation with tumors of the gastrointestinal tract. Galactosyl transferase isoenzyme-II (GT-II) is an antigen thought to correlate with malignancies of the pancreas, stomach, and colon. Finally, pancreatic onco-fetal antigen (POA) is a fetal protein that seems to have a high correlation to pancreatic tumors.

Prostatic acid phosphatase (PAP) is an enzyme classically associated with prostate cancer, and prostate-specific antigen (PSA) is a new and highly specific marker for prostate cancer. Human chorionic gonadotropin (HCG) is a placental antigen long known for its association with choriocarcinoma and is under investigation for correlation with testicular tumors. Alpha-fetoprotein (AFP) is an antigen associated with testicular germ-cell tumors, liver cancer, and gastric malignancies. Breast-cyst fluid proteins (BCFP) are tissue-associated antigens thought to correlate with breast carcinoma.

Beta-glucuronidase is a normal enzyme occurring abnormally in leptomeningeal carcinomatosis, as is lactic dehydrogenase (LAD). Calcitonin, a normal hormone, exhibits increased serum levels in thyroid carcinoma.

CONCEPT IX:
A carcinogen is a physical, chemical, or biological stressor that causes neoplastic change in normal tissue [15].

Carcinogens may act at the initial location of contact, in the organ where carcinogens have localized or accumulated, at the site of metabolism, or at the site of excretion. Co-carcinogens are stressors that work in conjunction with carcinogens to promote neoplastic change, although co-carcinogens do not themselves cause cancerous reactions. Carcinogens are classified into host and environmental factors [14]. Host factors include genetic, immunological, carcinogenic, and co-carcinogenic stressors [17]. A "cancer family" has certain characteristics [24]. There appears to be an increased incidence of adenocarcinoma, primarily in the colon and uterus. There appears to be an increased frequency of multiple primary malignancies, and the person in a "cancer family" seems to develop cancer at an earlier age than the population at large. There is a vertical transmission of cancer consistent with an autosomal dominant mode of genetic inheritance. Certain genetic disorders seem to increase host vulnerability for the development of specific types of cancer (see Tables 4.11 and 4.12).

Table 4.11.   Cancers Associated With Genetic Disorders [14]

Cancer Type	Associated Autosomal Dominant Disorder
Colon carcinoma	Familial polyposis coli
Sarcoma	Bilateral retinoblastoma
Fibrosarcoma	von Recklinghausen's neurofibromatosis
Neuroma	
Schwannoma	
Optic glioma	
Pheochromocytoma	
Basal cell carcinoma	Nevoid basal cell carcinoma syndrome
Ovarian carcinoma	

Table 4.12. Cancers Assoicated with Genetic Disorders [14]

Cancer Type	Associated Autosomal Recessive Disorder
Skin cancer	Xeroderma pigmentosum
	Albanism
Leukemias	Ataxia-telangiectasia
Carcinoma of stomach	
Brain tumors	
Acute monomyeloblastic leukemia	Fanconi's anemia

CANCER OF THE BREAST

Cancer of the breast appears to have a familial disposition, usually occurring in the same anatomical location among affected family members and occurring at an earlier age than in the general population. Approximately 15 percent to 30 percent of cases of breast cancer seem to have some type of genetic causation, and transmission appears to be in a dominantly inherited manner [4, 6].

If a woman has bilateral breast cancer, her female relatives have a 5.5 times greater risk of developing the disease than women in the general population [4, 7]. Relatives of a woman with bilateral disease have a higher risk than relatives of women with unilateral disease, irrespective of whether the client is premenopausal or postmenopausal. Sisters seem to have a greater risk than mothers [29]. If a woman develops bilateral breast cancer before menopause, her female relatives have a nine times higher risk, which translates to almost a 50 percent chance of developing the disease [4, 7]. However, risks for the female relatives of women with premenopausal breast cancer with unilateral disease are no higher than those for relatives of postmenopausal clients [29].

CANCER OF THE COLON

Cancers of the colon appear to have a familial disposition usually occurring in the same anatomical location among affected family members and occurring at an earlier age than in the general population [4]. The most frequently involved sites are the large and small intestines, stomach, pancreas, and esophagus. In 12 percent to 15 percent of persons with colorectal carcinoma there is a family history of the disease, and approximately 10 percent of persons with gastric carcinoma have a familial background for the malignancy.

CHILDHOOD CANCERS

Known genetic factors in childhood cancers fall into three categories [22]. First, single-gene defects are strongly related to the development of cancer in children. More than 150 single-gene disorders have been implicated in childhood carcinogenesis. Children with Down's syndrome (trisomy-21), for example, have a tenfold risk of developing leukemia during the first decade of life. Second, some birth defects may signal a high risk of specific childhood cancers. Examples include diverse genitourinary abnormalities associated with Wilms' tumor, cryptorchism and the linkage with testicular dysgenesis associated with testicular cancer, and the linkage of hemihypertrophy with adrenocortical carcinoma and hepatoma. Finally, a positive family history of cancer is particularly significant in the incidence of leukemia. When one of identical twins develops acute leukemia before age six, the risk for the other twin is 20 percent over the next few months [26]. The risk of leukemia development decreases with the increasing age at which the first twin is affected [46]. Fraternal twins and siblings of children with leukemia have a twofold higher risk than children in the general population [22].

IMMUNE SYSTEM DYSFUNCTION AS AN ETIOLOGICAL FACTOR IN CANCER

Dysfunction of the immune system may predispose to the development of cancer. Human immunity to cancer is a function of humoral factors (tumor-specific antibodies) and cellular factors (sensitized lymphocytes and macrophages). It is the occasional neoplastic cell which evades the host's immunodefensive system that results in clinical cancer.

When tested at the time of diagnosis, persons with cancer often have abnormal immune function. Persons with genetic immune system defects are more likely to develop leukemia or lymphoma than are persons who are immunocompetent [14]. Additionally, persons who have been purposefully immunosuppressed for organ transplants have an increased risk of cancer development. The overall risk for these individuals is 25 times higher than the general population, and reticulum cell sarcoma has a 300 to 700 times higher incidence than in the general population [14].

Several commonly occurring factors alter normal immune function, such as malnutrition, advancing age, and chronic disease. The physiological response to generalized stress includes thymicolymphatic involution, suppressing immunological capabilities [36].

ENDOGENOUS HORMONAL STATUS AS AN ETIOLOGICAL FACTOR IN CANCER

Endogenous hormonal status is thought to be a primary modifying factor in carcinogenesis by either promoting or inhibiting effects of environmental carcinogens. Hormonal changes in females, for example, seem to have a significant effect on the development of breast cancer. The age at which a woman delivers her first full-term infant appears to significantly correlate with the later development of breast cancer. The risk of women who deliver a full-term infant before age eighteen is one-third that of women whose first delivery is after age thirty-five. Nulliparous women exhibit an increased risk of breast cancer, and the incidence of breast cancer decreases as parity increases.

Lactation also seems to be related to the occurrence of breast cancer, since there is decreased incidence of the disease in populations of women who nurse for long periods of time. Early menarche increases the risk of breast cancer, and late menopause (after age fifty-five) carries a twofold higher risk than if the woman experiences menopause before age forty-five. Excretion of androgen metabolites have been found to be subnormal in women with breast cancer, and secretion of progesterone by the corpus luteum seems to exert a protective effect against breast malignancy. Women with hypoactive thyroid glands or who have had a thyroidectomy seem to experience an increased risk of breast cancer as compared to euthyroid women.

Animal studies show a significant relationship between pituitary prolactin and breast cancer [14]. Decreased serum levels of prolactin result in tumor regression, whereas increased serum levels lead to tumor growth.

PSYCHOLOGICAL STATUS AS AN ETIOLOGICAL FACTOR IN CANCER

Although research has not validated a direct causal relationship, certain psychological factors have been identified that may precipitate physiological stress, resulting in immunosuppression and increased host vulnerability to environmental carcinogenic stressors. The psychological responses of depression and despair following stressful life changes and significant losses may be psychogenically related to cancer. When a person experiences significant losses, the emotional responses of helplessness and hopelessness will lead to physiological dysfunction unless the person can cope successfully with the ''giving up'' experience [18]. The most consistent finding in research examining relationships between stressful life changes and the subsequent development of cancer has been the loss of a significant other weeks, months, or years prior to the onset of symptoms and diagnosis [10]. Median life change scores of women are consistently and significantly higher in women with abnormal Pap smears than in women with normal Pap results [44].

Certain lifelong personality traits seem to be consistently related to the development of cancer. Some characteristics may merely predispose persons to generally unhealthy states, such as failure of coping strategies, a decreased ability to express anger and generalized patterns of giving up, hopelessness, helplessness, anxiety, and depression [5, 8, 16]. However, the idea that a composite of certain personality traits may actually increase a person's vulnerability to the development of cancer is gaining credence [1]. These personality traits include lifelong tendencies toward denial and repression; impaired self-awareness and introspective capacity; poor outlets for emotional discharge; little aggressive self-expression; self-sacrificing and self-blaming behavior; and a tendency to experience hopelessness and helplessness in response to stressful life changes. A small amount of early life experience research also indicates that persons with cancer tend to exhibit a marked lack of closeness with parents [42].

DEMOGRAPHIC AND GEOGRAPHICAL FACTORS AS ETIOLOGICAL FACTORS IN CANCER [14]

Age seems to be related to the development of cancer since the general risk of cancer increases with advancing age. Certain types of cancer also have an increased incidence in certain age groups. *Sex* may be an etiological factor in the development of cancer since women may have an overall slightly greater risk for the disease than do men and since some cancers have a significant sex-related incidence. *Race* is an etiological factor as blacks have a greater risk than do whites. *Geographical location* may determine exposure to environmental carcinogenic stressors, and *cultural behavioral patterns* (e.g., smoking, consumption of alcohol, sexual behavior) may correlate with the development of cancer.

DIET AS AN ETIOLOGICAL FACTOR IN CANCER [14]

Dietary factors have been associated with up to 50 percent of malignancies in females and 30 percent in males in the United States [14]. Certain food additives and contaminants may be frankly carcinogenic. Aflatoxins, for example, are found in molds on grains and peanuts and are strongly linked with liver cancer. Nitrates and nitrites, used as food preservatives, are associated with gastric cancer, although only 10 percent of human nitrate consumption is traced to food additives. Artificial sweeteners have been related to bladder cancer in animal studies but this relationship has not been validated in human studies.

Excessive intake of fats has been linked with cancers of the breast, ovary, endometrium, prostate, and pancreas. Increased fat consumption stimulates the production and release of prolactin, thus possibly promoting the development of breast cancer. Increased consumption of fat and high levels of bile acid and bile acid metabolites are suspected of causing interactions thought to predispose to colon cancer. The carcinogen is suspected to be a metabolic derivative of bile acid degradation by the intestinal flora. The fat itself is not thought to be directly carcinogenic. Dietary deficiencies of specific trace elements and vitamins are thought to increase host vulnerability to carcinogenic stressors. Vitamins A and C, selenium, and zinc are currently being investigated.

TOBACCO AS AN ETIOLOGICAL FACTOR IN CANCER [14]

Tobacco is an environmental carcinogenic stressor that has been associated with 25 percent to 35 percent of cancer deaths in men and 5 percent to 10 percent in women. Tobacco has been associated with cancers of the lung, larynx, oral cavity, esophagus, and bladder. Most of the known carcinogenic agents in tobacco are found in the "tar," which is the aggregate of particulate matter in smoke after the removal of nicotine and water.

The risk of developing a tobacco-associated malignancy is affected by four primary factors: the duration of the smoking habit, the daily number of smoked cigarettes, the tar content of the cigarettes, and depth of inhalation of cigarette smoke. Cigar and pipe smokers have a lower risk for lung and larynx cancer than cigarette smokers unless smoke inhalation is deep, but the risk for oral cancer is the same for those who smoke cigarettes and who chew tobacco.

Tobacco and certain occupational carcinogens have a synergistic effect, thus increasing cancer risk. Smoking asbestos workers, for example, have an eight times higher risk of developing fatal bronchogenic cancer than do those smokers who do not work with asbestos. These same smoking asbestos workers have a ninety-two times higher risk of fatal bronchogenic carcinoma than do nonsmokers who do not work with asbestos.

ENVIRONMENTAL RADIATION AS AN ETIOLOGICAL FACTOR IN CANCER [14]

Environmental radiation is a known carcinogenic stressor because of its ability to penetrate and damage cellular DNA. Ultraviolet radiation from the sun has minimal ability to penetrate body tissues, thus leaving the skin most vulnerable to its effects. Ionizing radiation from X-rays and gamma rays can penetrate body tissues and has been associated with leukemia and solid tumors of the thyroid, breast, lung, and gastrointestinal tract. The carcinogenic potential of ionizing radiation is related to dose, particulate energy, and host factors. Less than 3 percent of human cancers have been related to ionizing radiation.

VIRAL INFECTION AS AN ETIOLOGICAL FACTOR IN CANCER [14]

Viral carcinogens have been clearly demonstrated in animals although no conclusive evidence has yet been documented in human cancers. Viruses are thought to contribute to the development of cancer by becoming incorporated into the host DNA or RNA. Genetic endowment, age, hormonal status, immunocompetence, and stress are thought to interact with and influence a person's vulnerability to oncogenic viruses.

Certain cancers have been theoretically linked to specific viruses (see Table 4.13). The Epstein-Barr virus is thought to be implicated in Burkitt's lymphoma, nasopharyngeal carcinoma, and Hodgkin's disease. The Herpes Simplex-2 has been related to the devleopment of cervical and prostatic cancers, and the Hepatitis-B virus may be linked to hepatocellular carcinoma. Although feline leukemia has been demonstrated to have a viral origin and is transmissible by the saliva and urine, a similar relationship has not been demonstrated in human leukemia [27]. In one study, however, 40 percent of persons with leukemia reported close social contact with other persons with leukemia prior to development of the disease. Among control subjects, only 13 percent reported similar contacts. The study results were

Table 4.13. Viruses Most Strongly Associated with Human Cancers [32]

Cancer	Primary Associated Virus Designation	Virus Group
Burkitt's lymphoma	Epstein-Barr (EBV)	Herpes
Nasopharyngeal carcinoma	Epstein-Barr (EBV)	Herpes
Cervical carcinoma	Herpes simplex-2	Herpes
Kaposi's sarcoma	Cytomegalovirus	Herpes
Acute myelogenous leukemia	Type C	Oncorna
Breast cancer	Type B	Oncorna

Source: F. Rapp and C. L. Reed, The Viral Etiology of Cancer: A Realistic Approach, *Cancer* 40 (1977): 421. Reprinted by permission of J. B. Lippincott and the author.

Table 4.14. Environmental Occupations and Carcinogenesis [14]

Occupational Carcinogen	Associated Malignancy
Asbestos fiber	Cancers of lung, esophagus, colon
	Mesothelioma
Coke oven emissions	Cancer of lung, kidney
Alpha-naphthylamine	Bladder cancer
4-Aminodiphenyl	Bladder cancer
Benzidine and salts	Bladder cancer
Vinyl chloride	Cancer of lung, brain
	Angiosarcoma of liver
Chloromethyl methyl ether (CMME)	Lung cancer
Bis (chloromethyl) ether	Lung cancer

statistically significant, raising the question of a communicable carcinogen involved in the development of leukemia [43].

OTHER ETIOLOGICAL FACTORS IN CANCER [14]

The consumption of alcohol is associated with cancers of the oral cavity, larynx, esophagus, and liver, with a fifteen-times greater risk if the drinker also smokes cigarettes. Occupational carcinogens are associated with 5 percent of all cancers. For example, workers who come into contact with certain chemicals and chemical by-products have increased risk of developing certain malignancies (see Table 4.14). The malignancies are usually organ-specific and found in small populations of workers, and may be rare types of cancer.

Although air pollution has been linked with carcinogenesis, the overall effect is minimal, owing to the dilution of particulate matter in the air and filtering by the respiratory tract. Specific drugs also seem to have carcinogenic effects related to dosage, duration of ingestion, and host factors. Alkylating antineoplastic agents are related to acute nonlymphoblastic leukemia, and arsenicals have been linked with squamous cell carcinoma of the skin. Cyclophosphamides, another group of anti-cancer drugs, have shown a relationship to subsequent development of leukemia and bladder cancer, and immunosuppressive agents seem to predispose the individual to histiocytic lymphoma. Estrogens increase the risk of adenoma and uterine carcinoma in premenopausal women and of uterine carcinoma in postmenopausal women. Androgens (17-methyl substitute) are associated with hepatocellular carcinoma. Finally, if a pregnant woman ingests diethylstilbestrol (DES), her female offspring have significant risk of clear cell adenocarcinoma of the vagina [13].

SUMMARY

It is not always valid to apply results of studies of animal research to humans because of several factors [15]. Human populations, for example, are heterogenous, whereas populations of research animals are almost always homogenous.

Human exposure to carcinogenic agents is usually intermittent and sporadic, whereas animal exposure during research is controlled; and human exposure to carcinogens is usually much less than that of research animals. Finally, tumor growth in animals does not necessarily predict the site and type of human tumors.

Tissues that are most vulnerable to malignant changes are either those surfaces at which demands are often made for repair of environmental-induced damage or those organs subjected to cyclic demands for function (see Table 4.15). Cancer is largely a reflection of patterns of damage inflicted by environmental stressors. Although the forms of environmental provocations are different, the neoplastic reactions are basically the same, and a large proportion of human cancers probably has an etiology of multiple factors. Seventy-five percent of all malignancies arise in tissues that constitute only a small percentage of the total number of body cells [40]. Cancer affects the homeostatic balance between external and internal influences; but once a sufficient level of neoplastic disorganization has been established, new conditions arise that result in further disorder and the familiar clinical cancer picture emerges.

CONCEPT X:
The hallmark of cancer is the proclivity of its cells to metastasize to distant sites, a complicated biological phenomenon influenced by a multitude of host/tumor interactions.

Table 4.15.   Persons at High Risk for Some Cancers [30]

Cancer Site	Stressors Resulting in High Risk
Cervix	1. Early sexual activity 2. Multiple sexual partners 3. Pregnancy factors
Colorectal	1. Multiple polyposis 2. Prolonged ulcerative colitis
Intraoral	1. Cigarette smoking 2. Tobacco chewing 3. Heavy consumption of alcohol
Lung	1. Cigarette smoking 2. Asbestos exposure 3. Uranium exposure
Skin	1. Outdoor exposure 2. Fair skin that sunburns easily
Stomach	1. Pernicious anemia 2. Atrophic gastritis
Thyroid	1. Ionizing radiation

The biochemical basis for metastasis is unclear. One factor may be that malignant cells are less adherent to one another than are normal cells, possibly related to reduced calcium in the walls of the cancer cells. The reduced adherence may also be related to their high negative surface charge, thereby resulting in a tendency for cancer cells to repel one another [31]. Decreased adhesiveness enables the cells to break away from the primary tumor, invade nearby veins and lymphatics, and then travel to distant sites and develop into secondary tumors.

The metastatic process begins with the invasion of tissues, blood vessels, and/or lymphatics by cells from a primary malignant tumor. After release into the circulation, most tumor cells die rapidly, with only about 0.1 percent surviving to form distant metastatic tumors [11]. After release into the circulation, most surviving tumor cells are arrested in the first encountered capillary bed. Some tumors, however, are able to remain at various sites in a dormant state for long periods of time [12]. Upon gaining access to lymphatics, tumor cells may be carried as emboli directly to a lymph node where they are arrested in the subcapsular sinus of one or more lymph nodes. Growth in the lymph node begins, with establishment of a new tumor growth in the lymph node itself. Tumor cells that are primarily lymphborne may enter the blood vascular system by way of venolymphatic communications in the interstitial spaces. Venous metastases are common in the lung since the pulmonary capillary bed is usually the first vascular sieve encountered by bloodborne tumor cells.

Following initial arrest in a lymph node or capillary bed tumor cells must invade the parenchyma and establish a microenvironment before they can grow into secondary tumors. The presence of micrometastatic disease at the time of diagnosis is the primary cause of treatment failure. Pulmonary metastases are the most common of all metastatic tumors since venous drainage of most areas of the body is through the superior and inferior vena cavae into the heart, making the lungs the first organ to filter malignant cells.

Liver metastases are among the most ominous signs of advanced cancer. The liver filters blood coming from the gastrointestinal tract, making it a primary metastatic site for tumors of the stomach, colorectum, and pancreas. Other malignancies reach the liver through arterial circulation. Of persons who die with cancer, 50 percent to 75 percent have metastatic disease in the liver, and it is estimated that hepatic failure is the direct cause of death in 40 percent of people with liver involvement [41].

Bone metastases represent the initial site of metastatic disease in a large proporiton of cancer cases and are generally ominous in terms of prognosis. Metastatic disease in the brain is both life-threatening and emotionally debilitating. Increased intracranial pressure may be lethal, and the loss of mentation and of motor function in addition to the original cancer is often an emotionally depleting burden.

Death from metastatic disease is usually the result of failure of an organ necessary for life [33]. Anorexia and cachexia secondary to disseminated cancer is a frequent cause of death. Infection, hematopoietic dysfunction, or paraneoplastic syndromes resulting from metastatic malignancy are also implicated as terminal events.

CONCEPT XI:
Prognosis is influenced by several tumor-related and host-related factors [30].

TUMOR-RELATED FACTORS

Tumor-related factors include specific characteristics of the tumor cells, degree of invasiveness, tumor size and location, and lymph node involvement. Undifferentiated malignancies with high cellular mitotic rates and rapid cell turnover have a poor prognosis in contrast to well-differentiated cancers with infrequent mitoses or slow growth rates. Malignant invasion of veins and venules is associated with a greatly decreased prognosis, and the size of tumor can usually be correlated with prognosis. The site of malignancy greatly influences prognosis. A tumor of the common bile duct or head of the pancreas, for example, becomes inoperable almost as soon as it begins to invade because it attaches itself to nearby vital structures which precludes curative surgery. In contrast, a tumor of the stomach may grow to a huge size and still be operable as long as it enlarges into the lumen.

Lymph node involvement is closely linked with prognosis. Persons with metastatic disease in the lymph nodes have five-year survival times only half that seen in persons without lymph node involvement. Prognosis progressively worsens as more lymph nodes are involved.

HOST-RELATED FACTORS

Host-related factors include both physiological status and state of mind. Immune system and nutritive status influence prognosis as does the individual's psychosocial state of health. The degree of general physical debilitation also influences prognosis.

CONCEPT XII:
Cure is defined as removal or destruction of a large enough percentage of the viable tumor cell population that the remaining tumor cells cannot reestablish clinically detectable disease.

Surgery and radiotherapy fail to effect a cure if the disease is systemic when first diagnosed because neither treatment modality can effectively kill distant or undetected metastases. Drug therapy is often not curative at the first clinical recognition of the disease, whether systemic or not, because the body burden of tumor usually exceeds the cell kill potential of most antineoplastic drugs. Thus, combined modality treatment is the most common—and usually the most effective—medical approach. Early detection of malignancies increases chance of cure.

CONCEPT XIII:
Most common causes of death in persons with cancer are, in descending order, infection, organ failure, infarction, carcinomatosis, and hemorrhage [21].

The most common fatal infections appear to be pneumonia, septicemia, and peritonitis. The majority of infections are caused by gram negative bacilli, such as *Escherichia coli, Klebsiella,* and *Pseudomonas aeruginosa.* A smaller proportion of fatal infections result from gram positive organisms, such as *Staphylococcus auerus, Clostridia,* and *Enterococcus.* Mixed gram positive and gram negative infections, fungal infections, and miliary tuberculosis have also been precipitants of fatal infections for persons with cancer. Necrotic or ulcerated tumors are directly responsible for the development of infection in the majority of persons with cancer. Neutropenia, radiotherapy-induced mucositis, tissue necrosis, perforations and adhesions, and operative procedures resulting in wound dehiscence and peritonitis have been implicated as factors in the development of fatal infections.

Organ failure causes a significant number of cancer-related deaths and most commonly results from dysfunction of the respiratory, cardiac, hepatic, renal, or central nervous systems.

Infarction of organs necessary for life often results in death for many persons with cancer. The most common sites of infarction are the lungs, heart, mesenteric arteries, or brain.

Carcinomatosis is the cause of death in a significant percentage of persons with cancer and is most often observed in persons with melanoma and breast carcinoma. These persons have no evidence of severe pathological processes other than advanced metastatic malignant disease. Severe emaciation and/or electrolyte imbalances contribute to the death. Postmortem examinations exhibit extensive dissemination of the malignancy to vital organs such as the heart, adrenal glands, pituitary gland, and brain.

Hemorrhage, usually secondary to thrombocytopenia, accounts for a significant number of cancer-related deaths. The most common sites for fatal hemorrhage are the gastrointestinal tract, brain, major blood vessels, and lung.

CONCEPT XIV:
To summarize, the background of most tumor development is sustained demand for growth combined with vulnerability to malignant change.

Sustained demand for growth may be either as repeated repair of damage or as hypertrophy for unfulfilled function. Vulnerability to malignant change is mediated by weakened or unstable growth control systems, genetic endowment, diminished host defense systems, and environmental carcinogenic stressors.

REFERENCES

1. Abse, D. W., Wilkins, M. M., van de Castle, R. I., Buxton, W. D., Demars, J., Brown, R. S., and Kirschner, L. G. Personality and Behavioral Characteristics of Lung Cancer Patients. *J Psychosom Res* 18:101, 1974.
2. Ackerman, L. V. and Rosai, J. *The Pathology of Tumors.* New York: American Cancer Society, 1972. Pp. 31–41.
3. American Cancer Society, *1983 Cancer Facts and Figures.* New York: American Cancer Society, 1982.
4. Anderson, D. E. Familial Cancer and Cancer Families. *Semin Oncol* 5:11, 1978.
5. Bahnson, M. and Bahnson, C. Development of a Psychosocial Screening Questionnaire for Cancer. *Cancer Detect Prev* 2:295, 1979.
6. Bakemeier, R. F., Cooper, R. A., and Rubin P. The Malignant Lymphomas, Multiple Myeloma, and Macroglobulinenua. In P. Rubin (Ed.). *Clinical Oncology for Medical Students and Physicians: A Multidisciplinary Approach* (5th Ed.). Rochester, NY: American Cancer Society, 1978. Pp. 228–244.
7. Buchman-Davidson, D. J. Is Breast Cancer the Same in Men and Women? *Cancer Nurs* 3:121, 1980.
8. Cohen, F. Personality, Stress, and the Development of Physical Illness. In G. Stone, F. Cohen, and N. Adler (Eds.). *Health Psychology.* San Francisco: Jossey-Bass, 1979. Pp. 77–111.
9. Cowen, D. R. Decreased Mutual Adhesiveness: A Property of Cells From Squamous Cell Carcinoma. *Cancer Res* 4:625, 1944.
10. Dohrenwend, B. and Dohrenwend, B. (Eds.). *Stressful Life Events.* New York: John Wiley and Sons, 1974.
11. Fidler, I. J. Immunologic Factors in Experimental Metastases Formation. In P. Rubin (Ed.). *Metastases and Disseminated Cancer.* New York: American Cancer Society, 1979. Pp. 8–11.
12. Fisher, E. R. and Fisher, B. Circulating Cancer Cells and Metastases. In P. Rubin (Ed.). *Metastases and Disseminated Cancer.* New York: American Cancer Society, 1979. Pp. 3–7.
13. Fuller, A. F. Jr. The DES Syndrome and Clear Cell Adenocarcinoma in Young Women. *Cancer Nurs* 1:201, 1978.
14. Gianella, A. Cancer Prevention: Carcinogenesis I. *Cancer Nurs* 5:133, 1982.
15. Gianella, A. Cancer Prevention: Carcinogenesis II. *Cancer Nurs* 5:221, 1982.
16. Greer, S. Psychological Attributes of Women with Breast Cancer. *Cancer Detect Prev* 2:289, 1979.
17. Hammond, E. C. The Epidemiological Approach to the Etiology of Cancer. *Cancer* 35:652, 1975.
18. Headley, D. B. Premorbid Psychological Factors of Cancer. *Biol Psychol Bull* 5:1, 1977.
19. Holley, R. W. A Unifying Hypothesis Concerning the Nature of Malignant Growth. *Proc Natl Acad Sci USA* 69:2840, 1972.
20. Houlihan, N. G. Leukemia: The Leukemia Process. *Cancer Nurs* 4:149, 1981.
21. Inagaki, J., Rodriguez, V., and Bodney, G. P. Causes of Death in Cancer Patients. *Cancer* 33:568, 1974.
22. Li, F. P. Host Factors in the Development of Childhood Cancer. *Semin Oncol* 5:17, 1978.
23. Lichtman, M. A. and Klemperer, M. R. The Leukemias. In P. Rubin (Ed.). *Clinical Oncology for Medical Students and Physicians: A Multidisciplinary Approach* (5th Ed.). Rochester, NY: American Cancer Society, 1978. Pp. 245–256.
24. Lynch, H. T., Krush, A. J., Thomas, R. J., et al. Cancer Family Syndrome. In H. T. Lynch (Ed.). *Cancer Genetics.* Springfield, IL: Charles C. Thomas, 1976. P. 355.

25. Megliola, B. Multiple Myeloma. *Cancer Nurs* 3:209, 1980.

26. Miller, R. W. Persons at Exceptionally High Risk of Leukemia. *Cancer Res* 27:2420, 1967.

27. Oberst, M. T. Research Highlights: Leukemia Carriers. *Cancer Nurs* 1:259, 1978.

28. Oppenheimer, S. B. *Cancer: A Biological and Clinical Introduciton.* Boston: Allyn and Bacon, 1982. Chapter 4.

29. Ottman, R., Pike, M. C., King, M., and Henderson, B. E. Practical Guide for Estimating Risk for Familial Breast Cancer. *Lancet* 2(8349):556, 1983.

30. Patterson, W. B. Principles of Surgical Oncology. In P. Rubin (Ed.). *Clinical Oncology for Medical Students and Physicians: A Multidisciplinary Approach* (5th Ed.). Rochester, NY: American Cancer Society, 1978. Pp. 21–27.

31. Prehn, R. T. and Prehn, L. M. Pathobiology of Neoplasia: A Teaching Monograph. *Am J Pathol* 80:529, 1975.

32. Rapp, F. and Reed, C. L. The Viral Etiology of Cancer: A Realistic Approach. *Cancer* 40:419, 1977.

33. Rubin, P. Metastatic Morbidity: The Less Common and Unusual Sites. In P. Rubin (Ed.). *Metastases and Disseminated Cancer.* New York: American Cancer Society, 1979. Pp. 170–176.

34. Rubin, P. Statement of the Clinical Oncologic Problem. In P. Rubin (Ed.). *Clinical Oncology for Medical Students and Physicians: A Multidisciplinary Approach* (5th Ed.). Rochester, NY: American Cancer Society, 1978. Pp. 1–10.

35. Selye, H. A Code for Coping with Stress. *AORN J* 25:35, 1977.

36. Silverberg, E. Cancer in Young Americans (Ages 15 to 34). *CA* 32(1):15, 1982.

37. Silverberg, E. Cancer Statistics, 1982. *CA* 32(1):15, 1982.

38. Simone, J. V. Leukemia. In American Cancer Society. *Proceedings of the National Conference on the Care of the Child with Cancer.* New York: American Cancer Society, 1979. Pp. 50–55.

39. Skipper, H. E. Kinetics of Mammary Tumor Cell Growth and Implications for Therapy. *Cancer* 28:1479, 1971.

40. Smithers, D. Epithelial Neoplasia: A Homeostatic Disorder. In L. C. Kruse, J. L. Reese, and L. K. Hart (Eds.). *Cancer: Pathophysiology, Etiology, and Management.* St. Louis: C. V. Mosby, 1979. Pp. 38–43.

41. Sullivan, R. D. Comment: Disseminated Cancer—Metastases to Liver. In P. Rubin (Ed.). *Metastases and Disseminated Cancer.* New York: American Cancer Society, 1979. Pp. 129–130.

42. Thomas, C. and Duszynski, P. Closeness to Parents and the Family Constellation in a Prospective Study of Five Disease States: Suicide, Mental Illness, Malignant Tumors, Hypertension and Coronary Heart Disease. *Johns Hopkins Med J* 134:251, 1974.

43. Timonen, T. T. and Ilvonen, M. Contact with Hospital, Drugs, and Chemicals as Aetiological Factors in Leukemia. *Lancet* 1:350, 1978.

44. Walters, C. M., Gallucci, B. B., Molbo, D. M., Pesznecker, B. L., and Holmes, T. H. The Association of Numerous Life Changes with Cervical Dysplasia and Metaplasia. *Cancer Nurs* 3:455, 1980.

45. Zeidman, I. Critical Comments. In P. Rubin (Ed.). *Metastases and Disseminated Cancer.* New York: American Cancer Society, 1979. Pp. 20–21.

46. Zuelzer, W. W. and Cox, D. E. Genetic Aspects of Leukemia. *Semin Hematol* 6:228, 1969.

PART II

TREATMENT AND NURSING CARE FOR THE CANCER PATIENT

Chapter 5

Nursing Care of the Surgical Oncology Client

CONCEPT I:
Oncologic surgery is one of the four major medical treatment modalities used to attempt reduction of the body burden of tumor.

CURATIVE SURGERY

The primary goal of curative oncologic surgery is to reduce the body burden of tumor to a very small quantity of cells [33]. If the tumor cell population can be decreased to very small amounts, the remaining malignant cells may then be destroyed by host immunological mechanisms, other systemic antineoplastic treatments, or a combination of both. Slowly proliferating cancers with long cell cycles are most amenable to successful surgical treatment. Other cancers that are highly cohesive and tend to metastasize late or not at all (e.g., basal cell carcinoma, chondrosarcoma, epidermoid carcinoma of the cervix) are often cured by surgery [27, 28]. Surgical cure rates tend to decrease as primary tumor size at the time of surgery increases [34].

DEBULKING SURGERY

Even if a malignancy cannot be totally resected, debulking surgical procedures decrease the tumor burden and consequently enhance the efficacy of radiotherapy, chemotherapy, and the client's immunological defenses. Since metastasis to regional lymph nodes occurs with most carcinomas and some sarcomas, the en bloc dissection of the tumor and the primary nodal drainage is usually performed for these cancers. Radical surgical procedures should be done only after careful assessment of possible cure or palliation; the accompanying physical and psychological trauma must be weighed against potential benefits of surgery.

PALLIATIVE SURGERY

Palliative surgery is used to decrease disease-related symptoms without attempting to surgically cure the cancer. About two-thirds of all clients with cancer are not curable because their disease is systemic when first detected [34]. Palliative oncologic surgery has three primary objectives: (1) to provide a higher level of comfort for the client, (2) to relieve distressing symptoms, and (3) to prevent the development of additional symptoms [3].

CONCEPT II:
Surgical removal of a primary tumor affects the client's immunological defenses [12].

It is generally accepted that malignant tumors elicit an immune response that is both humoral and cell mediated. Clinical data suggest that cell-mediated immunological responses are diminished by surgery, although humoral responses do not seem to be affected. Surgery has also been shown to diminish reticuloendothelial system activity and phagocytosis.

CONCEPT III:
Surgical removal of a primary tumor alters the growth patterns of metastatic lesions, probably by alteration of residual tumor cell kinetics.

As tumor mass increases, the growth fraction of viable tumor cells decreases [12, 32]. Large tumors generally contain a sizeable number of resting cells that are not dividing. Thus, the growth rate of the entire tumor mass slows. With surgical removal of the primary tumor, the growth fraction of residual tumor cells still within the client's body seems to increase [12]. Tumor cell generation time shortens, and metastatic tumor growth becomes more rapid. Nondividing, resting malignant cells apparently begin to actively divide and proliferate, thus becoming more vulnerable to postoperative radiotherapy and/or chemotherapy.

CONCEPT IV:
Several special surgical techniques are employed in the treatment of certain cancers [3, 27].

Electrosurgery uses the cutting and coagulating effects of high-frequency current applied by needle, disc, or blade electrodes and may be an alternative treatment for certain malignancies of the skin, oral cavity, and rectum. *Cryosurgery* is the application of liquid nitrogen by a probe to a tumor and may be used for treatment of cancers in the oral cavity, brain, and prostate. *Chemosurgery,* or *Moh's technique,* utilizes escharotic paste in combination with multiple, sequential frozen-section examinations in the attempt to achieve a surgical margin in certain skin cancers. *Laser surgery,* once hailed as an exciting and effective breakthrough in cancer treatment, has thus far been clinically disappointing.

CONCEPT V:
Surgical treatment failures are primarily the result of the presence of metastatic disease at the time of diagnosis.

Most malignant tumors are appropriately considered to be advanced disease at the time of diagnosis. A one-centimeter tumor, which is usually the size capable of physical diagnosis, has already progressed through thirty of its forty doublings, forty doublings being lethal to the client [12]. Very few tumors are detected when less than one centimeter in diameter.

Many cancers have microscopic or clinically apparent metastases at the time of diagnosis. Treatment failure rates of common cancers indicate the probability of metastatic disease at the time of diagnosis [12]:

1. 99 percent of clients with pancreatic cancer become treatment failures
2. 90 percent of clients with lung malignancy become treatment failures
3. 86 percent of breast cancer clients with four or more positive axillary nodes at the time of diagnosis become treatment failures
4. 70 percent of men with cancer of the prostate become treatment failures, and
5. 60 percent of clients with bowel cancer become treatment failures

Even when there is no clinical evidence of nodal involvement, microscopic metastases will be discovered in about one-third of persons diagnosed with cancer [27]. Malignant spread through blood vessels further reduces the likelihood of a surgical cure.

CONCEPT VI:
Preoperative nursing care of the surgical oncology client focuses on the reduction of anxiety, the enhancement of physical well-being, and teaching.

Anxiety seems to be more common and more severe in clients who do not have specific and accurate information about the impending surgery [35]. In order to decrease preoperative anxiety, nurses must assess and strengthen the client's available coping mechanisms. Continuity of care must be provided as much as possible in terms of personnel, procedures, and external environment. Nurses may reduce anxiety by facilitating client control over life events. This will reduce subjective feelings of helplessness, vulnerability, and anxiety. Additionally, if nurses will facilitate family support and availability, the client's anxiety will often decrease. The provision of accurate information regarding the purposes and procedures of diagnostic tests as well as the proposed surgery often reduces preoperative anxiety. During the preoperative period, concern about the disease itself often is replaced by concern about the impending surgery [35]. Honestly and clearly answering questions about the site, type, and extent of the surgery, as well as any expected bodily changes, will often reduce, not increase, the client's anxiety.

Enhancement of the client's physical well-being during the preoperative period will decrease the physical and psychological trauma associated with the surgery, decrease physical and psychological distress, and increase the client's coping abilities. Physical symptoms, such as pain, nausea and vomiting, bowel obstruction, diarrhea, fatigue, malnutrition, and weight loss, can be minimized. Stress-related symptoms, such as anorexia, insomnia, and headaches, can be decreased. Side effects of preoperative radiotherapy or chemotherapy increase the client's vulnerability to other postoperative physical and emotional problems. Thus, proper treatment of these side effects prior to surgery will directly and positively influence the client's response during the preoperative and postoperative periods.

Appropriate client teaching prior to surgery will reduce anxiety and helplessness. Nurses will be most successful if they formulate an individually tailored teaching plan. Level of knowledge and learning needs must be assessed, and goals must be established. A teaching environment that affords privacy and freedom from interruptions will enhance learning. Nurses must teach in fairly brief time periods, especially if the client's attention span is short or if the content is emotionally charged. Visual aids and examples are valuable tools in client teaching; by providing frequent and positive reinforcement, clients are likely to learn more quickly and the quality of learning will be increased. By evaluating the success of their teaching, nurses can determine areas needful of reinforcement.

Appropriate client teaching includes specific information about the surgical procedures as well as general postoperative behaviors expected of the client. Teach the techniques of coughing and deep breathing, incisional splinting, and range of motion exercises. Identify the kinds and purposes of technical apparatus to be used before and after surgery in order to reduce the client's apprehension about the use and meaning of the equipment.

CONCEPT VII:
Postoperative nursing care of the surgical oncology client includes physiological considerations.

WOUND ASSESSMENT

Wound assessment is a major postoperative physiological concern. Identify factors that increase the risk of wound complications. Poor vascularity to the surgical incision, for example, reduces oxygenation and nutrition of the injured tissue, delaying its repair and healing. Myelosuppression secondary to preoperative chemotherapy or radiotherapy increases the risk of infection, bleeding, and tissue hypoxia at the injured site. A final major factor in wound healing is obesity, which increases the risk of dehiscence and evisceration, especially in abdominal surgical wounds [15].

Hematoma Formation

Hematoma formation at the incision site may be a postoperative problem. Signs and symptoms include swelling and undue incisional pain. Nurses should monitor the appearance of undressed incisions for edema and discoloration and ensure the patency of any drains.

Infection

Wound infection usually occurs three to four days after surgery. Signs and symptoms include tachycardia, fever, wound inflammation, undue incisional pain, and leukocytosis. Since an increase in vital sign readings indicates infection, monitor the client's vital signs every four hours. Observe for leukocytosis and incisional inflammation. Monitor for alterations in the amount, color, odor, and consistency of drainage. Keep the incision site clean and dry, and administer antibiotics and special wound care as prescribed.

Dehiscence and Evisceration

Dehiscence and evisceration at abdominal wound sites may occur. Signs and symptoms include a sudden onset of serosanguinous drainage and the client may report a "popping sensation." Monitor the wound for alterations in the amount and color of drainage as well as for evidence that the incision may be "pulling apart." If dehiscence or evisceration occurs, notify the surgeon immediately and prepare the client for surgery. Absolute bedrest is necessary, and moist sterile towels should be placed over the wound site and extruded viscera.

PULMONARY ASSESSMENT

Pulmonary assessment is a major postoperative physiological concern. Identify factors that may increase the risk of pulmonary complications. For example, thoracic and upper abdominal operations predispose the client to the development of pulmonary complications, as does surgical interference with the respiratory tract. If the client has a history of obstructive pulmonary disease or heavy smoking, the development of pulmonary complications is more likely. Prolonged immobility and abdominal pain or distention increase the risk of pulmonary complications. Client anxiety about chest tubes or other postoperative technical apparatus usually decreases compliance with postoperative mobility and breathing exercises. Myelosuppression secondary to preoperative chemotherapy or radiotherapy increases the risk of pulmonary infection, bleeding, and tissue hypoxia. Impaired tissue healing secondary to malnutrition, disease process, and/or myelosuppression predisposes the client to the development of pulmonary complications. Finally, postoperative pain—especially in clients who have undergone thoracic or upper abdominal operations—often decreases the client's ability and willingness to successfully carry out postoperative coughing and breathing exercises as well as mobility.

Atelectasis

Atelectasis, or the collapse of a lobe or lung segment, may be a significant postoperative complication. Signs and symptoms include fever within forty-eight hours after surgery, tachypnea, moderate tachycardia, and decreased breath sounds over the affected area. Auscultate breath sounds every four hours for diminished air flow, and monitor for alterations in vital signs. Assist the client in coughing and deep breathing exercises, teaching the client to splint the incision to decrease discomfort. Administration of an analgesic before breathing exercises or ambulation will help the client to maximize his or her tolerance of these activities.

Aspiration Pneumonia

Aspiration pneumonia may be a postoperative pulmonary complication. Signs and symptoms include fever, tachycardia, tachypnea, dyspnea, hypotension, frothy and blood-tinged sputum, and decreased breath sounds. Monitor for alterations in vital signs every four hours, and notify the physician if the sputum becomes frothy or bloody. Auscultate breath sounds every four hours for diminished air flow. Administer antibiotics as prescribed.

Bacterial Pneumonia

Bacterial pneumonia may occur postoperatively. Signs and symptoms include fever with accompanying tachycardia and tachypnea, respiratory distress, and the auscultation of rales and/or areas of diminished air flow. Monitor vital signs every four hours for alterations indicative of bacterial pneumonia, and auscultate breath sounds every four hours for rales or areas of diminished flow. Administer antibiotics as prescribed.

Pulmonary Embolism and Infarction

Pulmonary embolism and infarction may occur seven to ten days after surgery and are medical emergencies. Signs and symptoms include tachycardia and tachypnea inconsistent with the degree of fever, sudden dyspnea and anxiety, hemoptysis, and pleuritic pain. Monitor vital signs every four hours for alterations indicative of pulmonary embolism and infarction, and observe for sudden dyspnea and anxiety. If signs of pulmonary embolism and infarction appear, notify the physician immediately. Maintain the client on strict bedrest and in Fowler's position. Administer oxygen, and administer anticoagulation therapy as prescribed.

URINARY SYSTEM ASSESSMENT

Urinary system assessment is a major postoperative physiological concern. Identify the factors that may increase the risk of urinary complications. Surgery performed on the urinary tract increases the client's risk for the development of urinary complications. Myelosuppression secondary to preoperative chemotherapy or radiotherapy increases the risk of urinary infection, bleeding, and tissue hypoxia. Reduced bladder capacity secondary to disease process, surgery, and/or radiotherapy predisposes to urinary complications. Impaired tissue healing secondary to malnutrition, disease process, and/or myelosuppression may contribute to urinary complications.

Urine Retention

Urine retention should be suspected if the client exhibits reduced urine output and bladder distention. Record accurate intake and output, observing for oliguria. Observe for bladder distention and accompanying lower abdominal pain. Insert a urinary catheter as prescribed.

Urinary Tract Infection

Signs and symptoms of infection of the urinary tract include fever, cloudy urine, and flank tenderness. Record accurate intake and output, observing for changes in the amount and characteristics of urine. Monitor vital signs every four hours for fever, and monitor the client's reports of pain. Maintain a fluid intake of at least three liters daily unless otherwise indicated, and administer antibiotics as prescribed.

Renal Failure

Acute renal failure is a serious and potentially life-threatening postoperative complication. Signs and symptoms include oliguria, hypertension, and signs of fluid overload. Record accurate intake and output, observing for oliguria. Monitor blood pressure every four hours, observing for hypertension. Administer diuretics, fluid restriction, and other medical therapies as prescribed.

GASTROINTESTINAL SYSTEM ASSESSMENT

Identify factors that may increase the client's risk of postoperative gastrointestinal system complications. For example, gastrointestinal surgical procedures predispose to the development of complications. Myelosuppression secondary to preoperative chemotherapy or radiotherapy increases the risk of gastrointestinal infection, bleeding, and tissue hypoxia. Impaired tissue healing secondary to malnutrition, disease process, and/or myelosuppression may contribute to gastrointestinal complications.

Paralytic Ileus

Signs and symptoms of a postoperative paralytic ileus include absent bowel sounds and a distended abdomen. Maintain nasogastric suctioning and/or an NPO status until bowel sounds are heard. Auscultate for bowel sounds every eight hours, and monitor for abdominal distention and tenderness. Assist the client with ambulation or provide turning every two hours in order to increase the client's mobility and decrease the risk and/or duration of paralytic ileus.

Postoperative Intestinal Obstruction

Signs and symptoms of this serious complication include vomiting, abdominal pain, the inability to pass feces or flatus, and abdominal distention. Monitor for the development of vomiting, abdominal pain, and/or abdominal distention. Record the frequency and characteristics of stools, and auscultate for absent bowel sounds. If intestinal obstruction has been diagnosed, provide nasogastric suctioning and intestinal decompression as prescribed.

Peritonitis

Peritonitis may occur secondary to the breakdown of internal sutures in abdominal surgeries. Signs and symptoms include abdominal pain, anorexia, nausea and vomiting, fever and chills, oliguria, thirst, paralytic ileus, hypotension, tachycardia, and tachypnea. Monitor the vital signs of clients at risk every four hours, and record accurate intake and output. Monitor the amount and characteristics of drainage, observing for alterations indicative of infection. Auscultate bowel sounds regularly. Administer intravenous fluids and antibiotics as prescribed, and provide oxygen as indicated.

PAIN ASSESSMENT

The type, site, and extent of the surgical procedure contributes to the client's postoperative pain experience. Other variables also influence the client's perception of pain, such as anxiety, environmental factors, and general physical condition. Signs and symptoms of acute postoperative pain include tachycardia, tachypnea, hypertension, pallor, dilated pupils, increased muscular tension, nausea, and guarding of the painful part. Assess the client's level of pain before administering analgesics, and evaluate the effectiveness of pain relief methods. Medicate the client promptly, adequately, and with the most effective agent. Medicate the client before the pain becomes intense, and provide distraction, relaxation, and rest to augment medications and thus decrease the pain experience. Further information regarding pain control and analgesic drugs may be found in Chapter 11.

CONCEPT VIII:
Postoperative nursing care of the surgical oncology client includes psychosocial considerations.

BODY IMAGE

Changes in body image may be difficult for the client to incorporate positively. Actual or perceived body changes usually precipitate grieving, and the actual or perceived reactions of others influence the client's ability to adapt to changes in body image.

Appropriate nursing measures will facilitate adaptation to changes in body image. By acknowledging the painfulness of the loss, nurses can help clients to accept their feelings as appropriate and acceptable. Ensure that the client may grieve in a safe, nonjudgmental environment. Identify and strengthen adaptive coping behaviors, and provide realistic yet hopeful client teaching regarding postoperative changes in life style and functioning. Strengthen the client's feelings of self-worth, and facilitate communication between the client and family.

ROLE CHANGES

The client may have difficulty adapting to the major and minor role changes that may occur after cancer surgery. The "sick role" may be incompatible with the client's self-concept, making it difficult for the client to even temporarily rely on caregivers for needed care. Appropriate nursing measures will facilitate adaptation to postoperative role changes. Encourage the client to express feelings about temporary or permanent role changes, and facilitate interdependence within the client/family unit. Counseling about changes in career, parenting, and/or roles as a spouse may help the client to adjust positively.

CONCEPT IX:
Surgical intervention is common for clients with colorectal malignancies.

The surgeon's choice of an operative procedure depends heavily upon the site of the malignancy. Carcinoma of the cecum or of the ascending, transverse, descending, or sigmoid colon may be resected and a primary anastomosis performed. Carcinoma of the rectum generally necessitates abdominoperineal resection with the formation of a permanent colostomy. Advanced or unresectable malignancies of the colon may require debulking surgery with a colostomy for relief of intestinal obstruction. An ileostomy is performed close to the ileocecal valve as surgical treatment for high intestinal malignancies [20].

PREOPERATIVE CARE

Preoperative care specific for colorectal surgery includes measures to reduce the risk of postoperative physiological complications. Two primary functions of the large intestine are to (1) provide a route for the excretion of waste products and toxic substances and (2) safely contain the microorganisms which, by fermentation, conclude the digestive process [7]. Thus, cleansing of the large bowel prior to surgery is an important measure to reduce the risk of postoperative infection. A low residue diet for several days prior to surgery and a clear liquid diet the day before surgery will reduce the amount of fecal material in the bowel. Bowel cleansing with laxatives and enemas will also help to reduce intestinal fecal material before surgery. Oral antibiotics, such as kanamycin or tetracycline, will decrease normal intestinal flora.

Preoperative measures to cleanse the bowel may cause decreased vitamin absorption. Supplemental vitamins may be temporarily necessary to compensate for this loss, and supplemental vitamin K is advisable because of the cleansed bowel's inability to synthesize its own vitamin K because of a decreased *E. coli* population [17]. Preoperative bowel cleansing may also increase the client's risk of dehydration since another major function of the large intestine is to conserve the water and electrolytes that are secreted into the gut during digestion [7]. Record accurate intake and output, observing for signs of dehydration, and supplement fluids and electrolytes as appropriate.

Preoperative care for the client facing colorectal surgery also includes measures to reduce anxiety and psychological discomfort. The combination of a diagnosis of cancer and impending ostomy surgery which will deprive the client of normal control over elimination represents a sizeable assault on self-image, frequently resulting in lowered self-esteem. Answering questions honestly and dispelling misconceptions will help to prepare the client for an ostomy. Since the client's self-concept and self-esteem after surgery seem to be related to (1) independence and perceived competence with ostomy self-care and (2) involvement in activities outside the home [43], teaching and counseling both before and after surgery is crucial for positive adaptation. Teach the client that the stoma will be edematous at first and will become smaller with time. The client should be made aware that all former activities except body contact sports can usually be resumed. Teach the client that satisfying sexual experiences are still possible after a colostomy. Physiological impotence does not occur. However, in men, there is a 50 percent chance that the presacral nerves will be resected, leaving the male client sterile but not impotent [17].

POSTOPERATIVE CARE

Postoperative care for colorectal surgical clients includes routine postoperative measures as well as specific interventions. Deep breathing and leg exercises are begun as soon as possible after recovery from anesthesia, and ambulation as tolerated is advised as quickly as possible. If a large internal dead space exists, the client will likely have an abdominal drain, which is generally shortened on the fifth postoperative day and removed on the seventh day after surgery [17].

If an abdominoperineal resection has been performed, drainage from the posterior perineal wound may be profuse for several days. The wound may be packed with gauze during surgery, and the packing is usually removed on the fourth or fifth postoperative day. The perineal defect is usually irrigated with 500 milliliters of potassium permanganate solution 1:10,000 twice daily to remove secretions and debris and to promote healing [17]. Observe the wound for bleeding or infection, and apply a sterile dressing after each irrigation, securing the dressing with a T- or Y-binder. Observe dressings every four hours for bleeding or drainage, and change or reinforce dressings as necessary. Administer transfusions of blood or plasma as prescribed to compensate for blood or fluid loss. After the abdominal wound has healed sufficiently, sitz baths will promote healing and cleanse the perineal wound of debris. Do not perform rectal temperatures or other rectal manipulations, and teach the client not to sit or lie upon rubber rings since wound edges may be pulled apart.

Nasogastric or gastrostomy tubes will be used for intestinal decompression until peristalsis resumes. Although the tube should not be routinely irrigated, a maximum of 30 milliliters of normal saline may be used for irrigation if the tube is not draining [17].

Gastric dilitation is a serious complication that may result in intestinal perforation or disruption of the intestinal anastomosis. Signs and symptoms include nausea and vomiting, abdominal pain, and abdominal distention. Medical treatment includes resumption of gastric decompression by nasogastric tube and withholding of oral foods and fluids until the situation is resolved.

The client may or may not return from surgery with a temporary ostomy bag in place. An ileostomy has continuous drainage of liquid stool, requiring use of a temporary collecting bag. A colostomy usually has no fecal drainage for two to three days, requiring postoperative dressings but no bag until feces begin to be expelled [16]. A loop colostomy is sometimes performed to protect the anastomosis when a low anterior resection is done. The colostomy is opened on the second postoperative day and usually closed in four to six weeks. The loop is covered with a large plastic collecting bag, and the glass rod that is used under the loop to support it is removed on the eighth postoperative day. The proximal stoma will drain liquid stool, whereas the distal stoma will drain only small quantities of mucus [17].

Postoperative diet progression is similar to other major abdominal surgeries. A clear liquid diet is resumed when peristalsis is auscultated and the nasogastric tube removed. As the diet advances, add buttermilk, soft cheeses, and yogurt as tolerated to repopulate intestinal flora.

Urinary complications occur in approximately 20 percent of clients [17]. Temporary urine retention resulting from surgical trauma to parasympathetic nerves is common. Urinary tract infections are also frequently seen, and prophylactic treatment with antibiotics may be prescribed.

Client teaching is a crucial part of nursing care for the client with a colostomy or ileostomy. The client who feels competent in ostomy care is more likely to adapt positively to surgically-induced body changes [43], so client teaching is of crucial importance. If bowel control is established early, psychological distress is minimized. An ileostomy is never irrigated [9], but colostomies may require irrigation for proper functioning. The lower the anatomical position of the colostomy, the less often will irrigations be necessary. With a loop (double-barrelled) colostomy, irrigate the proximal, or feces-draining, stoma. Irrigations are usually started by the nurse on the sixth or seventh postoperative day at the direction of the physician, using one-half liter of water for the first irrigation and one liter for the second. One to two quarts of water are recommended for succeeding irrgations [17]. Too large a quantity of water may cause prolonged return of the irrigant or abdominal cramps. Gentle abdominal massage may speed irrigant return. Use a number sixteen to eighteen French catheter [16], and insert the catheter four to eight inches into the stoma [23]. Never force the catheter if it meets resistance because of the danger of perforating the bowel. Use warm water (105° F.), placing the irrigation bag twelve to eighteen inches above the stoma, and irrigate the bowel at a moderate rate. Abdominal cramps may be precipitated by the use of water that is too hot or too cold or by filling the bowel too rapidly. Positioning the irrigation bag more than eighteen inches above the stoma may also cause abdominal cramping during the irrigation procedure. Prolonged instillation of the irrigant may be due to a partially blocked catheter.

The client must be taught not to perform digital dilatation of the stoma [20]. Digital dilatation may cause bleeding and mucosal injury. Stricture due to scarring may result.

The client must also learn proper skin care of the area around the stoma. This is of particular importance for the ileostomate because regulation of the ileostomy to achieve continence is not possible and enzymes in the fecal drainage are very irritating to the surrounding skin. Thus, an ileostomy must be covered by an appliance at all times. General skin care, however, applies to both ileostomates and colostomates. After removal of the bag, the area around the stoma must be washed with soap and water, then dried well. All traces of soap must be removed to allow proper adherence of skin preparations. Place a collar of tissue paper around the stoma to keep the skin clean and dry during the rest of the procedure. Apply tincture of benzoin around the stoma and allow to dry, or apply a Karaya gum ring around the stoma. The Karaya gum ring can be stretched to fit tightly around the stoma, and its soft edges will not injure the delicate tissue. Cut the opening of the new bag one-fourth inch larger than the stoma to allow expansion of the stomal tissue without injury. Remove the backing from the bag, applying a thin coat of cement to the sticky side of the bag and to the area around the stoma. After the cement has dried sufficiently (usually three to five minutes), apply the appliance to the skin. A small quantity of air in the bag is necessary to allow drainage flow. Close the open end with a rubber band or a clamp.

If skin excoriation around the stoma occurs, a Karaya gum ring may be safely applied over the irritated skin [16]. The ring will stick to the skin without cement. Cement may then be applied to the top of the ring to hold the bag in place, and the skin under the ring will be allowed to heal. The skin upon which the appliance bag itself rests may become irritated. Irritation may be prevented by frequent skin care, ensuring that the skin remains as clean and dry as possible. If a fungal infection develops, dusting the area with Mycostatin powder is advised [16].

The client must receive dietary instruction and must determine the effect of various foods on bowel habits. Diarrhea or constipation may result from an unbalanced diet or inadequate fluid intake. Gas-forming and odor-producing foods are generally avoided. These foods include milk, citrus fruit juices, eggs, fish, nuts, onions, cabbage, beans, asparagus, and turnips.

CONCEPT X:
For the client with an untreatable obstruction of the ureters or urethra or with irreparable bladder damage, an ileoconduit can prevent deterioration of renal function.

An ileoconduit is the surgical construction of a permanent urinary diversion [26]. One or both ureters are anastomosed to a segment of ileum which serves to transport urine to the external surface of the body. The proximal end of the ileal segment is sutured to the peritoneum to avoid herniation. The distal end of the ileal segment is then everted and sutured to the skin, forming an orifice similar to that of a colostomy. Intestinal peristalsis propels the urine toward the external body surface. A temporary urinary appliance is usually secured over the stoma during surgery.

PREOPERATIVE CARE

Preoperative nursing care of the client facing an ileoconduit includes a bowel-cleansing regime similar to that indicated for ostomy surgery. A low residue diet for several days prior to surgery and a clear liquid diet the day before surgery will reduce the fecal material in the bowel. Bowel cleansing with laxatives and enemas is also indicated for reduction of fecal material. Oral antibiotics, such as kanamycin, are indicated for the same reason as with ostomy surgery: to reduce normal intestinal flora [26]. As before, preoperative measures to cleanse the bowel may result in decreased vitamin absorption, necessitating supplemental vitamins. Vitamin K may also need to be supplemented because of the cleansed bowel's inability to synthesize its own vitamin K because of a decreased *E. coli* population [17]. Preoperative measures to cleanse the bowel may also result in an increased risk of dehydration. Record accurate intake and output, observing for dehydration, and supplement fluids and electrolytes as appropriate.

Preoperative care for clients who must have an ileoconduit construction includes measures to reduce anxiety and psychological discomfort. As with other surgeries, the client will be better able to cope with the trauma of this surgery if questions are answered honestly and misconceptions are dispelled. Teach the client that the stoma will be edematous at first and will become smaller in time. The client should be aware that all former activities, including sexual activity, are permissible as long as there is no danger of puncturing the collecting bag. Teach the client that bathing or showering with or without the appliance is permissible.

POSTOPERATIVE CARE

Postoperative care specific to ileoconduit construction includes appliance care and client teaching. A temporary appliance to collect urine will be used until stomal edema subsides. Empty the appliance whenever it contains approximately 100 milliliters of urine, or about every two hours, to avoid loosening of the appliance by the weight of the urine. Change the appliance only it if begins to leak or becomes uncomfortable.

Teach the client that urine characteristics will differ slightly from that which was stored in the bladder. Since the conduit is constructed from a small segment of intestine, a small quantity of mucus and perhaps some blood will appear in the urine and around the stoma [26]. Other changes in urine characteristics, as well as abdominal pain or swelling, should be promptly reported to the physician.

CONCEPT XI:
Mastectomy is a common surgical intervention for cancer of the breast.

In the United States, one of every eleven women will develop cancer of the breast in her lifetime, the statistics revealing that three women develop the disease every fifteen minutes [2]. If a woman has breast cancer, her risk of developing a secondary cancer in the other breast is five times greater than the risk of a breast malignancy in women who have never had the disease. If a mastectomy is performed, the affected woman develops cancer in the remaining breast 6.5 times per 100,000 risk-years of observation. In other words, thirteen secondary breast cancers would develop in a group of two hundred women surviving ten years, or in a group of one hundred women surviving twenty years [21].

Breast cancer remains the leading cancer killer of American women. In that hypothetical fifteen minutes in which three women develop the disease, one woman dies from breast cancer [2]. The relative five-year survival rate of women with breast malignancy during the 1960–1963 period was 63 percent, rising only 5 percentage points to 68 percent during the 1970–1973 period [1]. Thus, despite phenomenal advances in the treatment of many other types of cancer resulting in equally phenomenal leaps in survival rates, breast cancer has remained stubbornly resistant to old and new forms of medical treatment.

Breast cancer may be diagnosed by an operative biopsy (open or closed) or a fine-needle aspiration biopsy. The latter has considerable advantage over the former. It is less traumatic, can be carried out in a clinic or physician's office, and gives highly informative data. Although consistent reliability is highly dependent upon the skill of the operator, the fine-needle aspiration biopsy can achieve a definitive diagnosis in over 90 percent of breast carcinomas without the need for a surgical biopsy [9].

The overwhelming majority of American surgeons believe that mastectomy is the only treatment proven effective for breast cancer, and there is strong reluctance to abandon the mastectomy as the treatment of choice. There are several kinds of mastectomies, and each type carries its own implications for the woman's state of well-being, extent of mutilation, morbidity, and survival. The prerequisite for successful surgery is precise knowledge of the extent of the malignancy's anatomical spread. One leading expert contends that a segmental or simple mastectomy is indicated for true Stage I cancer, the classic Halsted radical mastectomy for true Stage II cancer, and partial dissection of the chest wall plus a radical mastectomy if the internal mammary nodes are histologically positive for cancer [30].

Before comparing the different types of mastectomies, a number of different factors must be acknowledged that profoundly influence the success or failure of *any* surgical treatment for breast cancer. First, the results of treatment are influenced more by nodal and distant spread of the disease than by local control of the malignancy [13, 37, 41]. Seventy-nine percent of clients with four or more positive lymph nodes at the time of surgery are treatment failures five years after radical mastectomy [12]. Lymphatic spread does not necessarily precede blood-borne dissemination of the malignant cells [31]. Since the "control" of solid tumors must include control of the primary tumor, lymph node disease, *and* distant metastases, it is readily apparent that to speak only of "local control" is an oversimplification of a highly complex matter. Second, the discovery of increasing numbers of very small cancers by means of new diagnostic techniques, especially mammography and fine-needle aspiration biopsy, results in more breast malignancies being found—and treated—in earlier stages of the disease. $T_1N_0M_0$ tumors have a much higher survival rate because the tumor can be removed before regional and distant spread has occurred. Currently, the five-year survival rate for early, localized breast cancer is 87 percent, whereas it is only 47 percent if the malignancy has spread to distant sites [1]. Third, there has been a more pressing demand from women for less mutilating surgical procedures, and clients have increasingly requested to be informed of the various possible treatments, including the more conservative surgical techniques.

Prior to the 1960s, the *classic Halsted radical mastectomy* was the treatment of choice in this country for nearly 100 years. The Halsted mastectomy generally includes removal of the breast, subcutaneous tissue, all axillary lymph nodes up to the apex of the axilla, as well as complete removal of the minor pectoral muscle and extensive removal of the major pectoral muscle. William Stewart Halsted developed the procedure, first publishing a description of it in 1894. For more than half a century, the merits of this type of mastectomy were undisputed. The Halsted radical mastectomy did not include removal of the internal mammary lymph nodes because it was thought that cancer of the breast was primarily a local disease. The Halsted radical mastectomy has the best five-year survival statistics among the various surgical procedures for breast cancer (see Table 5.1), although other surgical procedures have five-year survival statistics that are only slightly less than the Halsted radical mastectomy [29].

In 1948, two British surgeons reported the development of the *modified radical mastectomy*, which rapidly increased in usage, and now it is the most common surgical treatment for cancer of the breast. This technique calls for the same tissue dissection except that of the pectoral muscles. These muscles are left intact because the original surgeons did not believe that breast cancer was disseminated by the chest muscles; time has proven their assumptions to be correct. Survival statistics (see Table 5.1) are similar to those of the Halsted procedure [38].

Other, less well-known surgical treatments for breast cancer have been studied in the United States and Europe. *Local wide excision* (also called *lumpectomy* and *wedge excision*) is a procedure in which only the tumor mass itself and a small portion of the surrounding breast tissue is removed. The rest of the breast tissue, skin, muscles, and all lymph nodes are left intact, thus, there is minimal disfigurement and less surgical trauma. Unfortunately, since the first-station lymph nodes are not even biopsied and since most breast cancers are multicentric, a local wide excision cannot possibly eradicate the malignancy unless the "lump" is very small and has not begun to invade or metastasize. Postoperative irradiation is used in attempt to destroy lingering cancer cells, but the survival statistics (see Table 5.1) are disappointingly low [38].

Table 5.1. Five-Year Survival Rates, Various Mastectomy Types (Early Breast Cancer, Clinical Stages I, II)

Procedure	Reference	Five-year Survival
Extended radical mastectomy (Dahl-Iversen)	22	67%
	24	70%
	25	68%
	38	40%
	39	70%
Radical mastectomy (Halsted)	24	70%
	25	63%
	31	61%
	38	38%
	39	60%
Simple mastectomy (McWhirter)	22	66%
Quadrantectomy	42	89.6%

Quadrantectomy is the radical removal of the quadrant of the breast in which the primary tumor is located. The overlying skin and the fascia of the major pectoral muscle are removed, as are all axillary lymph nodes up to the axillary apex. When the primary tumor is located in one of the upper quadrants of the breast, the entire surgical procedure can be performed en bloc. If the primary is in one of the lower quadrants, a separate incision must be made for the axillary dissection. Surgical reconstruction of the breast is then done, with satisfactory cosmetic results in more than 70 percent of cases. Quadrantectomy is usually supplemented with radiotherapy and/or systemic chemotherapy, especially if axillary lymph nodes are clinically palpable or histologically positive for malignancy [42].

Simple mastectomy refers to the removal of only the breast, leaving the axillary lymph nodes and pectoral muscles intact (McWhirter's method). Today, the disease is clinically staged before simple mastectomy is performed and is generally done only if there are no palpable axillary nodes. Recurrence and survival rates are similar to those for the Halsted radical mastectomy [38]. Simple mastectomy is often combined with adjuvant postoperative radiotherapy, which is very effective in controlling nodal disease [14]. Cosmetic surgery is usually successful and satisfactory after simple mastectomy.

Partial mastectomy is thus termed because the tumor and two to three centimeters of surrounding tissue are removed, leaving behind some of the breast and half of the tissue, skin, and fascia. Despite the fact that the breast is partially saved, it is usually markedly disfigured. The disfigured breast can, however, usually be salvaged by later cosmetic surgery. A major argument opposing this procedure is the multicentricity of most breast cancers, thus leaving the woman vulnerable to cancer development in another part of the affected breast. This problem is partially solved by postoperative radiotherapy [38].

Table 5.2. Ten-Year Survival Rates, Various Mastectomy Types (Early Breast Cancer, Clinical Stages I, II)

Procedure	Reference	Ten-year Survival
Extended radical mastectomy (Dahl-Iversen)	22	42%
	39	54%
	40	62%
Radical mastectomy (Halsted)	18	44%
	39	33%
	40	44%
Modified radical mastectomy	19	41%
Simple mastectomy (McWhirter)	6	54%
	22	44%
Simple mastectomy plus radiotherapy	18	54% (Stage I)
		43% (Stage II)
Partial mastectomy	6	44%

The *extended radical mastectomy* (Dahl-Iversen technique) is the most mutilating of the surgical procedures for breast cancer. In this type of mastectomy, there is removal of the breast, subcutaneous tissue, all axillary lymph nodes, and both pectoral muscles, as well as dissection of the internal mammary nodes and dissection of nodes in the base of the neck. A portion of the rib cage must be removed in order to remove the latter two groups of lymph nodes. This technique was developed because of concern about the potentially malignant internal nodes being left in the woman's body [22, 38, 39]. Although it was hoped that the extended radical mastectomy would increase breast cancer survival rates, clinical trials have not supported this hope. Survival rates are surprisingly low when compared with other types of mastectomy (see Table 5.2), which may reflect in part a higher postoperative mortality because of the much greater trauma inflicted upon the body.

Prophylactic mastectomy is sometimes performed on women who carry a high risk for breast cancer, although this procedure is strongly opposed by many experts. Prophylactic mastectomy has been sometimes advocated in the following cases: (a) multiple persistent breast nodules, (b) a biopsy showing moderate to severe fibrocystic disease, (c) a family history of breast cancer, and (d) nodularity or cystic disease in one breast after a cancer has been found in the other [38].

Some breast malignancies are inoperable because of the expected high rate of recurrence [31]. The criteria for inoperability include the following:

1. Extensive edema of the skin over the breast
2. Satellite tumor nodules in the skin over the breast
3. Intercostal or parasternal tumor nodules
4. Arm edema
5. Biopsy-proven supraclavicular metastases
6. Inflammatory carcinoma, and
7. Distant metastases

The breast malignancy may also be considered inoperable if two or more of the following are present

1. Skin ulceration
2. Limited edema of the skin over the breast
3. Axillary nodes positive for malignancy on biopsy and larger than one inch in diameter, and
4. Fixation of axillary nodes to the skin or to deep structures in the axilla [31]

PREOPERATIVE CARE

Preoperative care of the mastectomy client includes measures to reduce anxiety and psychological discomfort. The client may experience a deep fear of the unknown and confusion about treatment alternatives [36]. Encourage her to question the surgeon about treatment alternatives, and help her to understand the meaning of test results. Client fears will often decrease if continuity of care is provided as much as possible and if family support and communication are facilitated. Answer the client's questions honestly, and provide appropriate teaching about postoperative medical and nursing management.

The client may also fear loss of personal control over her life. Facilitate her understanding of the tremendous importance of her role as a member of the treatment team. Teach postoperative exercises such as exercises for deep breathing, range of motion, and arm and shoulder mobility. Provide teaching about the client's role in postoperative symptom control, such as pain, nausea, and lymphedema. Provide teaching about her necessary involvement in maintaining optimal postoperative nutritional status, and facilitate the client's control over her environment.

The client may fear disfigurement and mutilation secondary to the surgery. Although immediate breast reconstruction has been shown to decrease psychological morbidity after mastectomy [8], not every case is amenable to breast reconstruction. Provide teaching about the surgical procedure as appropriate, since knowing what may be expected may reduce anxiety. Facilitate communication between the client and spouse or significant other.

POSTOPERATIVE CARE

Wound Complications

Mastectomy complications are usually related to wound problems [31]. During surgery, a stab wound is usually made near the axilla and a drain inserted [5], since accumulation of fluid beneath the skin flaps may cause dehiscence or infection. Very little incisional drainage should occur and dressings need not be extensive. Maintain patency of drains by emptying them at least every two hours or when they contain approximately 100 milliliters of fluid.

Wound infection may cause sloughing of the skin flaps. Monitor drainage for alterations in quantity, odor, color, or other characteristics. Observe the wound for inflammation during dressing changes, and monitor vital signs for alterations indicative of infection. Administer antibiotics and special wound care as prescribed.

Lymphedema of the affected arm secondary to impairment of lymphatic drainage is seen to some degree in almost two-thirds of cases [31], although lymphedema is less of a problem with the more conservative surgeries which result in less mutilation of the lymph system in the affected arm. Should lymphedema develop, routinely measure the circumference of both arms to determine the severity of edema. Teach the client to elevate the affected arm to facilitate gravity-induced drainage. The arm should lie above the client's head, each joint higher than the former. Apply pressure stockings to the affected arm as prescribed to facilitate drainage of fluid. Begin arm and shoulder exercises as prescribed (see Figure 5.1) as soon as possible to improve circulation in the arm and to prevent limitation of joint motion (frozen shoulder).

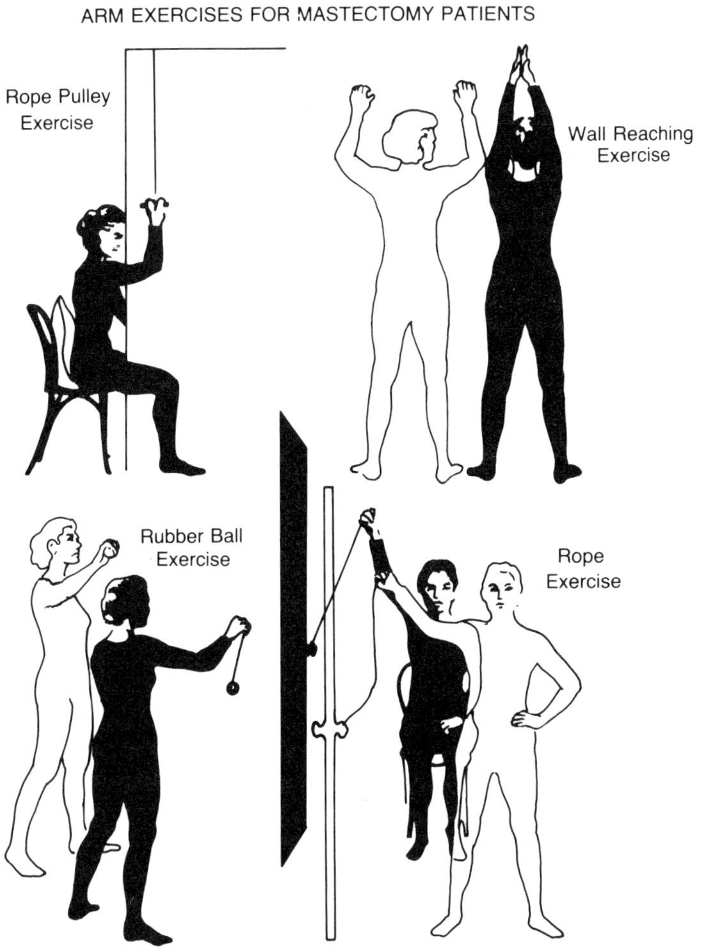

ARM EXERCISES FOR MASTECTOMY PATIENTS

Rope Pulley
Exercise

Wall Reaching
Exercise

Rubber Ball
Exercise

Rope
Exercise

Figure 5.1. Post-Mastectomy Exercises (Reprinted from *A Cancer Source Book for Nurses* (Rev. Ed.), page 76. Copyright © 1981, American Cancer Society. Used with permission.)

Teaching

Client teaching is a crucial part of postoperative nursing care for mastectomy clients. Teach those measures that are designed to prevent lymphedema in the affected arm:

1. Inform medical and nursing personnel that no injections, blood samples, or blood pressures are to be performed on the affected arm
2. Inform medical and nursing personnel that no intravenous lines or injections are to be performed on the affected arm
3. Wear a medical alert bracelet or necklace
4. Carry purses or heavy articles with the unaffected arm

5. Ensure that watches and jewelry are not too tight
6. Keep the affected arm and hand soft with skin cream
7. Wear gloves while using detergents or commercial cleaning agents
8. Protect the affected hand from burns or injuries when smoking, sewing, gardening, or doing housework
9. Wear oven mitts when reaching into the oven
10. Protect the affected hand and arm from sunburn
11. Report to the physician if the affected arm or hand becomes swollen, red, warm, or painful

BREAST SELF-EXAMINATION

Follow these simple steps:

Lie down. Put one hand behind your head. With the other hand, fingers flattened, gently feel your breast. Press ever so lightly. Now examine the other breast.

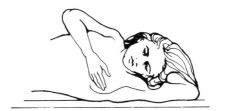

This illustration shows you how to check each breast. Begin where you see the A and follow the arrows, feeling gently for a lump or thickening. Remember to feel all parts of each breast.

Now repeat the same procedure sitting up, with the hand still behind your head.

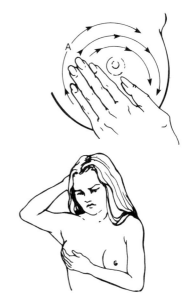

If you find a lump or thickening, make an appointment with your doctor immediately. Most breast lumps or changes are not cancer, but only a doctor can diagnose them.

Figure 5.2. Self Breast Examination (Reprinted from *A Cancer Source Book for Nurses* (Rev. Ed.), page 71. Copyright © 1981, American Cancer Society. Used with permission.)

Provide information about available prostheses, and provide teaching about pre-scribed postmastectomy irradiation or chemotherapy. Teach the client how to do postmastectomy exercises (see Figure 5.1) and regular breast self-examination on the unoperated breast (see Figure 5.2).

> **CONCEPT XII:**
> **Although head and neck malignancies constitute only a small percentage of all cancers, special consideration is warranted because of the drastic physical and psychosocial disruptions that often result from the disease and its surgical treatment.**

Devastating structural, functional, and psychosocial changes may result from surgery for head and neck cancers [11]. Routes of breathing and eating may be permanently altered, for example. Facial appearance may be radically changed, and the client's ability to communicate may be significantly impaired.

Adaptation to the alteration in body appearance and function depends upon the nature of the change, its meaning to the client, coping abilities, the response from significant others, and the assistance available to the client [4]. Specific client teaching may facilitate the major revisions in the client's self-care activity that are necessary, including techniques such as tracheostomy care, tube feedings, and oral irrigations. This teaching is of crucial importance because competence at self-care is a highly important aspect of the rehabilitation of this client population [10].

REFERENCES

1. American Cancer Society. *1983 Facts and Figures.* New York: American Cancer Society, 1982. P. 16.
2. American Cancer Society's National Task Force on Breast Cancer Control. Mammography 1982: A Statement of the American Cancer Society. CA 32:226, 1982.
3. Baldonado, A. A. and Stahl, D. A. *Cancer Nursing: A Holistic Multidisciplinary Approach.* Garden City, NY: Medical Examination Publishing Co., 1978. Pp. 79–86.
4. Blues, K. A Framework for Nurses Providing Care to Laryngectomy Patients. *Cancer Nurs* 1:441, 1978.
5. Carlson, L. D. Surgical Approaches to Cancer Management. In P. K. Burkhalter and D. L. Donley. *Dynamics of Oncology Nursing.* New York: McGraw-Hill, 1978. Pp. 110–135.
6. Crile, G. Jr. Management of Breast Cancer: Limited Mastectomy. In P. Rubin (Ed.). *Updated Breast Cancer.* New York: American Cancer Society, 1978. Pp. 19–23.
7. Cummings, J. H. Fermentation in the Human Large Intestine: Evidence and Implications for Health. *Lancet* 1(8335):1206, 1983.
8. Dean, C., Chetty, U., and Forrest, A. P. M. Effects of Immediate Breast Reconstruction on Psychosocial Morbidity after Mastectomy. *Lancet* 1(8322):459, 1983.
9. Dixon, J. M., Lamb, J., and Anderson, T. J. Fine Needle Aspiration of the Breast: Importance of the Operator. *Lancet* 2(8349):564, 1983.
10. Dropkin, M. J. Compliance in Post-operative Head and Neck Patients. *Cancer Nurs* 2:379, 1979.

11. Dropkin, M. J. Development of a Self-Care Teaching Program for Postoperative Head and Neck Patients. *Cancer Nurs* 4:103, 1981.

12. Fisher, B. Biological and Clinical Considerations Regarding the Use of Surgery and Chemotherapy in the Treatment of Primary Breast Cancer. *Cancer* 40:574, 1977.

13. Fisher, B. and Gebhardt, M. C. The Evolution of Breast Cancer Surgery: Past, Present, and Future. *Semin Oncol* 5:385, 1978.

14. Fisher, B., Montague, E., Redmond, C., and other National Surgical Adjuvant Breast Project Investigators. Comparison of Radical Mastectomy with Alternative Treatments for Primary Breast Cancer. A First Report of Results from a Prospective Randomized Clinical Trial. *Cancer* 39 (No. 6, Supplement):2827, 1977.

15. Friel, M. Concepts Relating to the Nursing Care of Surgical Oncology Patients. In D. L. Vredevoe, A. Derdiarian, L. P. Sarna, M. Friel, and J. A. G. Shiplacoff. *Concepts of Oncology Nursing.* Englewood Cliffs, NJ: Prentice-Hall, 1981. Pp. 227–269.

16. Gibbs, G. E. and White, M. Stomal Care. *Am J Nurs* 72:268, 1972.

17. Gutowski, F. Ostomy Procedure: Nursing Care Before and After. *Am J Nurs* 72:262, 1972.

18. Haagensen, C. D. Treatment of Curable Carcinoma of the Breast. In P. Rubin (Ed.). *Updated Breast Cancer.* New York: American Cancer Society, 1978. Pp. 24–29.

19. Handley, R. S. The Conservative Radical Mastectomy of Patey: 10 Year Results in 425 Patients. *Breast* 2:17, 1976.

20. Horowicz, C. Profiles in OPD Nursing: A Rectal and Colon Service. *Am J Nurs* 71:114, 1971.

21. Hubbard, T. B. Jr. Prophylactic Mastectomy for Prevention of the Second Primary. In P. Rubin (Ed.). *Updated Breast Cancer.* New York: American Cancer Society, 1978. Pp. 120–121.

22. Kaae, S. and Johansen, H. Five Year Results: Two Random Series of Simple Mastectomy with Post-operative Radiation Versus Extended Radical Mastectomy. *Am J Roentgenol* 87:82, 1962.

23. Katona, E. A. Learning Colostomy Control. *Am J Nurs* 67:534, 1967.

24. Koszarowski, T. Rational Approach to the Efficiency of Internal Mammary Lymph Node Dissection and Breast Cancer Cure. *Breast* 2:44, 1976.

25. Lacour, J. L., Bucalossi, P., Cacerse, J., Koszarowski, T., Rumeau-Rouquette, C., and Veronesi, U. Radical Mastectomy Versus Radical Mastectomy Plus Internal Mammary Dissection—5 Year Results of an International Cooperative Study. *Cancer* 37:206, 1976.

26. Murray, B. S., Elmore, J., and Sawyer, J. R. The Patient Has an Ileal Conduit. *Am J Nurs* 71:1560, 1971.

27. Patterson, W. B. Principles of Surgical Oncology. In P. Rubin (Ed.). *Clinical Oncology for Medical Students and Physicians: A Multidisciplinary Approach* (5th Ed.). Rochester, NY: American Cancer Society, 1978. Pp. 21–28.

28. Prescott, D. M. *Cancer: The Misguided Cell.* New York: Pegasus, 1973. Pp. 80–81.

29. Rubin, P. Introduction: The Search for the Ideal Surgical Procedure. In P. Rubin (Ed.). *Updated Breast Cancer.* New York: American Cancer Society, 1978. Pp. 17–18.

30. Rubin, P. Statement of the Clinical Oncologic Problem. In P. Rubin (Ed.). *Clinical Oncology for Medical Students and Physicians: A Multidisciplinary Approach* (5th Ed.). Rochester, NY: American Cancer Society, 1978. Pp. 1–10.

31. Savlov, E. Breast Cancer. In P. Rubin (Ed.). *Clinical Oncology for Medical Students and Physicians: A Multidisciplinary Approach* (5th Ed.). Rochester, NY: American Cancer Society, 1978. Pp. 63–74.

32. Schabel, F. M. Jr. The Use of Tumor Growth Kinetics in Planning "Curative" Chemotherapy of Advanced Solid Tumors. *Cancer Res* 29:2384, 1969.

33. Schabel, F. M. Jr. Concepts for Systemic Treatment of Micrometastases. *Cancer* 35:15, 1975.

34. Schabel, F. M. Jr. Surgical Adjuvant Chemotherapy of Metastatic Murine Tumors. *Cancer* 40:558, 1977.

35. Sutherland, A. and Orbach, C. Depressive Reactions Associated with Surgery for Cancer. In American Cancer Society. *The Psychological Impact of Cancer.* New York: American Cancer Society, 1974. Pp. 17–21.

36. Thomas, S. G. Breast Cancer: The Psychosocial Issues. *Cancer Nurs* 1:53, 1978.

37. Timothy, A. R., Overgaard, J., Overgaard, M., and Wang, C. C. Treatment of Early Carcinoma of the Breast. *Lancet* 2:25, 1979.

38. United States Department of Health and Human Services. *The Breast Cancer Digest.* Bethesda, MD: United States Department of Health and Human Services, NIH Publication No. 80:1691, 1980. Pp. 27–31.

39. Urban, J. A. Changing Patterns of Breast Cancer. *Cancer* 37:111, 1976.

40. Urban, J. A. Is There a Rationale for an Extended Radical Procedure? In P. Rubin (Ed.). *Updated Breast Cancer.* New York: American Cancer Society, 1978. Pp. 34–37.

41. Veronesi, U. Value of Limited Surgery for Breast Cancer. *Semin Oncol* 5:395, 1978.

42. Veronesi, U., Saccozzi, R., DelVecchio, M., et al. Comparing Radical Mastectomy with Quadrantectomy, Axillary Dissection, and Radiotherapy in Patients with Small Cancers of the Breast. *N Engl J Med* 305:6, 1981.

43. Watson, P. G. The Effects of Short-Term Postoperative Counseling on Cancer/Ostomy Patients. *Cancer Nurs* 6:21, 1983.

Chapter 6

Nursing Care of the Client Receiving Radiotherapy

RADIOTHERAPY AND RADIOBIOLOGY

CONCEPT I:
Radiotherapy is one of the four major medical treatment modalities used to attempt reduction of the body burden of tumor.

Radiotherapy has become an increasingly important tool in the treatment of malignant disease. Currently, radiation therapy is used in 50 percent of cancer clients, either as primary therapy, adjuvant therapy, or palliation [4, 11, 22]. The use of radiation as a treatment for cancer virtually dates from the time of the discovery of X-rays and radium. X-rays were first described by Roentgen in 1895, and radium was discovered by the Curies in 1896. The use of external beam radiation produced a positive response in a woman with carcinoma of the breast in 1896, and the first person to be cured of cancer by the use of radiation therapy was reported in 1899. In 1913, the first woman to be cured of cervical cancer by radiotherapy was reported.

In 1901, Becquerel observed that he had developed an area of ulceration on his abdominal skin next to a pocket in which he carried a tube of radium salts. This led to the first realization that ionizing radiation will damage normal tissue as well as malignant tissue. Before the 1930s, the results of radiation treatment were often inconsistent and nonreproducible. In 1934, the technique of protracted fractionation—or the division of the total dose of radiation into several sessions divided by periods of rest time—was developed and remains the basis for techniques of modern radiotherapy.

During the 1920s and 1930s, superficial (50–120 kV) and orthovoltage (120–300 kV) X-rays were used to treat both malignant and nonmalignant diseases. During the 1930s and 1940s, equipment was developed that was capable of delivering 500 to 800 kV, still orthovoltage X-rays. Megavoltage equipment emerged in the 1950s, with the Van de Graaff generator (2 MeV), the Cobalt-60 machinery (1.2 MeV), and the Betatron capable of delivering either photon or electron beams (10–40 MeV) being developed. In the 1960s, the photon or electron linear accelerator (2–40 MeV) was developed and remains the most advanced equipment for the delivery of radiation therapy.

CONCEPT II:

In order to provide effective nursing care to the client receiving radiotherapy, the nurse must first understand the principles of radiobiology.

The radiosensitivity of any tissue is in direct relationship to the cell-renewal characteristics of that tissue. Radiation therapy is most damaging to the cell during the period in its cycle when actual division (mitosis) takes place. Thus, radiotherapy is generally most effective against small, rapidly growing cancers and against those normal, noncancerous tissues with the greatest reproductive rates (e.g., skin, gastrointestinal epithelia, hair follicles).

Radiation capable of producing ions is called ionizing radiation, and radiotherapy is the use of these ionizing radiations to damage or destroy the malignant cells. The ionizing radiation may be electromagnetic (X-rays or gamma rays) or particulate (alpha or beta particles, neutrons). It may be spontaneously generated by radioactive elements or artificially produced by machines or nuclear reactions.

The atom consists of negatively charged electrons that orbit a positively charged nucleus. This nucleus consists of protons that carry a positive charge and neutrons that carry no charge. When an atom gains or loses an electron, it becomes an unstable ion. The unstable ion and the isolated charged particle become highly reactive and capable of further chemical reactions. In an attempt to regain stability, the unstable ion generates highly energetic nuclear particles (alpha, beta, and gamma waves); this generation of particulate energy waves is called radioactivity.

Atoms containing a large number of protons and neutrons have a greater likelihood of becoming unstable or radioactive. Atoms containing 209 or more protons and neutrons are naturally radioactive: for example, uranium, radium, thorium, and actinium. The half-life of a radioactive element is the time necessary for it to lose 50 percent of its radioactivity. Radioactivity will decrease in intensity over time, and the reduction of radioactivity occurs at a specific rate for each element (see Table 6.1).

The goal of radiotherapy in the treatment of cancer is to destroy tumor cells with minimum injury to the structure and function of adjacent normal tissues and organs. Radiation therapy in the treatment of cancer involves exposing a target area in the body to a radiation source. Since the target area or areas encompass relatively small percentages of body tissue, radiotherapy is not considered to be an appropriate primary treatment for disseminated or metastatic cancers.

Table 6.1. Half-Lives of Therapeutic Radioactive Materials [9,14]

Material	Half-Life
^{60}Co (Cobalt)	5.3 years
^{137}Cs (Cesium)	30.0 years
^{226}Ra (Radium)	1,602.0 years
^{32}P (Phosphorus)	14.3 days
^{131}I (Iodine)	8.05 days
^{222}Rn (Radon)	3.8 days

The roentgen is the unit of radiation that is delivered to the target area. The rad is the amount of energy absorbed by the irradiated tissues. The rem (*roentgen equivalent man*) describes the radiation dose required to produce a particular amount of biological damage.

Orthovoltage radiation consists of relatively low energy levels. Maximum absorption is at the skin or slightly below skin level. Therefore, when orthovoltage equipment is used, a full tumoricidal dose to underlying areas frequently results in excessive skin damage [18]. However, because the maximum radiation absorption with orthovoltage equipment is at skin level, this technique is still useful in the treatment of some skin cancers.

Megavoltage radiation is produced by Van de Graff generators, cobalt and betatron equipment, and linear accelerators. Megavoltage radiation consists of high levels of energy output and thus deeper tissue penetration. Radiation is delivered to deep tumors while the megavoltage beam pathway spares the skin and subcutaneous tissues. Megavoltage radiation has another significant advantage over orthovoltage therapy: the radiation beam is more precise with less lateral radiation scatter. Thus, it is more accurately administered and minimizes the amount of tissue that receives unnecessary radiation.

CONCEPT III:
The biological result of radiation occurs at the cellular level, disrupting the normal function and reproductin of both benign and malignant cells.

The ionization of living cells—either benign or cancerous—leads to physical and biochemical damage through chromosomal injury, the cessation or temporary suppression of cellular reproduction, blockage of immune responses, and/or cell membrane injury resulting in cellular deficits of oxygen and nutrients [21]. The biological impact of radiation is dependent upon the number and types of cells damaged rather than the type of radiation used. In other words, the degree and type of cell damage determines the extent of biological damage to the body as a whole.

Cells are most vulnerable to the damaging effects of ionizing radiation during the early phases of DNA synthesis and mitosis (actual division of the cell). Therefore, rapidly dividing, undifferentiated cells are most sensitive to radiotherapy; whereas slowly dividing, highly differentiated cells are most resistant. Ionizing radiation causes a strand breakage in DNA's double helix. The cell can often repair single strand breakage, but double strand breakage causes cell death.

CONCEPT IV:
Radiosensitivity and radioresistance vary according to tumor type.

The tumor's vulnerability to injury from ionizing radiation is determined by the amount of energy necessary for producing fatal cell injury and the number of tumor cells destroyed. A radiosensitive tumor is one that is destroyed by radiation in doses that are well tolerated by surrounding normal tissues [1]. The sensitivity of malignant cells to radiation is roughly equal to the sensitivity of the type

Figure 6.1 Radiosensitivity of Various Types of Tissue [21, 22]

HIGH RADIOSENSITIVITY
> Bone Marrow
> Lymphatics
> Gastrointestinal epithelium
> Mucous membrances
> Gonads

MODERATE RADIOSENSITIVITY
> Skin
> Salivary glands
> Kidney
> Liver
> Lung
> Growing bone cartilage

LOW RADIOSENSITIVITY
> Heart
> Brain
> Peripheral nerves

RADIORESISTANT
> Muscle
> Mature bone cartilage
> Connective tissue

of tissue from which they are derived. Generally speaking, the less differentiated the tumor, the more sensitive it is to radiation. Also, the tumor with a high growth fraction, or rapid proliferation, is generally more radiosensitive than slowly dividing cells.

A significant impact from radiotherapy is seen only if large numbers of tumor cells are destroyed and not rapidly replaced. Most tumor tissue can be destroyed by ionizing radiation, but the dose required for some malignancies is too toxic to surrounding normal tissue.

The cell's vulnerability to radiation damage is lessened if the cell is hypoxic. Many tumors contain hypoxic cells that may be appreciably more radioresistant than the other tumor cells or the surrounding normal cells [12, 21].

CONCEPT V:
Fractionation refers to a timing technique used in radiotherapy.

Radiotherapy is usually given in daily multiple doses with weekend rest periods over a specified length of time. Since normal cells are usually more efficient than malignant cells in compensating for the damage caused by ionizing radiation, fractionation allows for maximum repair of normal tissues during the course of treatment. Also, since the number of fatal double-strand breaks in the DNA helix increases with successive exposure to ionizing radiation, the technique of fractionation may enhance the tumor's vulnerability to radiotherapy.

EXTERNAL BEAM RADIOTHERAPY

CONCEPT VI:
External beam radiotherapy utilizes ionizing radiation to destroy malignant cells.

FACTORS INFLUENCING THE SUCCESS OF EXTERNAL BEAM RADIOTHERAPY

Tumor-Related Factors

Histological type may predict the sensitivity of the malignant cells to ionizing radiation. Undifferentiated cells are more radiosensitive than well-differentiated cells, and cells with a high growth fraction are more vulnerable to radiation damage. Some tumors have a combination of histological types and thus are less predictable regarding radiosensitivity.

The location of the tumor and its extent of spread influence the success of radiotherapy. The presence of distant metastases usually eliminates radiotherapy as a curative treatment modality, and the radiosensitivity of surrounding normal tissues may limit the use of ionizing radiation because of the risk of unacceptable radiation damage.

Large tumor masses are less successfully treated by radiotherapy. Bulky neoplasms often have an inadequate oxygen supply and a necrotic core that is more radioresistant than well-oxygenated malignant cells. Because of the extensive treatment fields necessary for large tumor masses, there is an increased risk of adverse radiation side effects.

Client-Related Factors

Severely debilitated clients are usually not appropriate candidates for vigorous radiotherapy. Also, the very young and the very old may be more vulnerable to radiation-induced side effects and toxicities.

CURATIVE EXTERNAL BEAM RADIOTHERAPY

External beam radiotherapy may be administered with curative intent (see Figure 6.2). Tumor curability is related to the tumor- and client-related factors as well as the overall radiosensitivity of the tumor. Because some malignancies are highly radiosensitive, external beam radiation is often the primary treatment of choice for these lesions.

Figure 6.2. Radiocurability of Common Malignancies [1, 15, 22]

HIGHLY CURABLE
Lymphoma
Seminoma of testes
Carcinoma of skin (basal cell epithelium, squamous cell)
Neuroblastoma
Retinoblastoma
Wilms' tumor
Squamous cell carcinoma of oral cavity, pharynx, larynx, and cervix
Pituitary lesions

MODERATELY CURABLE
Head/neck carcinoma
Bladder carcinoma
Prostate adenocarcinoma

LOW RATE OF CURE
Gastrointestinal cancers
Lung cancers
Bone sarcomas
Brain cancer
Melanoma

ADJUNCTIVE EXTERNAL BEAM RADIOTHERAPY

External beam radiotherapy may be used as an adjunct treatment to oncologic surgery and/or chemotherapy. Clinical data suggest that preoperative irradiation of the primary tumor can increase cure rates in certain tumor types, such as bladder, breast, and rectosigmoid cancers. Preoperative reduction in the size of rapidly growing tumors may decrease the extent of surgical resection, and the use of external beam irradiation may also reduce the risk of tumor cell seeding secondary to surgical manipulation. Surgery is generally delayed for several weeks after the completion of preoperative radiotherapy to reduce the risk of adverse side effects and to allow the repair of normal tissues so that healing of the surgical incision is possible.

Postoperative radiotherapy destroys residual but clinically undetectable malignant cells, thus reducing the risk of recurrence. Unresected lymph nodes are often treated with postoperative radiation. Postoperative external beam radiotherapy is usually delayed until after healing of the surgical wound.

PALLIATIVE EXTERNAL BEAM RADIOTHERAPY

Clients with advanced disease who are not candidates for extensive curative treatment may benefit from palliative radiotherapy, particularly for pain relief. Bone pain secondary to bony metastases is often dramatically relieved by external beam radiation [1, 20]. With both orthovoltage and megavoltage irradiation, bone is significantly more receptive to radiation energy than soft tissue. Radiation to the affected bone shrinks the tumor mass that is causing the pain, thus reducing pressure on afferent nerves. External beam radiotherapy is also moderately successful in relieving pain caused by stretching of the organ capsule, as in cancers of the parotid gland or liver. If a malignant tumor invades muscles or nerves and subsequently causes painful dysfunction, pain relief from radiotherapy is moderately successful.

Other distressing symptoms commonly seen in advanced malignant disease are frequently controllable by external beam irradiation. Bleeding, for example, can be readily relieved, as can a superior vena cava syndrome caused by tumor pressure on that blood vessel. Cough, hemoptysis, and shortness of breath secondary to tumor obstruction of major and minor bronchi often respond to radiation treatment. Neurological symptoms, ulcerations, and jaundice may also respond favorably to treatment with external beam radiotherapy.

CONCEPT VII:
The acute side effects of external beam radiotherapy result from the adverse effects of ionizing radiation on normal cells.

The acute side effects of external beam irradiation are dependent upon dose rate and time-dose fractionation rather than merely upon the total delivered dose. Adverse acute side effects are also influenced by the site and volume of tissue treated [16]. The adverse effects result primarily from the depletion of actively re-producing normal cells, which creates an imbalance in homeostasis. Therefore, the failure to maintain normal homeostasis causes the clinically observed adverse effects associated with external beam radiation.

Although occasionally severe enough to discontinue treatment, acute side effects are not generally used as criteria for termination of radiotherapy since a slight reduction in the daily dose increment will often alleviate unacceptable symptoms [4]. Repair of radiation damage by normal cells is dependent upon their positions in the cell cycle and upon the interval between fractions. Acute reactions will usually resolve soon after completion of the radiation treatment of when the daily dose increment is lowered and repopulation of normal tissue is unimpeded. The nursing and medical management of acute radiation side effects is usually symptomatic.

CONCEPT VIII:
Although significant skin reactions are much less common and less severe with the use of megavoltage radiation, skin care is still a primary nursing concern.

At one time, skin tolerance was the dose-limiting factor in radiation therapy, and dosage was determined by the degree of skin erythema that was produced. Acute, late, or chronic skin reactions were painful and disfiguring. Before the use of megavoltage equipment, external beam radiotherapy often produced severe radiodermatitis secondary to the skin's sensitivity to radiation and to the concentration of orthovoltage radiation at or slightly below skin level. The acute phase of this radiodermatitis consists of a progressive pattern of hyperpigmentation and erythema, edema, vesiculation, bullae, and ulceration and necrosis. The chronic phase is characterized by atrophy and wrinkling of the skin, telangiectasia, scleroderma on the feet and fingers, and the temporary or permanent loss of nails. The skin is especially vulnerable to radiation injury, and ulcerations often need excision and grafting. Before the use of megavoltage equipment, death resulting from severe radiodermatitis was not uncommon [11].

With modern megavoltage equipment and advances in radiation oncology, however, both the frequency and severity of skin reactions have dramatically decreased. Today, the term *radiodermatitis* is obsolete. Skin reactions are seldom significant because of the skin-sparing characteristic of high energy, megavoltage radiation. Although acute skin reactions are not entirely eliminated, the severity of these reactions is greatly reduced, and they are predictable, treatable, and seldom result in significant chronic skin changes [11, 17]. The chronic skin reactions most seen with high-dose megavoltage treatment include alopecia, telangiectasia, fibrosis, and minor changes in pigmentation [8, 14, 19, 31].

The term *altered skin integriy*, which is now used instead of *radiodermatitis*, implies a temporary, manageable situation with a potential for a return to unimpaired skin integrity. There is little consistency in the systems used to classify acute radiation-induced skin reactions, but the easiest is to simply describe the skin reaction as erythema, dry desquamation, or moist desquamation (see Table 6.2).

Another manner to describe acute skin reactions is in terms of degrees [16]. A *first-degree skin reaction* is characterized by alopecia secondary to the destruction of the hair follicles. Alopecia becomes evident about 18 days after radiotherapy begins, and the hair regrows in two or three months. *Second-degree skin reaction* results in erythema of the local irradiated area, with inhibition or destruction of the sweat glands. When the erythema subsides, a residual red pigmentation often remains and may be permanent. Dry desquamation and pruritus are common during a second-degree reaction. A *third-degree skin reaction* is characterized by erythema of a deeper red, moist desquamation with blisters, destruction of the sweat glands, and permanent alopecia. Ulceration is not generally associated with moist desquamation [10, 14, 23, 26]. A *fourth-degree skin reaction* is known as a "radiation burn." This severe skin reaction should not be seen, as it represents a technical mistake or an error in judgment. It is characterized by deeply colored erythema, deep blisters and ulceration, sloughing of the entire skin surface, and significant pain.

Skin reactions are more likely to occur and are usually more severe if areas of skin apposition and moisture are treated (for example, the axilla, groin, breasts, perineum). The warmth, moisture, and decreased aeration of these areas result in

Table 6.2. Acute Radiation-Induced Skin Reactions

Reaction	Skin is...
Erythema	Pink, dusky
Dry Desquamation	Flaking, scaly, itchy
Moist Desquamation	Painful, weeping, sloughing

an increased likelihood of skin reaction. Additionally, if radiosensitizing chemo-therapy such as Adriamycin or Actinomycin-D is used, there is a greater potential for significant acute skin reactions [11, 23, 24].

NURSING AND MEDICAL TREATMENT OF RADIATION-INDUCED SKIN REACTIONS

Current nursing and medical treatment of skin reactions heavily empha-sizes conservative measures. Treatment encompasses four goals: to decrease skin irritation, to reduce unintentional enhancement of skin reactions, to promote heal-ing, and to enhance comfort.

Skin irritation is lessened if the treatment area is not rubbed and does not come into contact with heat, cold, chemical irritants, tapes, or dressings. Chemical irri-tants include laundry detergents, perfumes and perfumed soaps, creams, deodor-ants, alcohol, and cosmetics. Assess the treatment site daily for erythema, blisters, and signs of skin breakdown. Keep the treatment area dry, and do not cover the treatment site with clothing in order to prevent continuous skin irritation and pos-sible subsequent skin breakdown. Do not shave the treatment area, and teach the client to avoid lying on the treatment site for prolonged periods of time.

Reduce unnecessary enhancement of skin reactions by avoiding the use of warm packs, heat lamps, menthol rubs, and powders or creams with a metal base. Al-though direct sunlight should be avoided during treatment and for varying periods of time after treatment, current authorities agree that exposure to sunlight is ac-ceptable if sunscreening agents are used and if a period of skin healing has been allowed [10, 23, 30].

Healing of the skin area and client comfort are promoted by appropriate cleans-ing and treatment of the affected skin. There is wide disagreement in the literature regarding the advisability of washing the irradiated skin. Those who advocate that the skin not be washed argue that wetting the area increases the potential for skin maceration and breakdown and that the treatment-portal markings are likely to be removed [5, 7, 23, 24, 25].

However, it is impractical to ask the client not to wash for lengthy periods of time, and gentle cleansing of irradiated skin increases client comfort, may promote healing, and is effective in prevention of infection. Healing of denuded skin areas is enhanced by moisture, which promotes the migration of epithelial cells from healthy tissue to areas of desquamation [10]. Thus, soaks, irrigations, and gentle washing of the treatment site with a nonperfumed, nonabrasive soap may speed healing of irradiated skin. Do not rub or scrub the skin area. Pat the skin dry with a soft towel after washing.

Authorities differ, however, on what solution is best to use for the cleansing of irradiated skin. Plain water [2, 3, 16, 30] or saline solution [2, 7, 13] are often recommended. Also, hydrogen peroxide combined with two to three parts water or saline is frequently advised [7, 10, 14, 19, 26, 29]. Considering the lack of agreement on what solution to use, or if washing should even be done, it is best to follow institutional policy.

If itching and peeling (dry desquamation) develop, keep the skin dry and well aerated. Apply mild lubricants as prescribed. Mild antiseptics such as Gentian Violet or dilute solutions of hydrogen peroxide may be beneficial [20]. If blisters (moist desquamation) develop, treatment goals are to speed healing, relieve itching and pain, and prevent infection. An ointment containing Vitamins A and D may enhance healing of the affected site, and topical steroid cream may be prescribed to relieve itching and pain. Keep the treatment area clean, and apply antibiotic ointments as prescribed to minimize the risk of infection.

CONCEPT IX:
External beam radiotherapy may cause other acute adverse effects on normal tissues or organs.

GASTROINTESTINAL TRACT

Irradiation of the mouth and oropharynx often results in stomatitis or esophagitis because of the destruction of epithelial cells in the mucous membranes. Stomatitis is characteristically heralded by erythema of the affected tissue and the inability to tolerate hot, cold, or spicy foods. The oral or esophageal ulcerations cause significant pain, often accompanied by an inability to swallow and a change in taste perception [28], contributing to decreased nutritional intake and possible malnutrition. Fungal infections occur frequently, usually characterized by the development of yellow-white patches on the tongue and oral mucous membranes. Irradiation of the salivary glands results in the production of thick saliva, leaving the client with the sensation of a dry mouth. This abnormally thick saliva does not clean the teeth and mouth as well as does normal saliva, so the client is further vulnerable to the development of infection or dental caries.

Irradiation of the mediastinum and/or stomach may result in esophagitis and nausea. Abdominal or pelvic irradiation often results in ulceration of the mucous membranes, bleeding, and/or diarrhea.

BRAIN OR NERVOUS TISSUE

Although the tissue of the brain and nervous system is usually radioresistant, acute side effects may occur. Nausea and vomiting may result from stimulation of the vomiting center in the brain. High doses of external beam radiotherapy may occasionally cause peripheral neuritis.

HEMATOPOIETIC TISSUE

Since hematopoietic tissue exhibits a rapid rate of cellular proliferation, it is especially vulnerable to external beam irradiation. Radiotherapy to a large area of hematopoietic tissue may result in anemia, leukopenia, and thrombocytopenia secondary to myelosuppression. These abnormalities are not common, however, unless large areas of bone marrow receive irradiation.

BONE

High doses of external beam radiation to bone may cause vascular damage, resulting in brittle and poorly oxygenated bone tissue. This causes the bone to be very vulnerable to either necrosis or pathological fractures.

REPRODUCTIVE ORGANS

In males, sperm production can be reduced by doses as low as 50 rad, and permanent sterility may occur with 1,000 rad [16]. Hormonal production, however, is not significantly altered in males.

In females, hormonal activity is often permanently altered by radiotherapy. Reduction or cessation of ovarian hormone production may occur, and temporary or permanent amenorrhea usually results.

RADIATION SICKNESS

Radiation sickness is a generalized illness that may occur during the course of external beam radiotherapy. Its primary cause is an increase of cell-death breakdown products in the blood, and the severity of the illness depends on the volume of tissue that is irradiated. Symptoms characteristic of this unusual condition include nausea, vomiting, fatigue, malaise, and weakness. Clients undergoing treatment for recurrent disease experience significantly more nausea and vomiting than do clients receiving radiation treatment for the first time, possibly because of larger treatment fields and higher radiation doses [27]. Nursing and medical management is usually symptomatic.

CONCEPT X:
Intermediate side effects of external beam radiotherapy are postulated to result from injury to cells that are of a slowly proliferating nature, possibly endothelium or connective tissue.

The intermediate side effects are related to time-dose fractionation characteristics as well as the total delivered dose. These intermediate side effects are usually mild in severity, temporary, without permanent sequelae, and responsive to curative nursing and medical management.

Radiation pneumonitis, for example, usually develops two to three months after completion of radiation treatments. The lung's tolerance of radiation is volume dependent and may be decreased by concomitant pulmonary disease, infection, or the use of Adriamycin or Actinomycin-D. The pulmonary inflammation associated with radiation pneumonitis may lead to fibrosis within the lung, inhibiting lung expansion and reducing vital capacity. The client with radiation pneumonitis is also vulnerable to the development of pulmonary infections. This intermediate side effect of external beam irradiation may be asymptomatic, but is most often associated with a dry, hacking cough and occasional mild exertional dyspnea.

Radiation-induced pericarditis may develop within a year after completion of radiotherapy. Symptoms include pleuritic chest pain, pericardial friction rub, electrocardiograph abnormalities, and cardiomegaly. Signs of tamponade are sometimes noted.

CONCEPT XI:
Late side effects of external beam radiotherapy may occur as early as a few months or as late as a few years after irradiation.

Late side effects are related to the total delivered dose of radiation, and they do not have a direct relationship to previous acute or intermediate reactions. Late reactions are chronic and not always amenable to correction. They include tissue necrosis, fistula development, and the formation of dense fibrotic tissue. Medical and nursing management is dependent upon the anatomical location of damaged tissue and is usually conservative because of the compromised blood supply in the involved areas.

CONCEPT XII:
Skilled nursing measures may prevent or minimize the side effects of external beam radiotherapy.

STOMATITIS, ESOPHAGITIS, DRY MOUTH

Assess the mouth daily for erythema or development of yellow-white patches indicative of fungal infection. Teach the client to avoid substances that irritate the damaged tissues, such as hot or spicy foods, smoking, toothpicks, hard-bristled toothbrushes, etc. Provide oral care after each meal and before sleep to remove food particles and to cleanse the teeth; a small amount of saline to rinse the mouth works well for this purpose. Administer artificial saliva as required to moisten the oral mucosa, and administer Viscous Xylocaine as prescribed before meals to reduce the pain associated with eating and swallowing. Antibiotics or antifungal agents should be medically prescribed to prevent or treat mucosal infection.

NAUSEA AND VOMITING

Nausea and vomiting caused by irradiation of the brain, mediastinum, or stomach may be prevented or minimized with a variety of simple nursing interventions. Avoid noxious external stimuli, such as unemptied bedpans or urinals, suction containiners within view of the client, etc. Remove lid covers from plates of food prior to entering the client's room. Provide six to eight small feedings per day of foods desired by the client, avoiding gas-forming foods. Provide ice chips and cabonated beverages as desired. Administer antiemetics before, not after, meals or as needed, and perform oral care frequently. Teach the client to take deep breaths during acute nausea. Monitor intake and output records, observng for dehydration, and monitor the client who is vomiting for signs of potassium deficit.

DIARRHEA, INTESTINAL ULCERATION, BLEEDING

Abdominal or pelvic irradiation may cause diarrhea, intestinal ulceration, and bleeding secondary to the destruction of the fragile mucosal cells. Assess for the number, frequency, and consistency of stools. Monitor for blood or mucous in the stools, and assess for accompanying cramping and pain. Assess for skin breakdown in or irritation of the perineum. Monitor bowel sounds twice daily for an increase in frequency. Provide the client with a bland, low residue diet, and ensure a fluid intake of two to four liters daily. Record accurate intake and output, monitoring for dehydration. Provide skin care to the perineum after every stool to minimize excoriation, and administer antidiarrheal medication as prescribed. If the client has significant diarrhea, monitor for signs and symptoms indicative of hypokalemia.

MYELOSUPPRESSION

Leukopenia

Leukopenia (low levels of circulating mature white blood cells) predisposes the client to infection. Septic phenomena are associated with a white blood cell count less than $2,000/mm^3$, and a white cell count of less than $1,000/mm^3$ is considered to be life-threatening. Therefore, the following infection precautions should be instituted if the white blood cell count is less than $2,500/mm^3$.

Monitor for temperature elevations every four hours, although *absence of fever does not rule out infection.* Use a private room for the client. Limit visitors and do not allow any ill persons (staff or visitors) to come into contact with the client. Avoid, however, strict isolation. Limitaton of visitors will minimize exposure to pathogens. Strict isolation, however, increases the client's subjective feelings of loneliness and may precipitate mental depression. Insist upon strict hand washing by both staff and visitors prior to contact with the client. Give mouth care every four hours and after meals, since oropharyngeal invasion by pathogens is common. Allow no cut flowers in the room, since standing water enhances the growth of *Pseudomonas* bacteria. Potted plants are permissible.

Allow no rectal manipulations of any kind in order to minimize the transmission of infectious organisms through the highly vascular rectal mucosa. Observe for signs of infection, realizing that signs of localized infection may not be present since the granulocytopenic client has less ability to localize infections. Signs of infection in the leukopenic client include:

1. Skin breakdown
2. Inflammation of intravenous site
3. Dental infection

4. Perirectal or vaginal infections
5. Sore throat
6. Localized edema or pain
7. Elevated temperature
8. Systemic signs of infection, such as malaise, fatigue, anorexia, and elevations in vital signs

Anemia

Anemia reduces the oxygenation status of the body and is reflected by an abnormally low hemoglobin level in the blood. Observe for pallor, fatigue, weakness, and shortness of breath upon exertion. Monitor the client's hemoglobin and hematocrit for falling levels. Provide a diet high in calories, protein, vitamins, and iron, and administer red blood cell transfusions as prescribed.

Thrombocytopenia

Thrombocytopenia (decreased numbers of circulating mature platelets) predisposes the client to bleeding. Hemorrhagic phenomena are associated with platelet counts of less than 50,000/mm^3, and a platelet count of less than 20,000/mm^3 is considered to be life-threatening. Therefore, the following hemorrhage precautions should be initiated if the platelet count falls below 50,000/mm^3.
Teach the client to avoid trauma of any kind. In particular, there should be NO:

1. Shaving except with an electric razor
2. Enemas, rectal manipulations, rectal temperatures
3. Douches
4. Toothpicks
5. Hard-bristled toothbrushes
6. Straining at stool
7. Intramuscular or direct intravenous injections
8. Aspirin or aspirin-containing products

Perform oral care with soft-bristled toothbrushes or oral swabs. Perform lab work by fingerstick, ear-lobe stick, or by a Hickman catheter. Prevent constipation and straining at stool by administering stool softeners as prescribed, since straining at stool increases intracranial pressure (the Valsalva maneuver) and may precipitate intracranial hemorrhage.

Apply firm manual pressure for ten minutes after subcutaneous injections, intravenous injections, or any invasive procedure (e.g., bone marrow aspiration, liver biopsy, etc.). Provide a soft diet, and lubricate the lips to prevent cracking and bleeding. Lubricate the nares with petroleum jelly if oxygen is being administered, since the drying effect of oxygen upon nasal mucous membrances may precipitate nasal bleeding. Observe for signs of bleeding, such as:

1. Epistaxis (nosebleed)
2. Hematuria (blood in urine)
3. Hematemesis (blood in emesis)

4. Hemoptysis (blood in sputum)
5. Melena or frank rectal bleeding
6. Bruises
7. Petechiae

Administer platelet transfusions as precribed.

RADIATION SICKNESS

The distressing symptoms of radiation sickness can be minimized or prevented by appropriate nursing measures. Schedule activities to allow for adequate rest periods, since malaise and fatigue are common secondary to anemia and to the increased serum levels of cell-death waste products. Encourage several small feedings per day, with a diet high in protein, carbohydrates, and vitamins, since anorexia may result from high levels of cell-death waste products. Encourage the client to drink two to four liters of fluid per day. Rapid cell death causes a significant increase in the level of serum uric acid, which must be excreted by the kidney. The client must be well hydrated to prevent crystallization of the uric acid within kidney tissue.

PATHOLOGICAL FRACTURES

Irradiation of bone may increase the client's vulnerability to pathological fractures. When moving clients at risk, support the long bones near the joints rather than in the middle of the bone. Ensure that enough staff are available to move debilitated clients safely.

RADIATION PNEUMONITIS

Radiation pneumonitis usually responds to symptomatic nursing and medical treatment. Assess breath sounds daily in clients at risk, since adventitious breath sounds are often the first sign of developing pneumonitis. If the client has a superimposed pulmonary infection, administer antibiotics as prescribed. Corticosteroids may be prescribed for clients with cough or dyspnea secondary to lung inflammation; however, it must be remembered that abrupt cessation of these drugs will result in an exacerbation of symptoms and often the development of pulmonary infiltrates in both irradiated and nonirradiated areas of the lung.

CONCEPT XIII:
Client teaching about external beam radiotherapy is a crucial part of nursing care.

An assessment of the client's knowledge about the disease process and radiation therapy is important to obtain prior to therapy. Reasons for the radiation therapy should be explained to the client and family, whether the reason be cure, adjunctive treatment, or palliation and symptom control. Duration of the therapy should be discussed, and the client and family should be reassured that the risks and side effects of radiotherapy have been minimized with modern equipment and technology. A brief tour of the treatment area is helpful.

The client should be told that the skin will be marked prior to the onset of treatment and that the markings should not be washed off. Teach the client how to care for irradiated skin areas. A diet high in protein and calories and a fluid intake of two to three quarts of fluid per day must be encouraged. Teach appropriate antiemetic measures to the client and family. The person undergoing radiation therapy should be assured that lethargy and fatigue are not uncommon during treatment and that frequent rest periods are helpful.

Instruct the client to maintain good personal hygiene and to avoid potential sources of infection. If he or she develops thrombocytopenia, trauma that may cause bleeding must be avoided. The physician should be notified promptly of any suspected infection, petechiae, or excessive bruising.

The client should be taught that the treatment procedure is, in itself, not painful. Although the client will be the only person in the treatment room while receiving external beam radiotherapy, he or she will be closely monitored by closed-circuit television and the staff will be immediately available should the need arise. Positioning of the body must be exactly maintained during the treatment. Although the treatment time may seem long, it is actually quite brief, usually lasting only a few minutes.

INTERNAL RADIOTHERAPY

CONCEPT XIV:
Internal radiotherapy utilizes ionizing radiation to destroy malignant cells.

Radioactive substances may be placed into a body cavity such as the chest, abdomen, or vaginal vault. Small sealed sources of radiation may be contained in needles, beads, seeds, or ribbons and placed directly into malignant tissue. Interstitial or intracavity radiotherpay is usually limited to treatment of gynecologic and occasional head and neck malignancies. Substances used in interstitial or intracavity radiotherapy include radium, cobalt, cesium, radon, gold, and iridium.

Internal radiotherapy carries significant but manageable hazards. While the applicator is implanted in the client, everyone near the client is exposed to potentially harmful radiation. The applicator can slip out of place inside the client and cause radiation damage to adjacent normal tissues and organs. The applicator may fall out of the client and expose hospital personnel to doses of radiation.

Intracavity radiotherapy is commonly used in the treatment of cervical carcinoma. The radioactive isotope, usually radium or cesium, is sealed within an applicator and placed within the vaginal vault. Clients usually have the applicator in place for forty-eight to seventy-two hours and must be isolated during this time.

Nursing staff must protect themselves from radiation exposure while caring for a client receiving internal radiotherapy. Distance, shielding, and time are the important factors in minimizing the nurse's radiation exposure [2, 6]. Work as far from the radiation source as possible, since intensity of radiation received by the nurse decreases with the greater distance between nurse and client. Whenever possible, utilize a lead shield between nurse and client. Making nursing care as time-efficient as possible will minimize the nurse's radiation exposure. A maximum of thirty minutes should be spent at the bedside unless a rolling lead shield is used [6]. Small doses of radiation can harm a fetus, so pregnant nurses should not be assigned to give nursing care to clients receiving internal radiotherapy treatment.

CONCEPT XV:
Inaccurate myths about internal radiotherapy still exist among health professionals.

Although the radioactive isotope is unstable, it is not explosive. Neither the client nor any of the body excretions become radioactive; and after the sealed source is removed from the body, no radiation remains. The nurse will not become radioactive by caring for a client with an internal sealed source of radiation.

CONCEPT XVI:
Skillful nursing measures will minimize or prevent distressing effects of internal radiotherapy utilizing an intravaginal applicator.

The client must be kept in a private room while receiving internal radiation. Restriction of movement by the client is necessary in order to prevent accidental dislodgment of the applicator. Once the applicator is in place, the client must be kept on strict bedrest until the applicator is removed. The head of the bed may be elevated ten to fifteen degrees, and the client can be propped with a pillow for short peridos of time. The client may not turn side-to-side or onto the abdomen. Do not give the client a complete bed bath while the applicator is in place, and do not bathe the client below the waist. Do not give the client a complete back rub, since she would have to be turned onto her abdomen. Active range of motion exercises with both arms and mild foot and leg exercises will minimize the hazards of immobility.

Monitor vital signs every four hours, observing for elevations in temperature, pulse, and respiration. Abnormal alterations in vital signs may signify pathology requiring medical intervention. Fever above 100° F. should be reported to the physician.

Monitor the client for rash, skin eruption, excessive vaginal bleeding, or vaginal discharge, as these conditons signify pathology that may require medical attention. Prevent dehydration, as the client receiving intravaginal irradiation is particularly vulnerable to the development of this condition. Record accurate intake and output, and ensure a fluid intake of at least three liters daily. Prevent constipation since the client receiving intravaginal irradiation is particularly vulnerable to development of paralytic ileus. Record number, frequency, and consistency of stool. Administer a stool softener as prescribed, and auscultate for hypoactive bowel sounds daily. Medicate the client for pain as necessary since immobility and apprehension will increase perception of physical discomfort associated with the intravaginal applicator.

Minimize unnecessary exposure of staff and visitors for the period of time that the radioactive isotope is in place [16]. Place a "Radiation in Use" sign on the door, and restrict visitors during the time that the client is receiving internal irradiation. Check the position of the applicator every four hours. If the loaded applicator or the radiation source falls out of the client, do not touch it. Instead, call the radiation therapy department and the attending physician at once. If the nurse touches the loaded applicator with bare hands, the result may be unnecessary radiation exposure or a radiation burn to the nurse.

CONCEPT XVII:
Skillful nursing measures after removal of the intravaginal applicator will increase the client's comfort.

Administer a Betadine douche and an enema as prescribed after removal of the applicator, and encourange the client to ambulate. Visitation restrictions and precautionary measures are no longer necessary. Advise the client to resume normal activities gradually, including sexual intercourse. Resumption of sexual intercourse is usually delayed for seven to ten days after the applicator has been removed [6]. Advise the client to notify the physician of the development of nausea, vomiting, diarrhea, frequent or painful urination, pain, or a temperature above 100° F.

CONCEPT XVIII:
Client teaching is a crucial part of nursing care to the client receiving internal radiation.

Clarify any misunderstandings or misinformation regarding the purpose and procedure of internal radiotherapy. Explain routines that will be carried out prior to insertion, during the time of irradiation, and after removal of the radiation source. Ensure that family and staff understand the necessary precautions that must be taken during the time of treatment.

REFERENCES

1. Abramson, N. Radiation Therapy—What Is It? In L. C. Kruse, J. L. Reese, and L. K. Hart (Eds.). *Cancer: Pathophysiology, Etiology, and Management.* St. Louis: C. V. Mosby, 1979. Pp. 153–156.
2. Baldonado, A. A. and Stahl, D. A. *Cancer Nursing: A Holistic Multidisciplinary Approach.* Garden City, NY: Medical Examination Publishing Co., 1978. Chapter 11.

3. Battles, C. Nursing Management of the Radiation Therapy Client. In L. Marino (Ed.). *Cancer Nursing.* St. Louis: C. V. Mosby, 1981.

4. Bloomer, W. D. and Hellman, S. Normal Tissue Responses to Radiation Therapy. In L. C. Kruse, J. L. Reese, and L. K. Hart (Eds.). *Cancer: Pathophysiology, Etiology, and Management.* St. Louis: C. V. Mosby, 1979. Pp. 170–175.

5. Bouchard, R. and Owens, N. Nursing Care of the Patient Receiving Radiation Therapy. In *Nursing Care of the Cancer Patient* (3rd Ed.). St. Louis: C. V. Mosby, 1976.

6. Breeding, M. A. and Wollin, M. Working Safely Around Implanted Radiation Sources. *Nurs 76* 6(5):58, 1976.

7. Clinical Practice Committee of the Oncology Nursing Society. Guidelines for Nursing Care of Patients with Altered Protective Mechanisms. *Oncol Nurs Forum* 9(2):115, 1982.

8. Glatstein, E. and Carter, S. The Chronic Toxicity of Cancer Treatment. In S. Carter, E. Glatstein, and R. Livingston (Eds.). *Principles of Cancer Treatment.* New York: McGraw-Hill, 1982.

9. Goodwin, P., Quimby, E., and Morgan, R. *Physical Foundation of Radiology* (4th Ed.). New York: Harper and Row, 1970.

10. Hassey, K. and Rose, C. Altered Skin Integrity in Patients Receiving Radiation Therapy. *Oncol Nurs Forum* 9:44, 1982.

11. Hilderley, L. Clinical Reviews: Skin Care in Radiation Therapy. A Review of the Literature. *Oncol Nurs Forum* 10:51, 1983.

12. Kaplan, H. S. Basic Principles in Radiation Oncology. *Cancer* 39:689, 1977.

13. Kelly, P. and Tinsley, C. Planning Care for the Patient Receiving External Radiation. *AJN* 81:338, 1981.

14. Leahy, D., St. Germain, J., and Varrichio, C. *The Nurse and Radiotherapy.* St. Louis: C. V. Mosby, 1979.

15. Meyskens, F. L. Human Melanoma Colony Formation in Vitro. *Prog Clin Biol Res* 48:85, 1980.

16. Ogi, S. Radiotherapy, Cancer, and the Nurse. In P. Burkhalter and D. Donley. *Dynamics of Oncology Nursing.* New York: McGraw-Hill, 1978. Pp. 136–158.

17. Peschel, R. and Fischer, J. Optimization of the Time-Dose Relationship. *Semin Oncol* 8:38, 1981.

18. Phillips, T. Principles of Radiobiology and Radiation Therapy. In S. Carter, E. Glatstein, and R. Livingston (Eds.). *Principles of Cancer Treatment.* New York: McGraw-Hill, 1982.

19. Rafla, S. and Rotman, M. *Introduction to Radiotherapy.* St. Louis: C. V. Mosby, 1974.

20. Rotman, M. Supportive and Palliative Radiation Therapy. In L. C. Kruse, J. L. Reese, and L. K. Hart (Eds.). *Cancer: Pathophysiology, Etiology, and Management.* St. Louis: C. V. Mosby, 1979. Pp. 182–187.

21. Rubin, P. and Poulter, C. Principles of Radiation Oncology and Cancer Radiotherapy. In P. Rubin (Ed.). *Clinical Oncology for Medical Students and Physicians: A Multidisciplinary Approach* (5th Ed.). Rochester, NY: American Cancer Society, 1978. Pp. 29–41.

22. Sarna, L. P. Concepts of Nursing Care for Patients Receiving Radiation Therapy. In D. L. Vredevoe, A. Derdiarian, L. P. Sarna, M. Friel, and J. A. G. Shiplacoff. *Concepts of Oncology Nursing.* Englewood Cliffs, NJ: Prentice-Hall, 1981. Pp. 154–205.

23. Schwade, J. and Lichter, A. Management of Acute Effects of Radiation Therapy. In S. Carter, E. Glatstein, and R. Livingston (Eds.). *Principles of Cancer Treatment.* New York: McGraw-Hill, 1982.

24. Smith, D. and Chamorro, T. Nursing Care of Patients Undergoing Combination Chemotherapy and Radiotherapy. *Cancer Nurs* 1:129, 1978.

25. Tealey, A. Radiotherapy and Hodgkin's Disease. In B. Peterson and C. Kellog (Eds.). *Current Practice in Oncologic Nursing, Vol. 1.* St. Louis: C. V. Mosby, 1976.

26. Varricchio, C. The Patient on Radiation Therapy. *AJN* 81:334, 1981.

27. Welch, D. Assessment of Nausea and Vomiting in Cancer Patients Undergoing External Beam Radiotherapy. *Cancer Nurs* 3:365, 1980.

28. Welsh, M. S. Comfort Measures During Radiation Therapy. *AJN* 67:1880, 1967.

29. Wilson, C. and Strohl, R. Radiation Therapy as Primary Treatment for Breast Cancer. *Oncol Nurs Forum* 9:12, 1982.

30. Yasko, J. Radiotherapy: A Patient/Significant Other Teaching Plan. In M. Donovan (Ed.). *Cancer Care: A Guide for Patient Education.* New York: Appleton-Century-Crofts, 1981.

31. Yasko, J. *Care of the Client Receiving External Radiation Therapy.* Reston, VA: Reston Publishing Co., 1982.

Chapter 7

Nursing Care of the Client Receiving Chemotherapy

CONCEPT I:
Chemotherapy is one of the four major medical treatment modalities used to attempt to reduce the body burden of tumor.

The goal of antineoplastic chemotherapy is to destroy all malignant tumor cells without causing excessive destruction of the client's healthy cells or disruption of normal cellular processes. Although there has been an intensive effort to identify and test more effective antineoplastic drugs, no chemotherapeutic agent is yet capable of meeting these goals. At the National Cancer Institute, thousands of chemical agents are tested annually. There are now over thirty drugs with significant anticancer activity available.

There are specific phases through which investigational drugs must pass. *Phase I* is the first administration of a new drug to human beings. Prior to Phase I administration, the drug has been extensively tested on animals. The goals of Phase I are (1) the establishment of a maximum tolerated dose on a given schedule, (2) establishment of toxicity patterns and determination of whether toxicities are predictable, tolerable, and reversible, and (3) specific evidence of antitumor activity. *Phase II* involves a determination of whether a new drug has antitumor activity worthy of further clinical evaluation. During *Phase III,* the drug is examined to determine if there are any unexpected activities or side effects. Phase III clinical trials also investigate new combinations of drugs. *Phase IV* involves the administration of an F.D.A.-approved drug to determine new uses.

CONCEPT II:
Understanding the basic concepts of chemotherapy is necessary for skillful oncology nursing.

Cancer chemotherapy alters a phase of the cell life cycle. The antineoplastic effects of chemotherapy are primarily due to the fact that more cancer cells than normal cells are participating in the reproductive cycle at any one time. Thus, more cancer cells are vulnerable to the lethal effects of anticancer drugs. In general, chemotherapeutic agents are most effective on cells in the proliferation phases of the cell life cycle.

Anticancer drugs work by the principle of *first-order kinetics.* A given dose of a given drug kills a constant *percentage* of the remaining body burden of tumor cells, rather than killing a certain absolute number of cells [2].

Chemotherapy destroys normal as well as malignant cells, and the toxic effects of anticancer drugs are a result of the destruction of normal cells. Those normal tissues that are most likely to exhibit adverse effects from the chemotherapy are those that normally reproduce rapidly: cells of the bone marrow, hair follicles, gastrointestinal mucosa, etc. Tolerance of chemotherapy is better with low tumor cell burden, less organ impairment, adequate nutrition, and greater resistance to infection.

CONCEPT III:
Combination chemotherapy consists of two or more drugs administered simultaneously or in a particular sequence to treat a specific cancer.

Combination chemotherapy has greater antitumor effectiveness than the use of single agents. When combination chemotherapy is used, there may be additive cell destruction without additive host toxicities. In combination chemotherapy, the drugs often complement one another by having different modes of action and different toxicities. Concurrent administration of drugs may be more toxic than sequential intermittent therapy [4].

Intermittent chemotherapy has more therapeutic benefit with lower cumulative toxicity. There is better client tolerance because intermittent therapy allows time for the repair of normal tissues in drug-free intervals between doses. Greater tumor cell kill usually results from high-dose intermittent chemotherapy than from continuous low-dose chemotherapy [2].

CONCEPT IV:
Antineoplastic drugs are classified as being either cell-cycle dependent agents or cell-cycle independent agents.

Cell-cycle dependent agents will kill cells only while they are in a specific phase of the cell life cycle. Cell-cycle independent drugs will kill cells whether they are dividing or in the resting (G_0) phase of the cell cycle.

CONCEPT V:
The administration of cancer chemotherapy requires special nursing skills.

Chemotherapy can be administered by several routes: oral, intramuscular, intravenous, intra-arterial, intrathoracic, and intrathecal (into the cerebrospinal fluid). Intravenous administration of chemotherapy is the most common; and although many clients have a Hickman subclavian catheter for the administration of chemotherapy, many other clients must depend upon the nurse's skill in peripheral intravenous drug therapy.

When giving intravenous chemotherapy by peripheral veins, use scalp vein needles (#23 or #25) if possible since they cause the least amount of damage to veins. Avoid administration of chemotherapy in the lower extremities because of the risk of phlebitis and thrombus formation. Always check the patency of the intravenous site with normal saline or sterile water in a syringe or intravenous tubing before *any* chemotherapy is given.

If no information is available, assume that the drug being given is a vesicant, causing severe local tissue necrosis if extravasated. Vesicant drugs should not be administered through an indwelling intravenous line that has been in place for six hours or more. The chances of extravasation at the insertion site increase with time. Vesicant drugs should be given in a superficial vein of the hand or forearm, with frequent checks for blood return. It is more difficult to recognize early signs of infiltration if deep veins or antecubital veins are used. If the nurse suspects extravasation of a vesicant drug, stop the drug at once and follow the institution's routine procedure for emergency treatment.

Nonvesicant drugs may be administered in any arm vein. Do not mix drugs together when giving combination chemotherapy. Many of the parenteral antineoplastic agents are highly unstable and thus untoward chemical reactions may occur if the drugs are mixed. Use at least three milliliters of sterile normal saline to flush between drugs and after the final drug.

Never administer Phase I agents or any drug with the potential of causing anaphylaxis by intravenous push. These drugs must be diluted and infused over thirty to sixty minutes or as prescribed.

CONCEPT VI:
Extravasation of vesicant drugs requires immediate treatment, although the procedure may vary in different institutions (see Figures 7.1, 7.2, and 7.3).

The extravasation of vesicant drugs may result in inflammation, ulceration, necrosis, loss of function, and possible amputation. The most severe reactions occur when immediate action is not taken.

Appropriate methods of administration will minimize the risk of extravasation. Dilute the vesicant drug in the appropriate amount of diluent to avoid high concentrations. Select an infusion site in the following order of desirability: Hickman subclavian catheter, forearm, dorsum of hand, wrist, antecubital fossa. Insert a butterfly needle into the peripheral vein with one venipuncture only. Use transparent tape distal to the needle to secure the butterfly tubing. Do not obscure the peripheral injection site by covering it with opaque tape. Administer five milliliters of normal saline and obtain a blood flashback to verify patency of the peripheral intravenous line. Observe for extravasation of normal saline. If extravasation of normal saline is obvious, select another site, preferably on the other arm. Administer the drug precisely at the prescribed rate. Ask the client repeatedly if there is any pain or burning. Follow the drug injection with at least five milliliters of normal saline to flush the tubing and needle. If multiple drugs are to be given, inject the nonvesicant agents first since nonvesicant drugs are least damaging to the vessels. If all drugs are vesicants, inject the one with the least amount of fluid volume first. Separate each administered drug with five milliliters of normal saline.

Prompt recognition of extravasation is necessary to minimize adverse effects. Pain, burning, and stinging at the injection site is often the first sign of extravasation. Swelling at the injection site indicates possible leakage of the fluid into sur-

Figure 7.1. Vesicant Drugs Commonly Associated with Severe Local Necrosis [16]

Actinomycin-D
Daunorubicin (Daunomycin)
Doxorubicin (Adriamycin)
Mechlorethamine (Nitrogen Mustard)
Mithramycin (Mithracin)
Mitomycin-C (Mutamycin)
Streptozotocin
Vinblastine (Velban)
Vincristine (Oncovin)
Vindesine

Figure 7.2. Drugs That are Irritants, Causing Burning or Inflammation Without Necrosis Upon Extravasation [16]

BCNU (Carmustine)
DTIC
Thio-TEPA

Figure 7.3. Drugs That are Nonvesicants and Devoid of Significant Vesicant or Irritant Effects [16]

L-asparaginase
Bleomycin (Blenoxane)
Cyclophosphamide (Cytoxan)
Cytosine Arabinoside (Cytarabine, Ara-C, Cytosar)
5-fluorouracil (5-FU)
6-mercaptopurine (6-MP)
Methotrexate
Cis-Platinum (Platinol)

rounding tissues, as does the inability to obtain a blood return through the intravenous tubing. If the nurse suspects extravasation, even in the absence of clinical signs, it is better to stop the drug infusion and consult the physician than to continue with the treatment. Protocols for the treatment of extravasation of anthracyclines and other vesicant drugs vary according to institution and physician. However, if standing prescriptions are not available, the physician should be contacted immediately.

One extravasation protocol [29] follows. Stop the infusion immediately, but do not remove the intravenous catheter or needle. Disconnect the syringe from the infusion needle. Attach a syringe containing 5 mEq of sodium bicarbonate and inject by the indwelling intravenous needle. Remove the infusion needle at this time. Inject hydrocortisone sodium succinate (Solu-Cortef) 100 mg. subcutaneously into the area of the infiltration. Apply hydrocortisone cream 1 percent and sterile dressings. Elevate the affected extremity and apply ice packs to the area for twenty-four hours.

There is disagreement in the literature as to whether ice packs or hot compresses should be applied to the site of extravasation [17]. Heat will produce vasodilation, facilitate fluid absorption, and decrease local drug concentration. Cold will produce vasoconstriction and decrease fluid absorption that may concentrate the extravasated drug at the site and potentiate local toxicity. If inflammation and induration of tissue continue despite local measures, surgical debridement and plastic surgery may be necessary.

CONCEPT VII:
Most antineoplastic chemotherapeutic drugs have common toxicities. Since they have the greatest effect on rapidly dividing cells, normal tissues with a high rate of proliferation usually exhibit significant adverse effects related to chemotherapy.

Myelosuppression can be a life-threatening toxicity of chemotherapy. When bone marrow function is suppressed, the amount and functional capabilities of platelets, white blood cells, and red blood cells may be seriously compromised. Bleeding secondary to thrombocytopenia, infection or sepsis secondary to leukopenia, and reduced tissue oxygenation secondary to anemia may be life-threatening. The "nadir" of the drug refers to the time when myelosuppressive effects are at their peak. The client is at greatest risk during and immediately after the nadir.

Gastrointestinal toxicities occur as a result of the drug's effect on the gastrointestinal mucosa. Nausea, vomiting, and diarrhea are common gastrointestinal toxicities. Stomatitis and mucositis may appear, ranging in severity from mild mouth inflammation to severe ulceration of the entire gastrointestinal tract.

Renal toxicity occurs as a result of the drug's damaging effects on kidney tissue. Renal toxicity is usually manifested by an increase in serum blood urea nitrogen (BUN) and creatinine and by a decrease in urinary creatinine clearance [33]. The client may ultimately experience renal failure.

Hyperuricemia may contribute to renal dysfunction and failure. This condition results when large numbers of tumor cells are killed, as with chemotherapy. Uric acid levels in the blood climb because of the high cell death. This high concentration of uric acid can crystallize in the renal tubules and cause permanent renal damage.

Hepatotoxicity may first exhibit itself by changes in liver enzymes. Steadily rising serum levels of the transaminases (SGOT, SGPT) and of CPK are often the first indication of impending liver damage.

Neurotoxicity is linked with the vinca alkaloid drugs. The first symptoms of peripheral neurotoxicity are decreased deep tendon reflexes progressing to complete loss of these reflexes with foot and wrist drop. Paresthesias may occur, and the client may eventually experience ataxia. This neurotoxicity may be reversible if the drug is discontinued at the first sign of diminished deep tendon reflexes or at the client's first report of numbness and tingling of the extremities [8].

Alopecia occurs as a result of the drug's effect on the rapidly proliferating hair follicles. Usually, hair will begin to regrow after chemotherapy has been discontinued. When the hair grows back, however, the texture and color may be different. Occasionally, the hair loss is permanent.

CONCEPT VIII:
Skillful nursing measures can minimize or prevent the distressing
adverse side effects of chemotherapy.

LEUKOPENIA

Septic phenomena are associated with a white blood cell count less than $2,000/mm^3$. A white blood cell count less than $1,000/mm^3$ is life-threatening. Therefore, the following infection precautions should be instituted when the white blood cell count is less than $2,500/mm^3$.

Infection precautions

Monitor for elevations in temperature every four hours, although *absence of fever does not rule out infection.* Observe for signs of infection, but realize that signs of localized infection may not be present since the granulocytopenic client does not have the capacity to produce pus and thus has little ability to localize infections. Watch for:

1. Skin breakdown
2. Infection or inflammation of intravenous sites
3. Dental infection
4. Sore throat
5. Perirectal or vaginal infection
6. Localized edema or pain
7. Elevated temperature
8. Systemic signs of infection, such as malaise, fatigue, and anorexia

Use a private room for the client and limit visitors, but avoid strict isolation. Do not allow any ill person to enter the client's room (staff or visitors). Limitation of visitors will minimize exposure to pathogens, but strict isolation increases the client's subjective feelings of isolation and may precipitate mental depression. Insist upon strict handwashing by *everyone* (staff and visitors) before contact with the client. Give mouth care every four hours and after meals, since oropharyngeal invasion by pathogens is common. Allow no cut flowers in the room, since standing water encourages the growth of *Pseudomonas* bacteria. Potted plants, however, are permissible. Allow no rectal manipulations of any kind in order to avoid transmission of infectious organisms through the highly vascular rectal mucosa. Administer lithium carbonate as prescribed to increase circulating granulocyte levels [31].

Leukocyte Transfusions

Administer leukocyte transfusions as prescribed. Ensure that the transfusion is ABO and Rh typed and cross-matched since there is some admixture of red blood cells in the solution of white cells, making an anaphylactic or hemolytic reaction possible. Obtain baseline data regarding vital signs, blood pressure, level of consciousness, and behavioral status before beginning the transfusion. Notify the physician if the client is febrile, although the transfusion is usually not postponed unless the fever exceeds 102° F.

Use a Y-type blood administration set with a standard blood filter. If an adverse reaction occurs, the Y-type set allows for rapid discontinuation of the leukocyte transfusion and the maintenance of a patent vein. Use normal saline as the second solution because normal saline will minimize cell lysis [23]. Fill the drip chamber above the filter to minimize cell damage resulting from the impact of the leukocytes against the filter mesh.

Administer the leukocyte transfusion over a two to four hour period. Stay with the client for the first fifteen minutes of the infusion, observing for signs of transfusion reaction (wheezing, urticaria, hypotension, shock). If these signs appear, discontinue the transfusion, maintain the patency of the vein with normal saline solution, and notify the physician.

Monitor vital signs twice during the first thirty minutes and then every thirty minutes for the rest of the transfusion. If the client has a febrile response, the temperature may rise to 105° F., resulting in shaking chills. In the client who is also thrombocytopenic, shaking chills are extremely dangerous, possibly resulting in central nervous system hemorrhage secondary to a rise in intracranial pressure. Parenteral meperidine (Demerol) will rapidly eliminate shaking chills. Treat the febrile client symptomatically with acetaminophen (Tylenol), a cool environment, and a slower rate of leukocyte infusion. The transfusion is usually not discontinued because of fever.

ANEMIA

Observe for pallor, fatigue, weakness, and shortness of breath upon exertion. Monitor hemoglobin and hematocrit for falling levels. Provide a diet high in calories, protein, vitamins, and iron. Administer transfusions of red blood cells as prescribed.

THROMBOCYTOPENIA

Hemorrhagic phenomena are associated with platelet counts less than 50,000/mm^3. Platelet counts less than 20,000/mm^3 are life-threatening. Therefore, the following hemorrhage precautions should be instituted when the platelet count falls below 60,000/mm^3.

Hemorrhage Precautions

Teach the client to avoid trauma of any kind. All of the following must be avoided:

1. Shaving (except with an electric razor)
2. Enemas, rectal temperatures, rectal manipulations
3. Constipation, straining at stool

4. Douches
5. Toothpicks
6. Hard-bristled toothbrushes
7. Intramuscular injections
8. Aspirin or aspirin-containing products

Oral care should be performed with soft-bristled toothbrushes or oral swabs. Perform lab work by finger-stick or through a Hickman catheter. Administer stool softeners as prescribed. It is very important to avoid constipation and straining at stool because the Valsalva maneuver raises intracranial pressure and may precipitate intracranial hemorrhage.

Apply firm manual pressure for ten minutes after subcutaneous injections, intravenous injections, or any invasive procedures. Provide a soft diet and lubricate lips to prevent cracking or bleeding. Lubricate the nares if oxygen is being used to prevent cracking and bleeding of the nasal mucosa. Observe for signs of bleeding, such as epistaxis, hematemesis, hematuria, hemoptysis, melena, frank rectal bleeding, bruises, or petechiae. Administer platelet transfusions as prescribed.

NAUSEA AND VOMITING

Nausea and vomiting are distressing adverse effects of chemotherapy that may be prevented or at least minimized by appropriate measures. Avoid noxious external stimuli, such as unemptied bedpans or urinals, suction containers within the client's view, etc. Remove lid covers from plates of hot food prior to entering the client room in order to allow the odor-laden steam to dissipate. Provide six to eight small feedings per day of foods desired by the client, avoiding gas-forming foods. Provide ice chips and carbonated beverages as desired by the client. Administer the prescribed antiemetic before the administration of chemotherapy, before meals, or as needed. Perform oral care frequently and at least after every meal or after each episode of vomiting.

Teach the client to take deep breaths during acute nausea. Observe for signs of potassium deficit. Monitor intake and output records, observing for dehydration. Prevent aspiration of emesis by elevating the head of the bed or performing oropharyngeal suctioning as needed.

STOMATITIS AND MUCOSITIS

Stomatitis and mucositis are distressing adverse effects of chemotherapy and may contribute to potentially life-threatening malnutrition and cachexia. Assess the client's mouth every eight hours for erythema or lesions. Monitor for complaints of oral burning, dry mouth, or sensitivity to hot, cold, or spicy foods. Check dentures to ensure a good fit; ill-fitting dentures may trap food particles or irritate the oral mucosa by rubbing or pressure.

Use soft toothbrushes or oral swabs for mouth care, which must be given frequently and at least after every meal and before sleep. Allow no toothpicks, and eliminate hot, cold, or spicy foods if not tolerated. Avoid commercial mouthwashes because of the irritating effects of the alcohol content. If a mouthwash is desired, use room temperature normal saline solution. Medicate with Viscous Xylocaine ten minutes before meals to provide enough local anesthesia to facilitate eating. The client should "swish and swallow" the Viscous Xylocaine.

Assess the mouth daily for the yellow-white patches indicative of a fungal infection. Keeping the mouth clean will often prevent the onset of infection. Antifungal antibiotics are prescribed to prevent or treat a fungal infection.

DIARRHEA

Assess for the number, frequency, and consistency of stools. Assess for blood and/or mucous in fecal material, and monitor for reports of cramping or abdominal pain. Assess daily for skin irritation or breakdown in the perirectal area. Monitor for hyperactive bowel sounds daily.

Provide a low-residue, bland diet, and ensure that fluid intake is at least two to four liters per day in order to prevent dehydration. The client with diarrhea must be on accurate intake and output records. Provide gentle cleaning and skin care to the perineum after every stool in order to minimize excoriation. Administer anti-diarrheal medication as prescribed.

RENAL TOXICITY

Renal toxicity may be a life-threatening effect of chemotherapy. Record accurate intake and output, monitoring for oliguria. Assess daily for dependent edema. Weigh the client daily, looking for an unexplained weight increase. Monitor breath sounds daily for rales and pulmonary congestion. Watch for increasing blood pressure. Assess for increasing levels of blood urea nitrogen (BUN) and serum creatinine. Monitor for decreasing levels of urinary creatinine clearance. Administer diuretics as prescribed.

HYPERURICEMIA

Hyperuricemia, if not prevented, may precipitate potentially fatal renal failure. Those persons with leukemia and lymphoma carry the highest risk for the development of this dangerous condition; these clients must therefore receive preventive nursing and medical care. Ensure adequate hydration by increasing fluids to at least three liters daily. Monitor serum uric acid for rising levels, and maintain accurate intake and output records in order to assess fluid status. Administer allopurinol (Zyloprim) as prescribed [2] to reduce purine metabolism and subsequent uric acid formation.

HEPATOTOXICITY

Monitor for elevations in liver enzymes (SGOT, SGPT, CPK, and alkaline phosphatase). Monitor for the development of jaundice in the skin and/or sclerae. Monitor for a decreasing level of consciousness in the client who has liver damage. If any of these signs appear, the physician should be notified.

NEUROTOXICITY

Tell the client to report the development of numbness or tingling of the fingers or toes. Assess for normal bowel and urinary elimination patterns. Monitor for a decrease in or loss of deep tendon reflexes. Watch for loss of fine motor control, arthritic symptoms in joints, somnolence, or lethargy. Monitor for hoarseness or complaints of jaw pain. Notify the physician of any signs of neurological toxicity.

ALOPECIA

Controversy exists regarding the effectiveness of antialopecia techniques, such as scalp tourniquets or ice turbans [34], and no antialopecia technique has proven to be consistently effective and safe. Teach the client that hair begins to regrow usually within two to six months but that hair color and texture may be different. Keep the room and bed clean and free of hair. Give emotional support, and suggest the use of wigs or scarves.

CONCEPT IX:
Antineoplastic drugs are divided into classifications according to mode of action (see Table 7.2).

Antimetabolites inhibit cell reproduction by interfering with the manufacture of protein. Alkylating agents interfere with DNA replication. Antineoplastic antibiotics are drugs that interfere with or inhibit DNA and/or RNA synthesis. The vinca alkaloids stop cell division at metaphase. Other drugs used in cancer chemotherapy have varying or unknown modes of action.

CONCEPT X:
The antimetabolites are a class of antineoplastic drugs that inhibit cell reproduction by interfering with the manufacture of protein.

The antimetabolites are cell-cycle specific (S-phase) agents. These drugs are dependent upon adequate hepatic function for degradation or inactivation of the drug. There are three subclassifications within the antimetabolite group of drugs: folate antagonists, pyrimidine analogs, and purine analogs.

Table 7.1. Chemotherapy Toxicity Criteria

Item	No Toxicity	1 + Toxicity	2 + Toxicity	3 + Toxicity	4 + Toxicity
HEMATOPOIETIC					
Hemoglobin gm%	≥10.0	9.0–9.9	7.0–8.9	5.0–6.9	< 5.0
WBC/mm^3	≥4,000	3,000–3,999	2,000–2,999	1,000–1,999	< 1,000
Platelets/mm^3	≥100,000	75,000–99,000	50,000–74,999	25,000–49,999	< 25,000
GENITOURINARY					
BUN mg%	≤20	21–40	41–60		≥100
Creatinine mg%	≤1.2	1.2–2.0	2.1–4.0		> 4
Creatinine clearance	normal	≥75 %	50–74%		<50%
HEPATIC					
SGOT	<40	41–60	61–200		>200
SGPT	<30	30–50	51–100		> 100
Bilirubin	<1	1–2	2.1–5.0		>5
				Clinical evidence of liver failure	
GASTROINTESTINAL					
Stomatitis	Normal	Erythema	Ulcers, but able to eat	Unable to eat because of ulcers	
Diarrhea	<3 stools daily	3–4 liquid stools daily, no dehydration	>4 liquid stools daily, needs IV hydration	Bloody diarrhea, needs IV hydration and/or blood	
Nausea/Vomiting	Normal	Nausea, no vomiting	Vomiting can be prevented by Rx <6 times daily	Vomiting >6 times daily despite antiemetics	
NEUROMUSCULAR	Normal	↓ DTRs and/or parasthesias	Absent DTRs, weakness, and peripheral nerve pain	Incapaciated, weakness to bedridden state, paresis	

Source: Reprinted from Southwest Oncology Group Chemotherapy Toxicity Criteria. Copyright (c) 1981. Southwest Oncology Group. Used with permission.

Table 7.2. Classifications of Antineoplastic Drugs

Classification	Drug
ANTIMETABOLITES	Methotrexate
	5-fluorouracil (5-FU)
	Cytosine arabinoside (Cytarabine, Ara-C, Cytosar)
	6-mercaptopurine (6-MP, Purinethol)
	6-thioguanine (6-TG, Thioguanine)
ALKYLATING AGENTS	Cyclophosphamide (Cytoxan)
	Thio-TEPA
	Mechlorethamine (Nitrogen Mustard)
	Chlorambucil (Leukeran)
	Carmustine (BCNU)
	Lomustine (CCNU)
	Semustine (Methyl-CCNU)
	Busulfan (Myeleran)
	Phenylalanine mustard (Alkeran)
	Cis-Platinum (Platinol)
	Dacarbazine (DTIC)
ANTINEOPLASTIC ANTIBIOTICS	Dactinomycin (Actinomycin-D)
	Mithramycin (Mithracin)
	Doxorubicin (Adriamycin)
	Daunorubicin (Daunomycin)
	Bleomycin (Blenoxane)
	Mitomycin-C (Mutamycin)
	Streptozotocin
VINCA ALKALOIDS	Vincristine (Oncovin)
	Vinblastine (Velban)
	Vindesine
HORMONES	
Corticosteroids	Prednisone
Androgens	Calusterone (Methosarb)
	Fluoxymesterone (Halotestin)
	Testolactone (Teslac)
	Testosterone proprionate (Oreton)
Estrogens	Chlorotianisene (TACE)
	Diethylstilbestrol (DES)
	Estradiol
	Ethinyl estradiol (Estinyl)
Antiestrogens	Tamoxifen citrate (Nolvadex)
Progestins	Hydroxyprogesterone caproate (Delautin)
	Medroxyprogesterone (Provera, Depo-Provera)
	Megestrol acetate (Megace)
ENZYMES	L-asparaginase (Elspar)
MISCELLANEOUS AGENTS	Hydroxyurea (Hydrea)
	Procarbazine (Matulane)
	Hexamethylmelamine (HMM)
	L-alanosine
	MGBG (Methyl-GAG)
	Dihydroxyanthracenedione (DHAD)

FOLATE ANTAGONISTS

Methotrexate

Methotrexate, a folate antagonist, blocks the reduction of folic acid to tetrahydrofolic acid by inhibiting an enzyme called folic acid reductase. This blockage impairs purine biosynthesis and inhibits the synthesis of DNA and thus cell reproduction [2]. Methotrexate is indicated for acute lymphoblastic leukemia; choriocarcinoma; breast, testicular, and head and neck carcinomas; sarcomas; and severe psoriasis, a nonmalignant skin condition [2, 5]. Administration is oral, intramuscular, intravenous, intrathecal, or into malignant effusions.

Methotrexate is excreted rapidly through the kidney and must be used cautiously in the presence of renal dysfunction. Since the drug is relatively insoluble in acidic urine, alkalinization of the urine is important to prevent renal damage. Drugs that interfere with tubular secretion may delay urinary clearance of methotrexate, thus decreasing excretion and increasing toxicities (probenicid, penicillin, sulfa drugs, phenylbutazone, salicylates).

Toxicities of methotrexate include myelosuppression (nadir day 7), gastrointestinal mucositis, nausea, and vomiting. Renal toxicity is a function of both serum concentration of the drug and duration of exposure. Hepatic dysfunction with transient elevation of enzymes and/or chronic cirrhosis may occur. Dermatitis (which may enhance any radiotherapy-induced skin toxicity) and alopecia are common. If the methotrexate is given intrathecally, neurotoxicities might be seen, with stiff neck, headache, fever, parasthesias, or encephalitis.

Specific nursing measures for methotrexate include interventions designed to minimize dermatitis. Keep the skin clean and dry. Assess daily for rashes, redness, or signs of skin breakdown. Avoid or minimize exposure to the sun, as sunlight potentiates the skin reaction.

High-Dose Methotrexate with Leucovorin Rescue

Methotrexate normally requires an active transport process to enter the cell, but it is thought that malignant cells may not have sufficient numbers of active transport sites on the cell membranes. With high doses of methotrexate, serum levels of the drug are high enough to force the drug into the cells through a passive transport mechanism [1]. Thus, methotrexate is forced into both normal and cancerous cells and can then exert its lethal effects. This alone, however, would ensure the death of normal cells as well as malignant cells. Leucovorin (citrovorum factor, folinic acid) is administered in varying doses to "rescue" normal cells from the lethal effect of high-dose methotrexate. It is thought that leucovorin selectively rescues only normal cells since the rescue drug utilizes the same active transport mechanism to enter the cell as does methotrexate [3]. Normal cells are able to transport the leucovorin across the cell membrane and thus neutralize the methotrexate. Malignant cells, because of insufficient numbers of active transport sites on the cell membrane, cannot take in the rescue drug, and thus the cancerous cells are killed by the methotrexate.

The toxicities associated with high-dose methotrexate with leucovorin rescue are serious and life-threatening. Adverse effects include myelosuppression, renal toxicity, pneumothorax, and hepatic dysfunction. Other distressing side effects are nausea and vomiting, diarrhea, stomatitis, alopecia, a maculopapular rash, and drug fever. There is a 6 percent mortality rate directly attributable to drug toxicity. Immediate causes of death include renal failure and myelosuppression with sepsis or hemorrhage [32].

It must be emphasized that the leucovorin rescue is a crucial part of this chemotherapeutic protocol. A delay in the administration of leucovorin for more than forty-two to forty-eight hours *or* missed doses of leucovorin may result in severe and/or irreversible methotrexate toxicity [1].

Renal toxicity may be prevented or at least minimized by careful nursing and medical measures. An intravenous pyelogram [IVP] must be obtained prior to the first course of treatment to rule out obstructed ureters and to establish the existence of two functioning kidneys. Before each course of therapy, ensure that serum creatinine is normal. Intravenous fluids should be given at a rate of two to three liters/m^2/day during high-dose methotrexate therapy and leucovorin rescue. This will ensure adequate hydration and help to maintain an alkaline urine. Alkalinization therapy should be given to maintain urine pH above 6.5 throughout the treatment [1]. Test urine pH at each voiding. Oral or intravenous sodium bicarbonate is used to alkalinize the urine. Monitor daily serum creatinine for rising levels. If serum creatinine levels increase more than 50 percent above the pre-methotrexate level, the risk of renal toxicity is greatly increased. Maintain accurate intake and output records, monitoring for oliguria. Leucovorin rescue therapy and alkalinization of the urine may be discontinued when serum methotrexate levels are below 5×10^{-8} [1].

Pneumothorax is most likely to occur within the first forty-eight hours after high-dose methotrexate is given. Monitor for diminished or absent breath sounds every eight hours for three days after administration of chemotherapy. Mark the Point of Maximal Intensity (PMI) on the client's chest and monitor for a shift in the PMI every eight hours for three days. Instruct the client to report any development of dyspnea or chest pain.

Table 7.3. High-Dose Methotrexate With Leucovorin Rescue: Frequency of Renal Toxicity With and Without Urine Alkalinization [24]

Number Evaluated	Increase in Serum Creatinine		
	25–50%	50%	Total
PER COURSE			
Nonalkalinized clients (73 courses)	18%	29%	47%
Alkalinized clients	11%	4%	15%
PER CLIENT			
Nonalkalinized clients (33 in number)	13%	60%	73%
Alkalinized clients (18 in number)	11%	28%	39%

Monitor for drug fever every four to eight hours. Administer acetaminophen (Tylenol) as necessary, usually when fever exceeds 101° F.

Maculopapular rash can occur with high-dose methotrexate therapy. Observe and record the color and distribution of the rash. Observe any surgical scars for inflammation or wound breakdown. Avoid or minimize exposure to the sun, as sunlight potentiates the skin reaction.

PYRIMIDINE ANALOGS

Cytosine Arabinoside

Cytosine arabinoside (Cytosar, Cytarabine, Ara-C) is an antimetabolite drug used in antineoplastic chemotherapy. Its mode of action is the inhibition of DNA synthesis. Cytosine arabinoside is indicated for acute myeloblastic or myelomonocytic leukemia; carcinomatous meningitis and leukemic infiltrations of the brain and meninges; and occasionally non-Hodgkin's lymphoma. Administration may be intravenous, subcutaneous, or intrathecal [2].

Toxicities associated with cytosine arabinoside include myelosuppression (nadir days 7–14), nausea and vomiting, transient elevations of liver enzymes, alopecia, and drug fever. Diarrhea or stomatitis is occasionally seen. Central nervous system toxicity is dose-related. Signs of central nervous system toxicity are nuchal rigidity (stiff neck), headache, and somnolence (see Table 7.4).

Specific nursing measures for cytosine arabinoside include measures to detect and treat central nervous system toxicity and drug fever. Monitor daily for nuchal rigidity, somnolence, and/or headache. Monitor for temperature elevation every four hours. Administer acetaminophen (Tylenol) as needed, usually when fever exceeds 101° F.

5-fluorouracil (5-FU)

The mode of action is inhibition of thymidylate synthetase and thus inhibition of DNA synthesis [2]. 5-fluorouracil in indicated for colon, breast, ovarian, and gastrointestinal carcinomas. Administration is most commonly by the intravenous route. Oral doses are not often given because of erratic absorption. Much

Table 7.4. Central Nervous System Toxicity With High-Dose Systemic Cytosine Arabinoside (ARA-C) [19]

Dose	Number of Clients	Number Exhibiting CNS Toxicity	Comments
24 g/m^2	12	0	—
36 g/m^2	19	3	Reversible
48 g/m^2	12	1	Reversible
54 g/m^2	6	4	May be irreversible

larger doses of 5-fluorouracil can be delivered by prolonged infusion over several days, and prolonged infusion also significantly reduces myelosuppression. 5-fluorouracil is rapidly metabolized to nontoxic forms by the liver.

Toxicities associated with 5-fluorouracil include myelosuppression, anorexia, nausea, mucositis, and diarrhea. The white blood cell nadir is days 9 through 14, lasting thirty days. Platelet nadir occurs between days 7 and 14. Alopecia is uncommon.

PURINE ANALOGS

6-mercaptopurine (6-MP, Purinethol)

The mode of action is interference with purine metabolism, thus disrupting nucleic acid synthesis [2]. 6-mercaptopurine is indicated for acute lymphoblastic and myeloblastic leukemias. Administration is oral, and 6-mercaptopurine is metabolized to nontoxic forms primarily in the liver.

Toxicities associated with 6-mercaptopurine include myelosuppression (nadir day 7), occasional nausea and vomiting, and hepatocellular dysfunction. To prevent hepatocellular dysfunction, the dosage should be reduced by at least 50 percent of normal when the client is concurrently receiving allopurinol [2]. The dosage should also be reduced in liver disease and renal failure.

6-thioguanine (6-TG, Thioguanine)

The mode of action is similar to that of 6-mercaptopurine, and it is indicated for acute lymphoblastic leukemia [2]. Administration is oral, and 6-thioguanine is metabolized to nontoxic forms primarily in the liver.

Toxicities associated with 6-thioguanine include myelosuppression (nadir 2–4 weeks), nausea, and stomatitis. There may be hepatotoxicity if 6-thioguanine is given in combination with cytosine arabinoside (Cytosar, Cytarabine, Ara-C). There is no need to decrease the dosage of 6-thioguanine if the client is also being treated with allopurinol [2], but the dosage should be reduced if liver disease is present.

CONCEPT XI:
The alkylating agents are a class of cell-cycle nonspecific antineoplastic drugs that injure DNA by cross-linking of strands, thus interfering with DNA replication [2].

CYCLOPHOSPHAMIDE (CYTOXAN)

Cyclophosphamide is indicated for lymphomas, chronic lymphocytic leukemia, acute leukemia, neuroblastoma, and breast and ovarian carcinoma. The drug is also useful in the treatment of lung cancer, especially oat cell carcinoma [2, 5]. Administration is oral or intravenous. Cyclophosphamide itself is inactive and must be activated in vivo by the liver. Since the drug is also detoxified by the liver, dosage should be adjusted in liver failure.

Toxicities associated with cyclophosphamide are myelosuppression, nausea and vomiting which usually begin six to eighteen hours after the drug is administered, alopecia, and hemorrhagic cystitis. The leukopenia nadir occurs between days 8 and 15 and lasts for seventeen to twenty-eight days.

Hemorrhagic cystitis is a dangerous side effect of this drug, but it is almost always preventable. A high urine output, large fluid intake, and frequent voiding for twenty-four to forty-eight hours after administration of the drug will nearly always prevent hemorrhagic cystitis. Force fluids to at least three liters daily or give intravenous hydration as necessary. Encourage frequent voiding, and check each voiding for the presence of blood with Hemastix for forty-eight hours after administration of the drug. Report any hematuria to the physician. Maintain accurate intake and output records to monitor fluid status.

THIO-TEPA (TRIETHYLENE THIOPHOSPHORAMIDE)

Thio-TEPA is less commonly used than other alkylating agents but is sometimes prescribed for treatment of lymphomas, malignant effusions, and breast and ovarian carcinomas [2]. Administration may be intramuscular, intravenous, or intracavity. Thio-TEPA is detoxified in the liver and excreted in the urine.

Toxicities associated with Thio-TEPA are delayed and prolonged because the drug binds to tissue and has a long half-life. Myelosuppression usually occurs, the nadir being between days 5 and 30. Other toxicities include nausea and vomiting, anorexia, drug fever, and intense pain with intramuscular injection. Persons with lymphoma are particularly at risk for profound hyperuricemia and hyperkalemia owing to massive lysis of malignant cells.

Monitor serum potassium and uric acid levels for elevation, and observe for signs of potassium excess. Monitor every four hours for temperature elevation. Administer acetaminophen (Tylenol) as necessary, usually when fever exceeds 101° F.

MECHLORETHAMINE (NITROGEN MUSTARD)

Mechlorethamine is indicated for treatment of chronic myelocytic leukemia, acute leukemia, lymphomas, and breast, lung, and ovarian carcinomas. The drug is highly unstable and may be administered intravenously or into a body cavity.

Mechlorethamine is a severe vesicant, so care must be taken with administration. Intracavity administration usually results in great pain, so the client should be medicated with an analgesic before mechlorethamine is administered into a body cavity.

Toxicities associated with mechlorethamine include myelosuppression (nadir days 4–10, duration 10–21 days), stomatitis, and alopecia. Severe nausea and vomiting usually begin within four or five hours after administration of the drug and generally last for twenty-four hours. Persons with leukemia or lymphoma are particularly vulnerable to the development of profound hyperuricemia and hyperkalemia owing to massive lysis of malignant cells. Monitor serum potassium and uric acid levels for elevations, and observe for signs of potassium excess.

CHLORAMBUCIL (LEUKERAN)

Chlorambucil is an oral drug used in the treatment of chronic lymphocytic leukemia, lymphocytic lymphoma and ovarian, breast, and testicular carcinomas [2]. It has a slow onset of action and a prolonged effect, even after the drug is discontinued.

Myelosuppression is often seen, and leukopenia may be delayed up to three weeks and lasts up to ten days after the last dose of the drug. Persons with leukemia or lymphoma are particularly vulnerable to the development of profound hyperuricemia and hyperkalemia owing to the massive lysis of malignant cells. Monitor serum potassium and uric acid levels for elevations, and observe for signs of potassium excess.

CARMUSTINE (BCNU)

Carmustine is an intravenous drug used in the treatment of lymphomas, melanoma, multiple myeloma, and carcinomas of the brain, colon, and stomach. It is one of the few antineoplastic agents that crosses the blood-brain barrier.

Carmustine is a vesicant drug, so care must be taken with intravenous administration. The drug is extremely painful upon intravenous injection, so medicate the client with an analgesic as necessary prior to injection.

Cumulative myelosuppression occurs four to six weeks after the drug is given and lasts one to two weeks. Nausea and vomiting usually occur two to six hours after administration of the drug. Persons with lymphoma are particularly vulnerable to the development of profound hyperuricemia and hyperkalemia owing to massive lysis of malignant cells. Monitor serum potassium and uric acid levels for elevations, and observe for signs of potassium excess.

LOMUSTINE (CCNU)

Lomustine is an oral alkylating agent that also crosses the blood-brain barrier. It is indicated for treatment of lymphomas, melanoma, multiple myeloma, and carcinomas of the brain, colon, lung, and kidney.

Lomustine causes myelosuppression with leukopenia (delayed up to six weeks and lasting one to two weeks) and thrombocytopenia (delayed up to four weeks and lasting one to two weeks). Nausea and vomiting usually begin within four hours after drug administration and last for twenty-four hours. Give lomustine on an empty stomach and implement other antiemetic measures. Stomatitis and alopecia may also occur. Persons with lymphoma are particularly vulnerable to the development of profound hyperuricemia and hyperkalemia owing to massing lysis of malignant cells. Monitor serum potassium and uric acid levels for elevations, and observe for signs of potassium excess.

SEMUSTINE (METHYL-CCNU)

Semustine is also an oral alkylating agent that crosses the blood-brain barrier. It is used in the treatment of lymphomas and brain tumors (metastatic or primary).

The myelosuppression nadir is three weeks and myelosuppression lasts one to two weeks. Nausea and vomiting are also common. Long-term treatment with semustine may result in renal damage or interstitial pulmonary fibrosis. Lymphoma clients are especially vulnerable to the development of profound hyperuricemia and hyperkalemia owing to massive lysis of malignant cells. Monitor serum potassium and uric acid levels for elevations, and observe for signs of potassium excess.

BUSULFAN (MYELERAN)

Busulfan is an oral alkylating agent indicated for use in the treatment of chronic granulocytic leukemia, polycythemia vera, and thrombocythemia. The metabolized drug is excreted in the urine.

Myelosuppression occurs, and the leukopenia nadir occurs at about day 10 and continues for two weeks after cessation of treatment. Other toxicities include nausea, vomiting, diarrhea, amenorrhea, and impotence. An Addison-like wasting syndrome may develop, with skin pigmentation, marked fatigue, and muscle wasting. Chronic, irreversible pulmonary fibrosis ("busulfan lung") may develop. Persons with leukemia are especially vulnerable to the development of profound hyperuricemia and hyperkalemia owing to massive lysis of malignant cells. Monitor serum potassium and uric acid levels for elevations, and observe for signs of potassium excess.

PHENYALANINE MUSTARD (ALKERAN)

Phenyalanine mustard is an oral antineoplastic drug, probably excreted by the kidney, which is used for multiple myeloma and carcinomas of the breast and ovary. Toxicities include delayed and severe myelosuppression and moderate nausea and vomiting.

CIS-PLATINUM (PLATINOL)

Cis-platinum is an important alkylating agent used in the treatment of carcinomas of the testes, ovary, bladder, ureter, and head and neck. Administration is intravenous. Urinary excretion of cis-platinum is slow; only 27 percent to 45 percent of the drug is excreted in the first five days after administration [10]. Toxicities are frequent and may be life-threatening.

Myelosuppression

Myelosuppression is transient and usually mild. The leukopenia nadir occurs between days 10 and 14, and the thrombocytopenia nadir is seen between days 17 and 21.

Nausea and Vomiting

Severe nausea and vomiting occur within one to four hours in virtually all persons receiving cis-platinum. The incidence and severity of nausea and vomiting increase with higher dosages of the drug. Usually nausea and vomiting subside within twenty-four hours, but occasionally nausea and anorexia will continue for as long as one week after treatment.

In view of the severe and sometimes intractable nausea and vomiting occurring with cis-platinum therapy, it is recommended that sedatives and potent antiemetics be administered just before cis-platinum is given. A large number of antiemetic drugs have been tested to try to control the severe nausea and vomiting but none seem to have any value in controlling this side effect. Concurrent administration of sedatives and potent antiemetics will usually allow the client to sleep through therapy and will often control nausea, but vomiting may still occur. Therefore, it is important to position the client so as to prevent aspiration of emesis and to have suction equipment at the bedside.

Nephrotoxicity

Nephrotoxicity is indicated by blood urea nitrogen (BUN) levels of more than 25 mg/100 ml. This toxicity can be life-threatening and dose-limiting. Evi-

Table 7.5. Nephrotoxicity of Cis-Platinum in Some Clinical Studies

Ref.	No. of Clients	Dose	Renal Function	Remarks
27	31	<50 mg/m^2	No changes	Courses spaced at least 14 days apart.
		50 mg/mls2	Mean BUN 31 mg/100 ml in 6/25 of courses	
		75 mg/m^2	Mean BUN 67 mg/100 ml in 2/14 of courses	Cumulative effect seen. Renal biopsies in 2 clients showed acute tubular necrosis.
		100 mg/m^2	Mean BUN 44 mg/100 ml in 11/18 of courses	Hyperuricemia in 16 cases following doses of 50 mg/m^2 or more
		200 mg/m^2	Acute renal failure in 1 client	*(continued)*

Table 7.5. Nephrotoxicity of Cis-Platinum in Some Clinical Studies, Continued

Ref.	No. of Clients	Dose	Renal Function	Remarks
20	21	3–7 mg/kg total course dose	Mean BUN 38.5 mg/100 ml Mean creatinine 2.2 mg/100 ml	Tubular necrosis in 2 autopsy cases. In 4 clients, persistent renal functional impairment noted.
		1.25–2.5 mg/kg total course dose	Increase in BUN in 9/19 of courses	In 2 clients, persistent renal functional impairment noted.
15	45	SINGLE-DOSE GROUP: 4–8 mg/m^2	No changes	—
		50 mg/m^2	Reversible nephrotoxicity in 3/3 of courses	
		75 mg/m^2	Reversible nephrotoxicity in 2/3 of courses	
		100 mg/m^2	Nephrotoxicity in 9/9 of courses	Tubular necrosis in 1 case. In 5 cases, probable irreversible nephrotoxicity occurred.
		5-DAY COURSE GROUP: 1.5–12.5 mg/m^2/day	No changes	
		18 mg/m^2 day	Nephrotoxicity in 1/5 of courses	Transient
		20 mg/m^2 day	Nephrotoxicity in 3/9 of courses	Acute tubular necrosis in 2 cases. In 4 cases, nephrotoxicity occurred after more than one course at the same dose
		24 mg/m^2/day	Nephrotoxicity in 2/3 of courses	Probable irreversible nephrotoxicity
7	10	SINGLE-DOSE GROUP: <1.95 mg/kg	No changes	
		1.95 mg/kg	Nephrotoxicity in 3/6 of courses	Reversible
14	1	5-DAY COURSE: 0.25 mg/kg/day	BUN 61 mg/100 ml, creatinine 5 mg/100 ml, creatinine clearance 29 ml/min	Acute tubular necrosis. 2 months posttreatment, stabilized creatinine clearance was 21.7 ml/min.

dence of acute tubular necrosis with tubular degeneration and interstitial edema has been observed [21]. The incidence and severity of nephrotoxicity appears to be related to the dosage of cis-platinum received by the client [7]. Elevations occur in the first seven to fourteen days. Renal toxicity seems to significantly increase with multiple courses of cis-platinum despite adequate hydration and diuresis [10]. See Table 7.8.

In view of the severe or fatal nephrotoxicity that may be induced by cis-platinum, it is imperative that adequate renal function be documented prior to each dose of the drug. Serum creatinine, blood urea nitrogen, and urinary creatinine clearance should be normal before cis-platinum is given. Administration of high-rate intravenous hydration for a minimum of twelve hours before cis-platinum administration and for twelve to twenty-four hours after the drug administration has been shown to decrease the client's risk of renal damage [21]. Fluid intake must be maintained at a minimum of two liters daily [10] to ensure a high urine volume flow. Maintain accurate intake and output records every eight hours to monitor for oliguria and fluid status. Occasionally, mannitol is used to promote diuresis, but the critical factor in preventing nephrotoxicity is the maintenance of high-volume fluid flow through the kidney.

Peripheral Neuropathy

Peripheral neuropathy similar to that caused by the vinca alkaloids may occur with high-dose cis-platinum therapy and may be a dose-limiting factor. The drug should be discontinued at the first sign of neuropathy and only resumed with great caution once resolution of the symptoms has been achieved [10].

Ototoxicity

Damage to the eighth cranial nerve has been reported with high doses of cis-platinum. The ototoxicity is usually mild and probably reversible, with tinnitus or high-frequency hearing loss being the most common symptoms.

Anaphylaxis

Anaphylaxis has been reported in some clients even though they have had previous cis-platinum therapy [10]. Symptoms are facial edema, wheezing, tachycardia, and hypotension. Treatment includes hydrocortisone, antihistamines, adrenaline, and supportive measures.

DACARBAZINE (DTIC)

Dacarbazine is the drug of choice for malignant melanoma. It is also used in the treatment of Hodgkin's disease, neuroblastoma, and some sarcomas. Administration is intravenous, and 40 percent to 50 percent of the drug is excreted unchanged by the kidney. Dacarbazine is inactivated by light. Protect the solution from exposure to light by covering the bottle or bag with an opaque sac and by wrapping aluminum foil or opaque tape around the intravenous tubing.

Dacarbazine is a vesicant, so care must be taken with intravenous administration. The drug causes myelosuppression, and leukopenia is exhibited for as long as five weeks after drug administration. Severe nausea and vomiting occur in virtually all individuals receiving dacarbazine. The nausea and vomiting usually begin within one to three hours and last one to twelve hours. Other toxicities include anorexia, a metallic taste sensation, parasthesias, alopecia, and facial flushing. A flu-like syndrome with an onset seven days after cessation of treatment and a duration of one to three weeks may occur. Advise treatment with rest, fluids, and acetaminophen (not aspirin or other salicylates). Persons with Hodgkin's disease are at risk for development of profound hyperuricemia and hyperkalemia owing to massive lysis of malignant cells. Monitor serum potassium and uric acid levels for elevations, and observe for signs of potassium excess.

CONCEPT XII:
The antineoplastic antibiotics are natural products that inhibit or interfere with DNA and/or RNA synthesis.

BLEOMYCIN (BLENOXANE)

Bleomycin's mechanism of action is thought to be inhibition of DNA synthesis [16]. It is indicated for treatment of lymphomas, reticulum cell sarcoma, lymphosarcoma, testicular carcinoma, and squamous cell carcinomas of the head, neck, and genital tract. Administration is subcutaneous, intramuscular, or intravenous. The metabolic fate of bleomycin has not been specifically determined. However, 20 percent to 40 percent of the drug is excreted in the active form by the kidney [11].

Toxicities associated with bleomycin include nausea, vomiting, anorexia, stomatitis, alopecia, and skin reactions. The skin dysfunction consists of rash, erythema, vesiculation, and hyperpigmentation. Drug fever often occurs within a few hours after bleomycin administration and lasting four to twelve hours. The client's temperature may rise to 105° F; treatment is symptomatic.

Anaphylaxis is a life-threatening complication and is most common in persons with lymphoma. It usually occurs after the first or second dose of bleomycin. Symptoms include hypotension, fever and chills, wheezing, and mental confusion. A test dose of five (5) units or less of bleomycin must be given prior to the full drug dose. Emergency equipment and drugs must be readily available.

Pneumonitis occurs in about 10 percent of individuals who receive bleomycin. The pneumonitis may progress to pulmonary fibrosis, which has a mortality rate of 1 percent [16]. Monitor breath sounds daily for the development of fine rales, which is the first sign of pulmonary toxicity, and watch for dyspnea. Clients who are receiving bleomycin therapy should receive only low oxygen concentrations during and after surgery in order to minimize the risk of postoperative pulmonary complications.

Bleomycin is not a vesicant. The drug is not toxic to bone marrow.

DACTINOMYCIN (ACTINOMYCIN-D)

The mechanism of action is inhibition of DNA-directed RNA synthesis [2]. Dactinomycin is indicated for use in the treatment of Wilms' tumor, rhabdomyosarcoma, methotrexate-resistant choriocarcinoma, and sarcomas. Administration is intravenous. Dactinomycin is excreted by the liver into bile, with only a small amount excreted in the urine.

Dactinomycin is a severe vesicant, so care must be taken with intravenous administration. Toxicities include myelosuppression, stomatitis, diarrhea, alopecia, and acne-like skin eruptions. Nausea and vomiting occur soon after administration and sometimes last several days.

DOXORUBICIN (ADRIAMYCIN)

Doxorubicin is an important antineoplastic antibiotic whose mechanism of action is the blockage of DNA biosynthesis. It has a wide spectrum of usage with particular effectiveness against sarcomas, breast carcinoma, lymphomas, and acute leukemia. Doxorubicin is administered intravenously and excreted by the liver into bile, with a small amount excreted by the kidney.

Doxorubicin is a severe vesicant, so care must be taken with intravenous administration. Myelosuppression is often severe. Leukopenia nadir occurs between days 10 and 15 with recovery by day 21. Other toxicities include severe nausea, vomiting, diarrhea, and stomatitis. Alopecia and skin changes (rash, hyperpigmentation) may occur. The client may void red-colored urine for one to two days after administration of the drug. Assure the client that the red-colored urine is not hematuria but rather a result of the red dye in the drug solution.

An extremely dangerous toxicity of doxorubicin is cardiotoxicity, which is a cumulative, dose-limiting factor. Characteristic signs and symptoms are sinus tachycardia, T-wave flattening, depression of the S-T segment, voltage reduction, and arrhythmias. Congestive heart failure with pulmonary edema may occur and has a mortality rate of 30 percent to 75 percent. An electrocardiogram must be performed before *each course* of doxorubicin therapy, assessing for signs of developing cardiotoxicity. Monitor for a high resting pulse, which is an early sign of this dangerous condition. If the cumulative, lifetime dose of doxorubicin exceeds 550 mg/m^2, monitor carefully for the development of congestive heart failure which may occur two weeks to six months after cessation of treatment [2].

DAUNORUBICIN (DAUNOMYCIN)

Daunorubicin is closely related in structure and action to doxorubicin. Its mechanisms of action is the blockage of DNA synthesis [2]. Daunorubicin is used in the treatment of acute lymphoblastic and myeloblastic leukemias. Route of administration is intravenous. Sixteen percent to 40 percent of the drug is excreted in the urine, and fecal excretion varies between 10 percent and 30 percent [26].

Daunorubicin is a severe vesicant, so care must be taken with intravenous administration. Toxicities are similar to those of doxorubicin: myelosuppression with leukopenia and thrombocytopenia nadir occurring between days 10 and 14 with recovery by day 21, stomatitis appearing by day 5, nausea, vomiting, diarrhea, alopecia, and cardiotoxicity. Nursing measures are identical to those for doxorubicin.

MITHRAMYCIN (MITHRACIN)

Mithramycin's mechanism of action is interference with the synthesis of RNA [2]. It is used in the treatment of embryonal cell carcinoma of the testis and is administered intravenously.

Mithramycin is a severe vesicant, so care must be taken with intravenous administration. Toxicities include thrombocytopenia, nausea, vomiting, anorexia, diarrhea, stomatitis, headache, and hepatic dysfunction. Nephrotoxicity may occur and is heralded by elevations in blood urea nitrogen (BUN) and serum creatinine. Hypocalcemia may also develop. Monitor serum calcium for abnormally low levels. Observe the client daily for tetany, carpopedal spasms, positive Chvostek's sign, and muscle cramps.

MITOMYCIN-C (MUTAMYCIN)

Mechanism of action is inhibition of DNA synthesis, probably by alkylation [2]. Mitomycin-C is used in the treatment of gastric and breast carcinomas. It is given intravenously and is inactivated primarily by the liver.

Mitomycin-C is a severe vesicant, so care must be taken with intravenous administration [9]. Toxicities include myelosuppression, nausea, vomiting, anorexia, stomatitis, drug fever, and alopecia. Interstitial pneumonia may occur, so the client should be assessed daily for the development of rales, wheezing, or dyspnea. Delayed renal damage resulting from glomerular necrosis is uncommon but often fatal [13].

Mitomycin-C is inactivated by light. Protect the solution from exposure to light by covering the bottle or bag with an opaque sack and by wrapping aluminum foil or opaque tape around the intravenous tubing. Discard any unused solution after six hours.

STREPTOZOTOCIN

Streptozotocin is an antineoplastic antibiotic with an unknown mechanism of action. It is indicated for use in the treatment of islet cell tumors of the pancreas and carcinoid tumors. Administration is intravenous, and 10 percent to 20 percent of the drug is excreted in the urine within one hour after administration.

Streptozotocin is a severe vesicant, so care must be taken with intravenous administration. Toxicities include occasional myelosuppression, nausea, vomiting, nephrotoxicity secondary to tubular damage, transient hepatic dysfunction with elevation of hepatic transaminases, and rare hypoglycemia.

CONCEPT XIII:
The vinca alkaloids are natural products, derived from the periwinkle plant.

Vinca alkaloids are cell-cycle specific drugs. They alter the appearance and function of the microtubules and the mitotic spindle, thus stopping cell division at metaphase [2]. Vinca alkaloids are metabolized by the liver and excreted in urine and feces.

VINCRISTINE (ONCOVIN)

Indications for vincristine include Hodgkin's disease, acute lymphoblastic leukemia, neuroblastoma, Wilms' tumor, and sarcomas. Administration is intravenous.

Vincristine is a vesicant drug, so care must be taken with intravenous administration. Toxicities include minimal myelosuppression (leukopenia nadir occurs at day 4), nausea, vomiting, anorexia, stomatitis, and alopecia. Persons with leukemia are especially at risk for the development of profound hyperuricemia and hyperkalemia owing to massive lysis of malignant cells. Monitor serum potassium and uric acid, and observe for signs of potassium excess.

Vincristine may cause severe neurotoxicity which may be fatal. Peripheral neuropathy is characterized by numbness and tingling in the extremities, loss of deep tendon reflexes, wrist and foot drop, ataxia, and possible paralysis with prolonged high-dose treatment. Central nervous system toxicity is heralded by orthostatic hypotension or cranial nerve dysfunction (jaw pain, hoarseness, vocal cord paresis, ptosis). Autonomic neuropathy is characterized by constipation, paralytic ileus, bladder atony, and incontinence or urinary retention. Any sign of neuropathy must be reported to the physician at once.

VINBLASTINE (VELBAN)

Vinblastine is structurally related to vincristine and has similar modes of action. It is used in the treatment of Hodgkin's disease and methotrexate-resistant choriocarcinoma. Administration is intravenous. Toxicities and nursing measures are the same as for vincristine.

VINDESINE

Vindesine is currently an investigational agent structurally related to the other vinca alkaloids. It is indicated for the treatment of metastatic malignant melanoma and has also been used in acute lymphocytic leukemia, Hodgkin's disease, non-Hodgkin's lymphoma, breast carcinoma, and non-oat cell carcinoma of the lung. Administration is intravenous. Toxicities and nursing measures are the same as for vincristine. Leukopenia is more common and more severe than thrombocytopenia. Vindesine's nadir occurs between days 6 and 8 and lasts ten to twelve days [25].

CONCEPT XIV:
Various hormones are used in the treatment of cancer and probably influence processes related to RNA-to-protein synthesis [12].

THE CORTICOSTEROIDS

Prednisone

Prednisone's specific cytotoxic action is not clear, but it is used in a wide variety of malignancies. Indications include acute lymphoblastic leukemia, lymphoma, disseminated breast carcinoma, intracranial metastases, and mediastinal and spinal cord compression syndromes [2]. Administration is oral.

Toxicities include gastric bleeding and ulceration, increased appetite and weight gain, diarrhea or constipation, abdominal distention, osteoporosis, and the Cushingoid state. Fluid and sodium retention and hypertension may develop. Prednisone may also cause hypokalemia, mood swings, euphoria, and immunosuppression.

THE ANDROGENS

Four androgens are sometimes used in the treatment of disseminated breast cancer: calusterone (Methosarb), fluoxymesterone (Halotestin), testolactone (Teslac), and testosterone propionate (Oreton). Calusterone and fluoxymesterone are oral drugs. Testolactone may be administered orally or by deep intramuscular injection, and testosterone propionate is given intramuscularly [2, 12].

Toxicities of the androgens include nausea, vomiting, anorexia, hypercalcemia, fluid retention, and edema. The drugs may also cause masculinizaton, increased libido, and hot flashes.

THE ESTROGENS

Four estrogens are sometimes used in antineoplastic chemotherapy: chlorotianisene (TACE), diethylstilbestrol (DES), estradiol, and ethinyl estradiol (Estinyl). Estrogens are indicated for use in the treatment of prostatic carcinoma and metastatic breast carcinoma with positive estrogen-receptor assay [2, 6]. Chlorotianisene and ethinyl estradiol are oral drugs. Diethylstilbestrol may be given orally or by intramuscular injection. Estradiol is a parenteral drug only, given by the subcutaneous or intramuscular routes.

Toxicities of the estrogens include nausea, vomiting, diarrhea, anorexia, hypercalcemia, fluid retention and edema, mental depression, and headache. The estrogens may also cause feminization in men.

THE ANTIESTROGENS

Tamoxifen Citrate (Nolvadex)

Tamoxifen citrate's mode of action is to compete with estrogen for binding sites in the target tissue. It is indicated for treatment of metastatic breast carcinoma with positive estrogen-receptor assay. Toxicities are mild, transient, and reversible. Tamoxifen may cause nausea, anorexia, transient leukopenia and thrombocytopenia, menstrual irregularities, vaginal bleeding, and hot flashes. Dizziness or headache may occur. A unique side effect of tamoxifen is known as "tumor flare," with tumor pain, bone pain, and significant hypercalcemia. Monitor the client carefully for this flare of pain, and observe serum calcium levels for elevations. Notify the physician if "tumor flare" occurs.

THE PROGESTINS

Three progestins are sometimes used in cancer treatment: hydroxy-progesterone caproate (Delalutin), medroxyprogesterone (Provera, Depo-Provera), and megestrol acetate (Megace). These drugs may be used in the treatment of prostatic, renal, and disseminated breast carcinomas [2, 12]. Hydroxyprogesterone caproate (Delalutin) and medroxyprogesterone (Depo-Provera) are intramuscular drugs. Medroxyprogesterone (Provera) and megestrol acetate (Megace) are oral drugs.

Toxicities include nausea, vomiting, anorexia, jaundice, fluid retention, headache, dizziness, and thrombotic disorders. Amenorrhea, breakthrough bleeding, and decreased libido may also occur.

CONCEPT XV:
One enzyme is currently in use in antineoplastic chemotherapy: L-asparaginase (Elspar).

L-asparaginase is cell-cycle nonspecific. The drug is thought to hydrolize asparagine, an amino acid necessary for cellular reproduction. Certain malignant cells are unable to synthesize their own asparagine and therefore must obtain it from the body's extracellular pool. L-asparaginase depletes the body's extracellular pool of asparagine, thus reducing the amount available for malignant proliferation. The drug is used in the treatment of acute lymphoblastic leukemia. It is given intravenously, but its metabolism and fate in the body are unclear. L-asparaginase does not cross the blood-brain barrier.

L-asparaginase may cause a severe and life-threatening anaphylactic reaction, the likelihood of which *increases* with continuing administration of the drug. For this reason, L-asparaginase is rarely given in an outpatient setting. A test dose must always be given prior to the full dose, and close scrutiny of vital signs and client condition is imperative during and for twenty-four hours after drug administration. Emergency equipment and drugs should be readily available.

L-asparaginase may induce hyperglycemia and diabetes mellitus. Monitor serum glucose levels for elevations, and test urine for sugar during therapy. Monitor for the development of polyuria, polydipsia, and polyphagia. Any indication that this condition has developed should be promptly reported to the physician.

Pancreatitis may also develop as a result of therapy with L-asparaginase. Monitor serum amylase levels for elevation. If amylase levels rise, the physician must be notified and the drug dosage altered.

Other toxicities associated with L-asparaginase include renal failure, somnolence, fatigue, confusion, headache, drug fever, and coagulation abnormalities. Nausea and vomiting are severe and often last for twenty-four hours despite potent anti-emetics.

CONCEPT XVI:
Several miscellaneous drugs are used in antineoplastic chemotherapy.

HYDROXYUREA (HYDREA)

Hydroxyurea is similar in structure and action to the antimetabolites. It is cell-cycle specific, inhibiting DNA synthesis at the S-phase [2]. Hydroxyurea is indicated for use in the treatment of chronic granulocytic leukemia, renal carcinoma, and melanoma. Administration is oral, and the drug is well-absorbed from the gastrointestinal tract and excreted unchanged in the urine.

Toxicities associated with hydroxyurea include myelosuppression (nadir between days 1 and 2 with rapid recovery), mild nausea and vomiting, stomatitis, and teratogenesis. Persons with leukemia are vulnerable to the development of profound hyperuricemia and hyperkalemia owing to massive lysis of malignant cells. Monitor serum levels of potassium and uric acids for elevations, and observe for signs of potassium excess. In addition, ensure that all clients of child-bearing age are fully informed about the mutagenic effect the drug may have on future offspring.

PROCARBAZINE (MATULANE)

Procarbazine's mechanism of action is unclear, but it is thought that the drug injures cellular DNA in some manner [2]. Procarbazine is a mild monoamine oxidase inhibitor [22]. Administration of the drug is by the oral route, and metabolism and fate in the body are unknown. Procarbazine is used in the treatment of Hodgkin's disease.

Although procarbazine is a monoamine oxidase inhibitor, it is a mild one. Therefore, it is not necessary for clients to strictly avoid consumption of foods that are high in tyramine. The drug will, however, cause a distressing Antabuse-like reaction following the ingestion of alcoholic beverages [22]. Other toxicities include myelosuppression, nausea, vomiting, headache, dizziness, confusion, and alopecia.

HEXAMETHYLMELAMINE (HMM)

The mechanism of action is unknown. Hexamethylmelamine is indicated for treatment of lymphomas and carcinomas of the breast and ovary. Administration is oral. The drug is well-absorbed from the gastrointestinal tract, metabolized in the liver, and excreted in the urine.

Toxicities associated with hexamethylmelamine include moderate myelosuppression, severe nausea, vomiting, and anorexia. Neurotoxicity may develop with long-term daily therapy [2].

L-ALANOSINE [33]

L-alanosine is an investigational antineoplastic antibiotic derived from *Streptomyces alanaosinicus*. The drug has both antitumor and antiviral activity. The mechanism of action is the inhibition of cell division through disruption of the synthesis of RNA, DNA, and protein. It is indicated in the treatment of acute lymphocytic or nonlymphocytic leukemia. Administration is by intravenous infusion.

The most common side effect of L-alanosine is stomatitis/mucositis, and this reaction is dose-limiting. Infusion of the drug should be discontinued at the first sign of mucositis.

Other toxicities associated with L-alanosine include anaphylaxis, myelosuppression, nausea, vomiting, diarrhea, parasthesias, headache, drug fever, malaise, and skin rash. Hypertension or hypotension may also occur.

MGBG (Methyl-GAG)

MGBG is indicated for a number of malignancies. It is used as initial chemotherapy in inoperable or disseminated carcinomas of the kidney, esophagus, or pancreas. MGBG may also be prescribed after initial chemotherapy in lymphoma, multiple myeloma, and carcinomas of the breast, colon, and head and neck. Administration is by intravenous infusion or deep intramuscular injection. Excretion of MGBG is delayed, probably because of accumulation in human tissue. Sixty percent of the intravenous dose is found to be excreted through the urine and less than 20 percent through the feces over a three-week period of time [18].

Severe local tissue irritation will occur if MGBG is extravasated during intravenous injection or if the drug is not injected deeply enough during intramuscular administration. MGBG may cause significant hypoglycemia, so the client's serum glucose must be monitored carefully. Serum glucose levels less than 50 mg/100 ml are considered to be a 4+ toxicity.

Other toxicities associated with MGBG include myelosuppression, nausea, vomiting, anorexia, diarrhea, stomatitis, and mucositis. Skin rash may also occur.

DIHYDROXYANTHRACENEDIONE (DHAD)

DHAD is an investigational agent. Its mechanism of action is inhibition of DNA and RNA synthesis. It is used in the treatment of acute leukemia and is administered by intravenous infusion. The drug disappears rapidly from the plasma; in fact, DHAD has been detected only in three-minute blood samples. Less than 1 percent is detectable in the urine twenty-four hours after administration. Initial studies indicate a rapid distribution, a half-life of eight minutes, and an elimination half-life of two hours. Most of the drug seems to be excreted through the biliary system [28].

DHAD is a severe vesicant, so care must be taken with intravenous administration. Myelosuppression is a dose-limiting factor. The myelosuppression nadir occurs near day 9, and the bone marrow suppression lasts for ten to twelve days. DHAD also causes occasional nausea and vomiting, and green urine.

CONCEPT XVII:
Specific criteria are utilized to define the response of leukemia to chemotherapy [28].

BONE MARROW (200 CELLS)

Degree of Abnormality A-1

Promyelocytes and blasts must be less than 10 percent of the total nucleated cells in the bone marrow sample. Lymphocytes must be less than 20 percent. Granulocytes (white blood cells), erythrocytes (red blood cells), and platelets must be essentially normal in appearance.

Degree of Abnormality A-2

Promyelocytes and blasts must be less than 25 percent of the total nucleated cells. If the lymphocytes are equal to or less than 50 percent, this rating may be given if no blasts or promyelocytes are observed in the bone marrow sample.

PERIPHERAL BLOOD

Degree of Abnormality B-1

Hemoglobin must be greater than 11 grams/100 ml with no transfusions during the preceding two weeks. The circulating granulocyte level must be 1,000 to 9,000/mm^3. Platelets must be greater than 100,000/mm^3, and there may be no blast cells in the peripheral blood.

Table 7.6. Toxicities of Common Chemotherapeutic Drugs

Drug	Vesicant	Anaphylaxis	Myelosuppression	Nausea, vomiting	Diarrhea	Constipation	Stomatitis	Alopecia	Fever	Neurotoxicity	Hepatotoxicity	Nephrotoxicity	Hyperuricemia	Hyperkalemia	Lung Toxicity	Cardiotoxicity	Skin Toxicity	Other
Adriamycin	X		X	X			X	X								X	X	Red urine
Alkeran			X	X														
BCNU			X	X								R						Painful injection
Bleomycin		X		X	X		X	X	X						X		X	Headache
Busulfan			X	X		X							R		R			Amenorrhea
CCNU			X	X		X									R			
Chlorambucil			X	X									R		R			
Cis-Platinum	X		X	X						R		X						
Cyclophosphamide			X	X			X	X				X						Hemorrhagic cystitis
Cytosine			X	X			X	X		R	X	X						
Dactinomycin	X		X	X		X	X	X										Acne
Daunomycin	X		X	X		X	X	X								X	X	Red urine
DHAD	X		X	R		X	X	X										Green urine
DTIC			X	X		X		X		X								Flu syndrome
5-FU			X	X		X	X	R		X			R					Malaise

Continued

Table 7.6. Toxicities of Common Chemotherapeutic Drugs, Continued

Drug	Vesicant	Anaphylaxis	Myelosuppression	Nausea, vomiting	Diarrhea	Constipation	Stomatitis	Alopecia	Fever	Neurotoxicity	Hepatotoxicity	Nephrotoxicity	Hyperuricemia	Hyperkalemia	Lung Toxicity	Cardiotoxicity	Skin Toxicity	Other
HMM			X	X						R								Teratogenesis
Hydroxyurea			R										X	X			X	Headache
L-alanosine	X		X	X			X		X	X								Hyperglycemia
L-asparaginase	X		X				X		X		X							Jaundice
6-mercaptopurine		X	X				X				X							
Methotrexate		X	X	X			X	X		R	X	X				X		
HDMTX + Leucovorin		X	X	X			X	X	X		X	X	R	R		X	X	Pneumothorax
Methyl-CCNU		X	X								R	R					R	
MGBG	X	X	X	X		X	X			X	X						R	Hypoglycemia
Mithramycin	X	X	X	X		X	X		X		X	X						Hypocalcemia
Mitomycin-C	X	X	X	X		X	X							X				
Nitrogen mustard	X	X	X	X		X	X	X	X				R					
Procarbazine		X	X	X				X										Mild MAO-I
Streptozotocin	X	R	R	X							X	X						Hyperglycemia
6-thioguanine		X	X			X	X											
Thio-TEPA		X	X	X			X		X			R	R					
Vinblastine	X	X	X	X	X	X	X	X		X		R	R					Headache
Vincristine	X	R	R	X	X	X	X	X		X		X	R					
Vindesine	X	X	X	X	X	X	X	X		X								

X common   R uncommon or rare

Degree of Abnormality B-2

Hemoglobin must be equal to or greater than 9 grams/100 ml with no transfusions during the preceding two weeks. The circulating granulocyte level must be greater than 1,000/mm^3, and promyelocytes and blast cells must be less than 5 percent.

PHYSICAL FINDINGS

Degree of Abnormality C-1

There must be no evidence of leukemic infiltration. The spleen, lymph nodes, and bone must be normal and without evidence of leukemic involvement.

Degree of Abnormality C-2

Physical findings may not exceed the following criteria. Hepatomegaly may not be greater than three centimeters below the right costal margin at the mid-clavicular line. Splenomegaly may not be greater than three centimeters below the left costal margin. No lymph node may exceed two centimeters in greatest diameter.

CLINICAL FINDINGS (SYMPTOMS)

In *degree of abnormality D-1*, no symptoms attributable to leukemia are evident. In *degree of abnormality D-2*, the client exhibits moderate incapacitation resulting from leukemia. In *degree of abnormality D-3*, the client is totally incapacitated by leukemia.

RATING OF RESPONSE TO THERAPY

Complete remission has been achieved if each of the categories has a degree of abnormality of 1 (A-1, B-1, C-1, and D-1). Leukemia is considered to be in *partial remission* if a degree of abnormality of 2 is present in any one category and a degree of abnormality of 1 in the other three categories. A *partial response* rating is obtained if the client has at least one number rating lower in at least three of the categories than at the time of initiation of therapy. Clients will be considered a *treatment failure* when there is insufficient change to raise the rating to that of partial response or partial remission. Finally, the client may experience a *relapse from remission*. Remission is considered to be terminated when there is change sufficient for a degree of abnormality rating of 3 to exist in any one or more of the categories.

Figure 7.4. Response of Leukemia to Chemotherapy

COMPLETE REMISSION
    A-1
    B-1
    C-1
    D-1

PARTIAL REMISSION

A-1	A-1	A-1	A-2
B-1	B-1	B-2	B-1
C-1	C-2	C-1	C-1
D-2	D-1	D-1	D-1

PARTIAL RESPONSE
    At least 1 number rating lower in at least 3 categories than before chemotherapy

TREATMENT FAILURE
    Insufficient change in disease to increase rating to partial response or partial remission

RELAPSE FROM REMISSION
    Rating of 3 in one or more categories

CONCEPT XVIII:
Specific criteria are utilized to define the response of solid tumors to chemotherapy [18].

COMPLETE REMISSION

For complete remission to be achieved, all of the following criteria must be met. There must be disappearance of all clinical evidence of active tumor for a minimum of four weeks. The skeletal survey and/or bone scan must have clear improvement, and all lytic lesions must exhibit reossification. In clients who have had bone disease, bone pain must be absent without analgesic medication. No pathological fractures are evident, and no new bone lesions must occur. The client must be free of any symptoms attributable to the malignancy.

PARTIAL REMISSION

For partial remission to be achieved, all of the following criteria must be met. There must be a 50 percent or greater decrease in the sum of the products of all diameters of measured lesions, and no simultaneous increase in the size of any lesion must occur. No new lesions may appear. Clients with liver metastases must have at least a 30 percent reduction in the sums of measurements below the costal margins.

STABLE DISEASE

Stable disease is defined as a steady state or a response less than partial remission. No new lesions may appear, and symptoms may not worsen.

PROGRESSION OF DISEASE

Progression of the disease occurs if the following factors occur. Any measurable lesion will exhibit at least a 50 percent increase in size, or new lesions will appear. Uncontrolled hypercalcemia develops, and there is clearly progressive skeletal involvement as manifested by an increasing number of lytic lesions.

RELAPSE

The client is in relapse if either of the following occur: new lesions have appeared, or there is reappearance of old lesions in clients who have previously experienced complete remission.

Figure 7.5. Response of Solid Tumors to Chemotherapy

COMPLETE REMISSION
No clinical evidence of active tumor (minimum 4 weeks)
Improved bone scan, reossification, no new bone lesions
No bone pain
No fractures
No symptoms of disease

PARTIAL REMISSION
50% + decrease in sum of products of all diameters of lesions
No increase in size of any lesion
No new lesions
Liver: minimum of 30% decrease in sums of measurements below costal margins

STABLE DISEASE
Steady disease state or response less than partial remission
No new lesions
Symptoms may not worsen

PROGRESSION
50% increase in size of any lesion, or new lesions occur
Hypercalcemia
Progressive skeletal disease

RELAPSE
Either new lesions have appeared; or
Old lesions have reappeared

CONCEPT XIX:
Appropriate client teaching prior to chemotherapy will reduce anxiety and feelings of helplessness.

Assess the client's level of knowledge and learning needs, and establish learning goals. Ensure that the teaching environment affords privacy and freedom from interruptions. Teach in brief time periods. This is especially important if the

Figure 7.6. Sample Teaching Sheet for Chemotherapy.

SAMPLE TEACHING SHEET FOR CHEMOTHERAPY
Vincristine

Another name for vincristine is Oncovin. Your physician has prescribed vincristine for you in order to kill cancer cells throughout your body. This drug is a natural product derived from the periwinkle plant. Vincristine works by stopping cell division, and it is broken down in your liver and excreted through the urine and bowel movements. Vincristine is only given intravenously (IV).

Side effects of vincristine are not usually severe. Its damaging effects on the bone marrow, white cells, red cells, and platelets are generally minimal. It does the greatest damage to the bone marrow on about the fourth day after you have received the drug. Therefore, during this time and for several days afterwards, you should be especially careful to avoid contact with people who are sick, to avoid any risk of causing yourself to bleed, to get plenty of rest and sleep, and to eat a well-rounded nutritious diet.

Nausea, vomiting, loss of appetite, and sores in your mouth sometimes occur. If your physician has prescribed medication for nausea and vomiting **and** if you are experiencing these symptoms, it may be wise to take the antinausea medication thirty minutes before you eat. If you notice that your mouth is very dry or if it is uncomfortable for you to eat very hot, very cold, or spicy foods, these may be early signs that sores are developing in your mouth. Consult your physician right away so that medication can be prescribed before the problem becomes serious.

Sometimes, vincristine will cause hair loss. Usually, this is only a temporary side effect, and your hair will grow back within a relatively short time. When your hair regrows, it may be a different texture or color than before. Scarves, wigs, and toupees can help you to manage this temporary side effect.

It is important to drink plenty of fluids (2–4 quarts per day) while you are receiving vincristine. A large amount of urine flow will help to move the drug properly through your kidneys. The fluid does not have to be plain water; you may also drink juice, tea, 7-Up™, etc.

Tell your nurse or physician at once if you experience any of the following:

1. numbness or tingling in your fingers or toes.
2. dizziness or fainting
3. stumbling or difficulties with walking
4. difficulty in urinating
5. jaw pain, hoarseness, drooping of the eyelids
6. constipation

The above symptoms might indicate that the dosage of vincristine needs to be changed slightly.

Vincristine is an anticancer drug that has been approved by the Federal Drug Administration. This means that it has been through thousands of tests before it was available for use with human beings. It is an extremely effective anticancer drug, and it is relatively safe for you to take.

client's attention span is short, if the client is emotionally distressed, or if the client is in pain. Use visual aids and examples, and provide frequent positive reinforcement. Evaluate the success of the teaching and thus determine areas needful of reinforcement.

REFERENCES

1. Akahoshi, M. High-dose Methotrexate with Leucovorin Rescue. *Cancer Nurs* 1:319, 1978.
2. Bakemeier, R. F. Principles of Medical Oncology and Cancer Chemotherapy. In P. Rubin (Ed.). *Clinical Oncology for Medical Students and Physicians: A Multidisciplinary Approach* (5th Ed.). Rochester, NY: American Cancer Society, 1978. Pp. 42–50.
3. Bertino, J. R. Rescue Techniques in Cancer Chemotherapy: Use of Leucovorin and Other Rescue Agents After Methotrexate Treatment. *Semin Oncol* 4:203, 1977.
4. Catane, R., Lichter, A., et al. Small Cell Lung Cancer: Analysis of Treatment Factors Contributing to Prolonged Survival. *Cancer* 48:1936, 1981.
5. Chang, J. C. and Wergowske, G. Correlation of Estrogen Receptors and Response to Chemotherapy with Cyclophosphamide, Methotrexate, and 5-Fluorouracil (CMF) in Advanced Breast Cancer. *Cancer* 48:2503, 1981.
6. Dao, T. L., Sinha, D. K., Nemoto, T., and Patel, J. Effect of Estrogen and Progesterone on Cellular Replication of Human Breast Tumors. *Cancer Res* 42:359, 1982.
7. DeConti, R. C., Toftness, B. R., Lange, R. C., et al. Clinical and Pharmacological Studies with Cis-diammine-dichloroplatinum (II). *Cancer Res* 33:1310, 1973.
8. Donley, D. L. Chemotherapy and the Nurse's Role. In P. Burkhalter and D. L. Donley. *Dynamics of Oncology Nursing.* New York: McGraw-Hill, 1978. Chapter 16.
9. Duvall, E. and Baumann, B. An Unusual Accident During the Administration of Chemotherapy. *Cancer Nurs* 3:305, 1980.
10. Eustace, P. History and Development of Cisplatin in the Management of Malignant Disease. *Cancer Nurs* 3:373, 1980.
11. Fujita, H. and Kimura, K. Blood Level, Tissue Distribution and Inactivation of Bleomycin. *Prog Antimic Anticancer Chemother* 2:309, 1970.
12. Goth, A. *Medical Pharmacology: Principles and Concepts* (10th Ed.). St. Louis: C. V. Mosby, 1981. Pp. 702–710.
13. Hanna, W. T., Krauss, S., Regester, R. F., and Murphy, W. M. Renal Disease After Mitomycin C Therapy. *Cancer* 48:2583, 1981.
14. Hardaker, W. T. Jr., Stone, R. A., and McCoy, R. Platinum Nephrotoxicity. *Cancer* 34:1030, 1974.
15. Higby, D. J., Wallace, H. J. Jr., et al. Cis-diammine-dichloroplatinum (NSC-119875): A Phase I Study. *Cancer Chemother Rep* 57:459, 1973.
16. Hoffman, D. M. Bleomycin: A Review of Its Use and Guidelines for Administration. *Cancer Nurs* 1:335, 1978.
17. Ignoffo, R. J. and Friedman, M. A. Therapy of Local Toxicities Caused by Extravasation of Cancer Chemotherapeutic Drugs. *Cancer Treat Rev* 7:17, 1980.
18. Knight W. III. Evaluation of MGBG in Solid Tumors and Refractory Hematologic Malignancies, Phase II. Southwest Oncology Group Protocol #7860, December 9, 1980.
19. Lazarus, H. M., Herzig, R. H., et al. Central Nervous System Toxicity of High-Dose Systemic Cytosine Arabinoside. *Cancer* 48:2577, 1981.
20. Lippman, A. J., Helson, C., et al. Clinical Trials of Cis-diamminedichloroplatinum (NSC-119875). *Cancer Chemother Rep* 57:191, 1973.

21. Madias, N. E. and Harrington, J. T. Platinum Nephrotoxicity. *Am J Med* 65:307, 1978.

22. Maxwell, M. B. Reexamining the Dietary Restrictions with Procarbazine (An MAOI). *Cancer Nurs* 3:451, 1980.

23. Patterson, P. Granulocyte Transfusion: Nursing Considerations. *Cancer Nurs* 3:101, 1980.

24. Pitman, S. W. and Frei, E. Weekly Methotrexate-Calcium Leucovorin Rescue: Effects of Alkalinization on Nephrotoxicity; Pharmacokinetics in the CNS; and Use in CNS Non-Hodgkin's Lymphoma. *Cancer Treat Rep* 61:695, 1977.

25. Quagliana, J. Vindesine in Adults with Metastatic Malignant Melanoma, Phase II: Pilot Study. Southwest Oncology Group Protocol #7930, December 7, 1979.

26. Reich, S. D. Daunorubicin: A Brief Review. *Cancer Nurs* 3:465, 1980.

27. Rossof, A. H., Slayton, R. E., and Perlia, C. P. Preliminary Clinical Experience with Cis-diamminedichloroplatinum (II) (NSC-119875, CACP). *Cancer* 30:1451, 1972.

28. Saiki, D. and Von Hoff, D. Evaluation of DHAD in Acute Leukemia, Phase II. Southwest Oncology Group Protocol #8032, October 22, 1980.

29. Satterwhite, B. E. What to Do When Adriamycin Infiltrates. *Nurs 80* 10(2):37, 1980.

30. Southwest Oncology Group. *Southwest Oncology Group Chemotherapy Toxicity Criteria.* San Antonio, TX: Southwest Oncology Group, 1981.

31. Stein, R. S., Howard, C. A., Brennan, M., and Czorniak, M. Lithium Carbonate and Granulocyte Production: Dose Optimization. *Cancer* 48:2696, 1981.

32. Von Hoff, D. D., Penta, J. S., Helman, L. J., and Slavik, M. Incidence of Drug-Related Deaths Secondary to High-Dose Methotrexate and Citrovorum Factor Administration. *Cancer Treat Rep* 61:745, 1977.

33. Weick, J. Evaluation of L-Alanosine in Acute Leukemia, Phase II. Southwest Oncology Group Protocol #8051, April 14, 1981.

34. Welch, D. and Lewis, K. Alopecia and Chemotherapy. *Am J Nurs* 80:903, 1980.

Chapter 8

Investigational Treatment Modalities

IMMUNOTHERAPY

CONCEPT I:
The immune system is a protective mechanism that defends the individual against potentially harmful invaders (see Figure 8.2.)

The immune system in the human being is characterized by memory, specificity, and the ability to recognize elements foreign to "self." All cells have antigens on their surfaces. A foreign antigen is recognized as "not self" and stimulates an immune response. After initial exposure to a foreign antigen, the person becomes sensitized to that specific antigen because certain cells have the ability to remember, recognize, and respond to that specific foreign antigen when it enters the body.

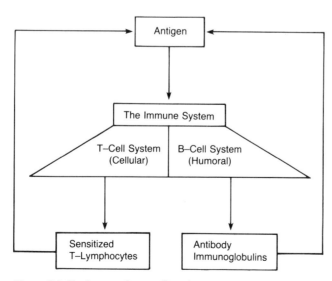

Figure 8.1. The Immune System: Overview.

INNATE IMMUNITY

Innate immunity is the body's first line of defense [12]. A healthy person is protected from potentially harmful invaders by several nonspecific immune mechanisms. Innate immunity is present from birth and is genetically endowed. Innate immune mechanisms do not depend on prior exposure to specific antigens. There are four mechanisms of innate immunity: mechanical barriers, chemical barriers, fever, and the inflammatory response. Mechanical barriers include mucous membranes and the skin. Chemical barriers include saliva, tears, gastric juices, and perspiration. Fever is a protective bodily response to temperature-dependent microorganisms. The inflammatory response is a protective system of blood and tissue phagocytes that engulf and destroy foreign invaders. Small neutrophils (microphages) and larger monocytes (macrophages) are the blood-borne phagocytes; histiocytes and reticulocytes are tissue macrophages.

ACQUIRED IMMUNITY

Acquired immunity is the body's second line of defense against pathogens and other foreign invaders. Both forms of acquired immunity—cellular and humoral—develop simultaneously and are not usually functional until a few months after birth. Both cellular and humoral immunity involve lymphocytes that become activated in response to initial and subsequent exposures to specific foreign antigens. This activation results in the eventual destruction of the antigen.

Cellular Immune System

The cellular immune system is mediated by thymus-dependent (T-) lymphocytes that become sensitized after initial exposure to the antigen. In response to subsequent invasion by the same antigen, the sensitized T-lymphocytes release lymphokines, enzymes, and enzyme precursors that inhibit the antigen's activity and facilitate its destruction by the phagocytic cells. Sensitized T-lymphocytes are also able to directly destroy the antigen.

Cell-mediated immunity provides defense against fungi, parasites, viruses, cancer cells, and foreign tissue. This immune system, for example, is responsible for the "rejection" of organ transplants by recognizing the foreign tissue as "not self."

T-lymphocytes can be specifically identified by laboratory testing [30]: (1) the E-rosette test (surface receptors for sheep erythrocytes), (2) cytotoxic destruction by specific antiserum, (3) live cell membrane immunofluorescence by specific thymus antiserum, and (4) blast transformation by phytohemagglutinin (PHA). Cellular immunity cannot yet be successfully transferred from one person to another. In other words, one cannot obtain cellular immunity through immunizations.

Humoral Immune System

The humoral immune system actually is comprised of two subsystems: the antibody system and the complement system. The antibody system is mediated by B-lymphocytes (also called Bursa-equivalent lymphocytes) which are the precursors of plasma cells. In response to recognition of a foreign antigen, B-lymphocytes differentiate themselves into plasma cells that then secrete antibodies into the blood. Antibodies are proteins which bind with the specific antigen that stimulated the antibody production. After the antibody has bound itself to the antigen, the antigen can then be phagocytized.

Antibodies are antigen-specific and belong to a group of immunoglobulins. Immunoglobulins are divided into five classes: IgM, IgG, IgA, IgE, and IgD. During the first exposure to the antigen, there is a primary antibody response predominantly of the IgM group. Later exposure to the antigen results in a secondary antibody response predominantly of the IgG class. This secondary response is longer in duration and involves greater quantities of antibodies. IgM, IgG, and IgA primarily defend the body against bacteria and viruses. IgE is the "anaphylactic antibody" and is responsible for allergic reactions. The role of IgD is unknown at the present time.

The complement system involves various enzyme precursors that facilitate destruction of the antigen.

The humoral immune system may produce different types of antibody-antigen reactions. Precipitation is a reaction between a soluble antigen and an insoluble antibody, thus forming precipitates. Agglutination is a reaction between a particulate antigen and the antibody, thus forming clumps. If opsonization occurs, the antigen and antibody undergo chemical changes that result in the surface of the antigen becoming sticky. Complement fixation is a series of enzymatic changes that eventually result in lysis of the antigen. The humoral immune system provides protection against bacteria and some viruses.

B-lymphocytes can be specifically identified by laboratory testing [30]: (1) surface immunoglobulin identification by live cell fluorescence, (2) the EA-rosette test (sheep erythrocyte antibody rosette formation), and (3) Pokeweed mitogen blast transformation. Humoral immunity can be transferred between human beings.

Actively acquired humoral immunity may be induced by an overt or subclinical infection. Some infections induce lifetime immunity (e.g., chicken pox, measles, mumps), whereas other infections fail to produce lasting immunity (e.g., the common cold, influenza). Actively acquired immunity may also be deliberately produced by immunization (vaccination).

Humoral immunity may also be passively transferred from one individual to another. Passively acquired immunity may, for example, be transferred naturally from mother to fetus or to a breast-fed infant by the passage of maternal antibodies across the placental barrier or in colostrum. Humoral immunity may also be passively acquired by the transference of factors from the lymphoid cells of an immune person to a nonimmune person. This type of immunity is called "adoptive immunity" and is currently under investigation.

NATURAL KILLER CELLS

A third component of the immune system has been tentatively identified: NK (Natural Killer) cells [23]. The existence of NK cells was discovered from the observation that animals have some natural resistance to tumors and that this re-

Table 8.1.   Cells Involved in the Immune Process

Acquired Immunity	Innate (Inherited) Immunity
B-lymphocytes (humoral system)	Neutrophils (blood microphages)
T-lymphocytes (cellular system)	Lymphocytes
? NK (Natural Killer) cells	Histiocytes (tissue macrophages)
	Monocytes (blood macrophages)

sistance is apparently not mediated by either T- or B-lymphocytes. Natural Killer cells can be enhanced or suppressed but not to a great extent. Production of NK cells seems to be stimulated by viral infections, possibly through bodily production of interferon. NK cells are probably a type of lymphocyte.

Null Cells

Null cells may participate in killer T-cell function, or they may act as precursors to B-lymphocytes. Null cells are currently without identifiable surface markers [30]. See Table 8.1 and Figure 8.2.

CONCEPT II:
When a normal cell undergoes malignant transformation, it often experiences biochemical changes that result in new antigens on the cell's surface [13, 24].

Although current knowledge of the biochemical nature of these antigens is very limited, they are sufficiently different that they are recognized as "not self" by the body, causing an immune response. If the cellular antigen is highly specific for that individual tumor, it is called a tumor-specific antigen. If the cellular antigen is commonly found among several different types of malignant cells, it is called a tumor-associated antigen. Both types of malignant cell antigens are recognized as "not self" and stimulate the immune response in most people.

Although the immune response to tumor antigens involves both cellular and humoral immunity [8, 13], it seems to be the cellular division that predominates in antitumor activity [13]. Cellular immunity is mediated by sensitized T-lymphocytes that either directly kill the "not self" cell or release lymphokines to attract and activate phagocytes against the "not self" cell. The humoral division, which is the result of B-lymphocyte activity, induces production of antitumor antibodies. The humoral immune response may be stimulated directly by tumor cell antigens or indirectly by the appearance of sensitized T-lymphocytes. Once coated with antibody, the tumor cell—recognized as "not self"—can be engulfed and destroyed by phagocytic cells. Complement fixation of the tumor cell damages the cell membrane and causes cell death. Most solid tumors are relatively unaffected by circulating antibodies and, under some circumstances, it is even possible for the combination of tumor cell antigen and antibody to enhance tumor growth [13].

DEVELOPMENT OF IMMUNE CELLS

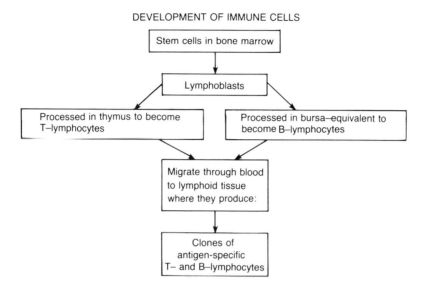

IMMUNE CELL RESPONSE TO ANTIGENS

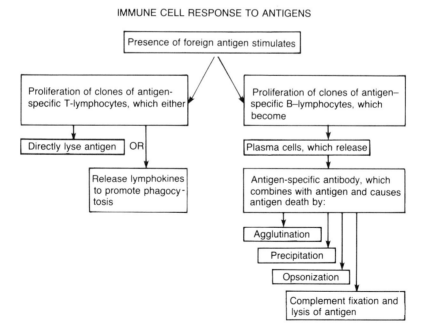

Figure 8.2. Steps in the Immune Process

CONCEPT III:
Based on the identification of tumor-specific or tumor-associated antigens, immunological techniques may be used as diagnostic tools in some malignant diseases since normal adult tissues do not have these antigens (see Table 8.1).

Carcinoembryonic antigen (*CEA*) is a tumor-associated antigen that is associated with colon, stomach, pancreatic, lung, and breast cancers [3, 24]. CEA is often found in small amounts in the serum of persons without any evidence of cancer, but higher levels of the antigen occur in individuals with advanced malignancies. Levels decrease with successful antineoplastic therapy and subsequent tumor regression.

Alpha-fetoprotein (*AFP*) was first observed in the serum of individuals with hepatoma but now is also associated with teratoma-cell malignancy of the ovary and testis [8]. AFP is also often found in small amounts in the serum of persons without any evidence of cancer. Higher levels of AFP occur in individuals with advanced malignancies, and levels decrease with successful antineoplastic therapy and subsequent tumor regression.

Human chorionic gonadotropin (*HCG*) has been found to be significantly elevated in more than 70 percent of persons with pleural and ascitic effusions secondary to choriocarcinoma and ovarian, lung, and breast cancers [9]. *Erythrocyte-rosette-positive T-cell markers* may have value in diagnosing and/or providing prognostic data in persons with common acute lymphocytic disease [3].

Other tumor antigens are being investigated for their usefulness in providing diagnostic and/or prognostic information by acting as tumor markers. *Beta-glucoronidase* and *lactic acid dehydrogenase* (*LAD*) are normal enzymes occurring abnormally in leptomeningeal carcinomatosis. *Colon mucoprotein antigen* (*CMA*) and *colon-specific*

Figure 8.3. Human Malignancies with Demonstrable Tumor Antigenicity [13, 24].

Childhood neuroblastoma
Retinoblastoma
Leukemia
Burkitt's lymphoma
Liposarcoma
Osteogenic sarcoma
Renal cell carcinoma
Wilms' tumor
Malignant melanoma
Basal and squamous cell carcinomas of the skin
Carcinomas of:
  parotid gland
  thyroid
  esophagus
  lung
  breast
  stomach
  colon

antigen (CSPA) are antigens that are apparently specific for colon cancer. *Tennessee antigen (Tennagen)* is a recently discovered glycoprotein associated with colorectal cancers, and *zinc glycinate marker (ZGM)* is a tissue-associated antigen found to correlate with malignancies of the gastrointestinal tract. *Pancreatic oncofetal antigen (POA)* is a fetal protein found to have an apparently high correlation with pancreatic cancer. *Prostate-specific antigen (PSA)* is a newly discovered, highly specific antigenic marker for prostate cancer.

CONCEPT IV:
Although it has not been definitely established that cancer develops as a result of immune system failure, innate or induced immunosuppression may contribute to tumor development.

The theory of immune surveillance states that a person's natural immunity prevents cancer cells from developing into tumors. Development of small numbers of mutated malignant cells may be a common occurrence in most people, but a normally functioning immune system will immediately recognize the abnormal cancer cells as foreign ("not self"). An immune response will then be initiated to destroy the abnormal malignant cells.

Immunodeficiency or immunosuppression may allow proliferation of tumor cells that would have otherwise been destroyed by immune surveillance [8, 13, 27]. Renal transplant recipients, who receive high doses of immunosuppressive medications to prevent cell-mediated rejection of the transplanted kidney, exhibit a very high incidence of cancer. Children with congenital immunosuppressive conditions have a high incidence of malignancy, especially lymphoma. These high risks of cancer may be related to immunosuppression. The kind, duration, and intensity of the immune system dysfunction may be important variables that influence the possible development of malignancy.

The normal immune response can only control tumor growth up to approximately ten million cells [13]. A tumor that is one centimeter in diameter (the smallest size that is usually clinically detectable) represents one billion cells. Therefore, once a tumor can be detected, its growth has far surpassed normal immune system control. At this point, one may safely assume that the immune system has been overwhelmed by the malignancy.

The evidence that a relationship exists between immunity and the development and progression/regression of cancer is growing. There is an increased incidence of malignant disease among persons who are naturally immunodeficient or who have experienced induced immunosuppression [8, 13, 28], and growing tumors apparently suppress the immune response [8, 13, 23, 28]. Persons who are anergic (lack the ability to generate an immune response) have a poorer prognosis and a more rapid tumor growth. The development of rapidly progressive recurrent disease for as long as ten to twenty years after successful initial treatment of a primary tumor strongly suggests that the person's defenses inhibited tumor growth during the disease-free interval. Lymphocytes can infiltrate solid tumors and cause spontaneous remission of the cancer, and metastases sometimes regress after the surgical removal of the primary tumor.

It has also been indicated that a growing solid tumor may shed soluble tumor-associated antigens into the blood. There, they circulate as free antigens or as antigen-antibody complexes. These tumor antigens can inhibit T-lymphocyte destruction of the cancer cells in vitro and may have a similar effect in vivo; this effectively blocks the immune response that might have otherwise destroyed the malignancy. A growing cancer often results in a nonspecific, generalized immunosuppression in the ill person. The extent of the immunosuppression seems to correlate with the amount of tumor burden, and it may be reversed by removal of the growing tumor [27, 37].

CONCEPT V:
Immunotherapy is an attempt to stimulate the person's immune system.

Nonspecific generalized augmentation of the person's immune system can cause tumor destruction, and biochemical alterations of the surfaces of tumor cells may render them more immunogenic (capable of causing an immune response). However, immunotherapy still has a poorly defined role in cancer treatment.

There are several predisposing factors that apparently are necessary in order for immunotherapy to be successful. Tumor cells must have specific cell surface antigens [8]; otherwise, stimulation of the person's immune system will be ineffective. The tumor burden must also be small since the immune response, even under optimal conditions, is not capable of eradicating a large tumor burden [1, 8, 24]. If the tumor burden is large, it must first be reduced to a minimum by surgery, radiotherapy, or chemotherapy. The client must exhibit immunocompetence or exogenous immunity must be provided, and tumor cells must be vulnerable to attack by the immune system.

Generally used as an adjunct treatment, immunotherapy may be used either to stimulate a specific immune response against the malignancy or to produce a generalized enhancement of the client's immune functioning. The conventional treatment modalities serve to decrease the body burden of tumor, and then immunotherapy attempts to stimulate the immune system to kill any remaining malignant cells. Timing of immunotherapy is an important factor in its effectiveness. Concomitant chemotherapy may impair the person's ability to mount an immune response and thus inhibit the immune system.

Specific immunotherapy uses tumor antigens to stimulate a specific immune response against the cancer, turning an "immunological spotlight" on the tumor. The client's general immune function is not necessarily enhanced by this immunological spotlight. Specific immunotherapy uses substances that are antigenically related to the tumor. These include (1) killed tumor cells from the same person or from another person with a similar tumor, (2) tumor cells that have been altered in the laboratory to make them more immunogenic, and (3) antigen preparations extracted from tumor cells. Nonspecific immunotherapy uses a variety of agents to stimulate a general enhancement in overall immune functioning. There are three main classifications of immunotherapy—active, passive, and adoptive—that correlate with the three types of acquired immunity.

CONCEPT VI:
Before immunotherapy is begun, there should be an assessment of the person's immune status through evaluation of skin tests and blood samples [10].

Assessment of the client's immune status is done before initiation of immunotherapy. Baseline data is obtained and the tests are repeated intermittently during immunotherapy to detect any change in immune response. An increase in the client's immune response could indicate a desirable response to immunotherapy, whereas a decrease in immune response may indicate recurrence or progression of the malignancy and a poorer prognosis.

DNCB SKIN TESTS

Skin tests using the agent DNCB (dinitroclorogenzene] will stimulate the cellular immune response in approximately 65 percent of persons with cancer. DNCB 2,000 micrograms is applied on the forearm as a sensitizing dose. Two weeks later, the person's immune memory is challenged by the topical application of three smaller doses of DNCB (100, 50, and 25 micrograms). A delayed hypersensitivity reaction is characterized by erythema and swelling or induration at the original test site. Erythema alone is not a positive reaction. A positive reaction consists of both erythema and induration, and the induration or wheal must be at least five millimeters in diameter. A positive reaction is definite evidence of the person's ability to initiate a specific cellular immune response.

DELAYED SKIN HYPERSENSITIVITY TESTS

Cellular immunocompetence can also be demonstrated by a positive reaction to the intradermal administration of four to six antigens commonly encountered in the environment. These are called delayed skin hypersensitivity tests. Antigenic agents commonly used include:

1. Dermatophytin, a fungus
2. PPD, or the "tuberculin test"
3. Mumps, a virus
4. Streptokinase and/or Streptodornase, enzymes
5. Candida, a fungus
6. A normal saline control

Areas of erythema and induration are measured after twenty-four and forty-eight hours to give an index of the client's immunocompetence. As with DNCB, erythema alone is not a positive reaction. Criteria for positive skin test reactivity are the same as for DNCB testing. Unless the person reacts positively to at least two substances, he or she is considered to be anergic (incapable of mounting a cellular immune response). Anergic clients have a poorer prognosis for their malignancies than do clients who can generate a cellular immune response.

BLOOD TESTS

Evaluation of blood samples will give an index of the client's humoral immunocompetence. Blood tests include (1) total protein, (2) protein electrophoresis, and (3) quantitative immunoglobulin assays.

CONCEPT VII:
In active immunotherapy, antigens are administered in an attempt to stimulate the client's body to produce antibodies or sensitized lymphocytes to destroy the malignancy.

The goal of active immunotherapy is either to elicit a specific immune response against the tumor or to nonspecifically potentiate the client's overall immunocompetence. Thus, active immunotherapy may be either specific or nonspecific in nature.

ACTIVE SPECIFIC IMMUNOTHERAPY

Active specific immunotherapy consists of the administration of tumor-specific or tumor-associated antigens in the form of tumor-cell vaccines [14]. A vaccine is a solution of antigenic material given to stimulate a specific immune response to the tumor cells. The tumor cells used in vaccines are usually irradiated prior to administration to the client in order to prevent subsequent new tumor growth. The vaccines are usually injected intradermally in small doses. Tumor-cell vaccines include (1) autologous vaccine produced from the client's own tumor cells, (2) allogenic vaccine produced from a mixture of tumor cells from people with the same type of cancer, and (3) modified vaccine produced from tumor cells that have been biochemically altered in the laboratory.

ACTIVE NONSPECIFIC IMMUNOTHERAPY

Active nonspecific immunotherapy consists of the administration of antigens other than those prepared from tumor cells and is currently the most widely used form of immunotherapy. Its rationale is that certain bacterial substances can enhance the client's generalized immunocompetence. Although the exact mechanism of action is unknown, active nonspecific immunotherapy seems to increase the person's immunological response to a wide variety of antigens including those produced by cancer [27]. The agents used in this type of immunotherapy are called nonspecific immunopotentiators, meaning that they cause a general enhancement of the immune response.

BCG

BCG (bacillus of Calmette and Guerin) is used in active nonspecific immunotherapy and is the same attenuated form of the living bovine tubercle bacillus (*Mycobacterium bovis*) used to immunize humans against tuberculosis. Investigation of BCG for use in cancer immunotherapy began about twenty years ago when it was observed that children who had been vaccinated against tuberculosis had a decreased incidence of leukemia.

BCG is a potent immunological agent capable of increasing the client's immune responses to a wide variety of tumor-specific antigens [27]. A great part of its immunological activity may be the result of the induction of a local delayed hypersensitivity reaction within the tumor itself. Despite its use in antineoplastic immunotherapy, BCG seems to have no direct antitumor activity itself. Instead, its purpose is to increase the ability of the client's immune system to destroy "not self" malignant cells.

BCG has several profound effects on the macrophages involved in the immune response. Macrophages become more active in engulfing and destroying foreign substances, and the quantity of macrophages is increased. Increased quantities of lymphokines are synthesized and released by the macrophages. In addition, in laboratory tissue cultures, the BCG-activated macrophages will sometimes destroy malignant cells, leaving normal cells unharmed [29].

BCG has been used in the treatment of malignant melanoma. Scarification and intralesional BCG applications have produced regressions of cutaneous but not visceral melanomas; and BCG plus DTIC chemotherapy in persons with levels III, IV, and V melanomas result in significantly fewer relapses and better two-year survival rates. Effective and sometimes prolonged palliation of cutaneous melanoma metastases has been obtained with the use of BCG. Intralesional injection of BCG has resulted in complete tumor regression in up to 90 percent of lesions in immunocompetent clients, and concomitant regression of uninjected nodules located within the same lymphatic region occurs in 15 percent to 20 percent of these individuals [33].

Lung cancer has been treated with BCG. When BCG was instilled intrapleurally in persons with Stage I lung carcinomas, there was a significantly reduced rate of local treatment failure and a significantly increased survival rate (9 recurrences in 22 persons not receiving BCG as opposed to 0 recurrences in 17 persons receiving BCG). However, no difference in local failure or client survival was noted in BCG treatment of more advanced lung carcinomas [25].

BCG has also been used to treat childhood and adult leukemias, Hodgkin's disease, basal and squamous cell skin cancers, certain colorectal cancers, carcinomas of the head and neck, bladder and kidney cancers, and breast cancer. BCG immunotherapy remains an adjunctive antineoplastic treatment for these types of cancer.

Varying strains of BCG are supplied for use and may be administered orally, intravenously, or by intravesical, intradermal, or intralesional injection. BCG may also be administered by scarification which is actually a special type of intradermal application.

Intralesional BCG is not effective in anergic individuals [33] and is associated with more severe toxicities than the other routes of BCG administration. Intradermal injection may be done either by the tine technique or by scarification.

The tine is a square grid with thirty-six prongs and is used to puncture the skin twice. BCG solution is then applied to the broken skin and massaged into the area with the flat edge of a needle since a thorough admixture of blood and BCG will assure adequate uptake of the drug [8]. A cool air flow, such as a hair dryer set on low speed, may be directed to the area until the blood and BCG solution have thickened. The application of some type of occlusive dressing for twenty-four hours will prevent drainage of the BCG solution from the treatment area.

The scarification technique may be used instead of the tine technique to provide intradermal injection of BCG. Prior to scarification, a topical anesthetic should be applied to the treatment site to reduce pain. Scarification consists of a ten-by-ten scratch grid made with the cutting edge of an eighteen-gauge needle at the bevel while holding the skin taut. The needle is held at a forty-five-degree angle, avoiding the point of the needle. Enough pressure must be used to penetrate the intradermal layer of skin and induce slight capillary oozing. Free-flowing bleeding is not desired. BCG is then applied, massaged, and thickened, and an occlusive dressing is applied as in the tine technique. Scarification is usually done at sites of major lymph drainage and generally is restricted to the administration of BCG only. Healing of BCG treatment sites is slow and usually results in a permanent scar.

Adverse local reactions associated with BCG vary with the route of administration, the type of BCG strain, and the strength of the BCG solution. With intradermal administration, local reactions are classified as to type and severe reactions may necessitate a dosage change. A Type-0 reaction consists of a treatment site with no visible change. A Type-1 reaction consists of a small local maculopapular rash without pustules; if pustules are present, the reaction is classified as Type-2. A Type-3 reaction consists of a large local maculopapular rash with pustules, and a Type-4 reaction is characterized by pustules with confluent erythema and swelling. A Type-W reaction consists of open, weeping areas at the treatment site. A Type-R reaction is characterized by a diffuse rash. Type-4, Type-W, and Type-R reactions are considered to be severe reactions.

Intradermal BCG often causes pain at the treatment site, and draining, tender ulcers may form. Although the incidence of infection at the ulcerated sites is low, BCG abscesses may drain for as long as three months.

Intravesical administration of BCG into the bladder may result in hematuria. Intralesional administration may cause severe local abscess formation and severe systemic reactions.

Immunotherapy with BCG may also result in systemic side effects. Shaking chills and fever may occur but usually subside within twelve to forty-eight hours. Flu-like symptoms may occur [10], and regional lymphadenitis is common [10, 27]. Although uncommon, active tuberculosis, a systemic BCG infection, or granulomatous hepatitis may occur. Clients with hepatic dysfunction may exhibit a slight elevation in serum alkaline phosphatase and SGOT [4, 10]. Pancytopenia and osteomyelitis may also occur [17].

The administration of BCG—a protein foreign to the body—may result in an anaphylactic reaction [10, 17, 33]. A mild anaphylactic response is characterized by fever and urticaria. A severe anaphylactic response, however, may be life-threatening and is characterized by dyspnea, cyanosis, hypotension, tachycardia, and seizures. A severe anaphylactic reaction is more common with intravenous BCG.

MER

Active nonspecific immunotherapy includes the use of MER, the methanol-extracted residue of the tubercle bacillus. MER is currently being investigated for use in the treatment of malignant melanoma [14].

Cellular immunity is more profoundly stimulated when MER is given intradermally, although it may also be given by intralesional or intravenous injection. Injections are very painful and a residual stinging sensation may persist for several minutes. MER is also more toxic to surrounding normal tissues than is BCG. The total dose is generally less than 0.5 mg and usually given in increments [8].

Do not dilute the MER until the original solution is thoroughly mixed, thus ensuring accurate dosage. Although either sterile water or sterile normal saline may be used as the diluent for MER, the normal saline is less traumatizing to surrounding tissue and less painful.

Healing of the MER treatment site is very slow and marked scarring occurs. Adverse local, systemic, and anaphylactic side effects similar to those seen with BCG may occur with MER therapy [10]; however, MER will not cause active tuberculosis infections.

Corynebacterium parvum

Active nonspecific immunotherapy includes the use of *Corynebacterium parvum* [8, 27, 29], a bacterial substance. *C. parvum* is given by subcutaneous or intravenous injection, and it has been shown to shrink liver and lung cancers. Side effects are similar to those seen with BCG. *C. parvum* may also cause bronchospasm, hypertension or hypotension, and leukopenia [8].

Levamisole

Active nonspecific immunotherapy includes the use of Levamisole [1, 10, 14]. Levamisole is an anthelmintic drug used in veterinary medicine, and studies in human beings have shown that the drug enhances cellular immunity. Its mechanism of action is thought to be an alteration of nucleotides in lymphocyte membranes. Levamisole is currently under investigation as an antineoplastic treatment for Hodgkin's disease, head and neck cancers, and breast carcinoma. It is administered by mouth every two weeks and is less toxic than BCG, MER, or *C. parvum*. The most common adverse effects of Levamisole are nausea, vomiting, and diarrhea.

Thymosin

Thymosin is a hormone derived from thymus glands of calves and is sometimes used in active nonspecific immunotherapy [1, 10, 14]. It has been shown to increase the number of circulating T-lymphocytes in some people. Clinical trials with Thymosin are being done in clients with disseminated cancers, lung cancers, and cellular immunodeficiency. Local reactions are similar to those seen with BCG. Moderate to severe pruritis at the treatment site often occurs.

NovoPyrexal

NovoPyrexal is a highly purified preparation of *Escherichia coli* used in active nonspecific immunotherapy. It is currently being tested in persons with malignant melanoma. NovoPyrexal is administered intravenously, and systemic reactions similar to those observed with BCG therapy may occur. Hemorrhagic necrosis of normal tissue may also occur after the administration of NovoPyrexal [10].

Interferon

Interferon is a substance produced by human leukocytes when they are infected by a virus. To qualify as interferon, the substance must be a protein that exerts nonspecific antiviral activity in at least homologous cells [29]. The nonspecific antiviral activity must effect cellular metabolic processes involving the synthesis of both RNA and protein. Any protein can be considered to be interferon if it interferes with viruses in a general way through cellular metabolic synthesis of RNA and protein.

Laboratory studies indicate that interferon has an inhibitory effect on DNA and protein synthesis and thus may directly inhibit tumor growth [23]. Interferon is being used as an investigational agent in the treatment of lymphoma and malignant melanoma. It is administered intravenously. Systemic reactions similar to those

Table 8.2.   Nonspecific Immunotherapeutic Agents

Agent	Route of Administration	Adverse Side Effects
BCG	Intradermal -tine technique -scarification Intralesional	Local and systemic reactions
	Intravenous	Anaphylaxis Active TB infection Hepatic dysfunction
	Intravesical	Hematuria Pyuria
	Oral	Nausea, vomiting, diarrhea, mucositis
MER	Intradermal	Local and systemic reactions
	Intravenous	Anaphylaxis
Pseudomonas vaccine	Subcutaneous	Local and systemic reactions
	Intravenous	Anaphylaxis
Mixed bacteria vaccine	Subcutaneous	Local and systemic reactions
	Intravenous	Anaphylaxis
Levamisole	Oral	Nausea, vomiting, diarrhea
Thymosine	Subcutaneous	Local reactions, pruritis
NovoPyrexal	Intravenous	Systemic reactions Hemorrhagic necrosis of normal tissue
Interferon	Intramuscular	Systemic reactions Nausea and vomiting Myelosuppression in 3–10 days
Poly-ICIC	Intravenous	Systemic reactions Nausea and vomiting

seen with BCG may occur, and nausea and vomiting may be seen. Profound myelosuppression in three to ten days often occurs with interferon therapy.

Poly-ICIC

Poly-ICIC is an investigational agent that seems to stimulate the person's own leukocytes to produce interferon [14]. It is administered intravenously and may cause systemic reactions similar to those seen with BCG. Poly-ICIC may also cause nausea and vomiting.

SIDE EFFECTS COMMON TO ALL AGENTS

Active immunotherapy has adverse side effects common to all agents currently being used [8]. Nausea, vomiting, anorexia, fever, and chills are frequent but usually subside within twelve to forty-eight hours. Standard medical and nursing interventions for gastrointestinal dysfunction and fever and chills should be instituted if the client develops these common symptoms.

CONCEPT VIII:
Passive immunotherapy consists of the passive transfer of antitumor immunity from one person to another.

Passive immunotherapy may be achieved by the transfusion of immune serum from another person. The serum contains antitumor antibodies from an individual with cancer that is in remission. The serum is transfused into another cancer client with a growing tumor of the same type. A possible side effect is anaphylaxis secondary to the infusion of foreign proteins [14].

Passive immunotherapy also includes the transfusion of antitumor lymphocytes [8, 14]. The lymphocytes are mechanically separated from other blood components and then sensitized in vitro to the tumor cells. When these sensitized lymphocytes are then transfused intravenously into the client, they should eradicate the malignant cells that have persisted after other modes of therapy have been implemented. This procedure has been used in clients with chronic lymphocytic leukemia, resulting in a temporary decrease in leukemic cells [1].

Passive immunotherapy is used only infrequently, probably because its effects are transient and short-lived. This is because the foreign antibodies and lymphocytes both induce an immune response in the recipient that brings about their own destruction.

CONCEPT IX:
Adoptive immunotherapy consists of the attempt to transfer tumor immunity at the informational level itself, free of foreign cells.

In adoptive immunotherapy, the client accepts passive immunity and then "adopts" and maintains it. It is not known whether the conveyed information is tumor-specific or whether the agents nonspecifically promote some portion of the client's immune system. Unlike intact lymphoid cells, the agents are nonimmuno-genic and thus do not cause an immune response in the client that would destroy them.

Adoptive immunotherapy may be achieved by the infusion of transfer factor. Transfer factor is an extract from human lymphocytes that contains all of the cell's immunological memories [14]. It can be isolated and extracted from the lympho-cytes of cancer clients who are in remission or who have been cured of a specific tumor. This factor may assist a person with the same kind of malignancy to mount a cellular immune attack against the tumor. Transfer factor has been shown to transfer positive skin test reactivity to specific antigens (such as PPD) when pre-pared from the lymphocytes of a skin test-positive person and given to a skin test-negative person [22]. Thus, immune information is transferred from one person to another. Transfer factor seems to affect only cellular immunity with no demonstra-ble effect on antibody production [23].

Adoptive immunity may also be achieved by the infusion of immune-RNA [14, 29]. Immune-RNA can be extracted from lymphocytes that have been sensitized to cancer cells. Immune-RNA carries an immune message that seems to promote an immune response within the recipient. For example, the immune-RNA from lym-phocytes of humans who have been cured of malignant melanoma appears to be able to stimulate the client's own lymphocytes to attack melanoma cells. Thus, immune information is transferred from one person to another.

CONCEPT X:
Although it is unlikely that immunotherapy alone will cure persons with large body burdens of tumor, the future prospects for immunotherapy are exciting.

Immunotherapy may be used more often as an effective adjuvant to on-cologic surgery, especially for clients with metastatic disease. Conservative surgical resection could be employed to decrease the tumor burden followed by postopera-tive immunotherapy to control smaller foci of metastatic disease at distant sites. It is also theoretically possible to develop a vaccine prepared from purified tumor-specific antigens in order to prevent certain types of cancer from developing [26, 28].

HYPERTHERMIA

CONCEPT XI:
Hyperthermia used alone or in combination with radiotherapy is currently an investigational treatment modality.

The use of heat as a treatment for cancer was introduced in the late nine-teenth century [21]. Significant regression of unresectable tumors in clients who had experienced high fevers was reported as early as 1893, and many of the clients survived for quite a long time without recurrence of their widespread cancer [6].

Induced, sustained fevers of more than 39.4° C. (103° F.) apparently resulted in subjective and objective tumor regression [7]. In the 1930s, hyperthermia was again used as a treatment modality by elevating the systemic temperature of thirty-two clients with advanced cancer to 41.5° C. for twenty-four hours, resulting in tumor regression [37].

Between the 1930s and the 1960s, little use was made of hyperthermia. In the 1960s, systemic hyperthermia was induced by placing cancer clients in a paraffin wax bath and administering heated air through an endotracheal tube, raising body temperature to approximately 41.8° C. [32]. Clients tolerated the hyperthermia treatment well and had significant palliation with both clinical and radiological evidence of tumor regression. The most significant tumor regressions occurred in soft tissue sarcomas, gastrointestinal malignancies, and malignant melanomas. In those clients upon which an autopsy was performed after death, tumor necrosis was evident in most sites.

Another group of cancer clients was exposed to local heat plus radiation to the tumor [11]. The exposed tumor was heated by microwave to approximately 60° C. for fifteen minutes. Various doses of radiation were used. Two of the five subjects experienced long-term survival and retained function of the affected area.

In the 1960s, both local and systemic hyperthermia were used to perfuse tumors with blood heated to temperatures up to 43° C. Clients with melanoma of the extremities experienced a 50 percent positive response rate, and tumor control was maintained for periods of seven to twenty-eight months [5].

Since the 1970s, some findings regarding hyperthermia have indicated that it may be an effective antineoplastic treatment. Hyperthermia alone is tumoricidal [5, 20, 21, 36] and can kill tumor cells in vitro. Cell kill seems to be related to the degree of temperature and the duration of the hyperthermia. Temperatures in the range of 42° to 45° C. are apparently cytotoxic with little or no dependence on levels of cellular oxygenation. Systemic hyperthermia with a body temperature between 41.5° C. and 41.8° C. is tolerable and safe, as is local or regional hyperthermia in the range of 38° to 43° C.

CONCEPT XII:
Hyperthermia appears to work in part through inhibition of cellular repair [18].

Selective heat on tumor cells may inhibit repair because of the higher rate of anaerobic metabolism found on the cellular level and/or the subsequent lower pH (increased acidity) within the tumor [5]. Malignant cells are more vulnerable to damage by temperatures in the 42° to 44° C. range than are normal cells [31].

Hyperthermia may be induced by hot water baths, ultrasound, diathermy, microwaves, radio frequency generators, and inhalation of heated air. Localized hyperthermia by intra-arterial perfusion or microwave heating is under investigation.

CONCEPT XIII:
Hyperthermia has been used in conjunction with radiotherapy or chemotherapy because of the synergism that is present when any two treatment modalities are given together.

Clinical results are greater when radiotherapy and hyperthermia are used concurrently, and tumor damage is perhaps twice that of surrounding normal tissues [16]. When heat is applied to growing cells in vitro, the cells become more sensitive to the damaging effects of radiotherapy during the S (synthesis) phase of the cell cycle [35]. One of the greatest reasons for radiotherapy failure is tumor radioresistance, and hyperthermia seems to reduce the tumor's resistance to radiotherapy.

Inhibition of in vivo repair of sublethal damage caused by radiotherapy has also been demonstrated when hyperthermia is added to the treatment protocol [2, 20]. It has been shown, for example, that poorly oxygenated breast cancer cells that are heated become more sensitive to radiotherapy [16]. Although hyperthermic perfusion of melanomas has had inconsistent results, the combination of hyperthermia and radiation has resulted in greater tumor cell kill [19, 33].

Regional hyperthermia combined with chemotherapy is now under investigation in the treatment of melanoma. Prewarmed blood containing melphalan has been perfused regionally into areas of melanoma involvement, raising the skin and muscle temperature of the involved area to 38° to 40° C. The local tumor response rate has been 80 percent as compared to 38 percent with melphalan treatment alone [36].

CONCEPT XIV:
Hyperthermia will be useful clinically only if tumoricidal doses can be tolerated by normal tissues.

Normal tissue tolerance to hyperthermia, especially in the skin and spinal cord, must be carefully documented before hyperthermia will be used more widely. Careful assessment and management of fluid and electrolyte balance is essential, as is the prevention or treatment of hyperuricemia secondary to tumor cell death. The major limitations of hyperthermia at present include knowledge of the fundamental biological phenomena that occur during hyperthermia and the design of adequate equipment to accomplish hyperthermia.

BONE MARROW TRANSPLANTATION

CONCEPT XV:
Bone marrow transplantation involves changing the client's immune status by replacing diseased or deficient bone marrow [15].

Bone marrow transplantation is currently under investigation in persons who have acute leukemia, severe aplastic anemia, and certain immunodeficiency diseases. Because the client must have a matched donor, two tests of histocompatibility are necessary before bone marrow transplantation is initiated. Tissue typing involves matching of antigens that are present on leukocytes and fixed tissue (human leukocyte antigen, or HLA). Since the chance that a sibling has inherited the same configuration of human leukocyte antigen as the client is one in four, siblings are the most common donors. Identical twins are ideal donors. When it is determined that two people have compatible tissue types, they are said to be HLA-matched.

Mixed lymphocyte culture (MLC) is a test of histocompatibility in which T-lymphocytes from both the client and the prospective donor are mixed together. T-lymphocytes are the cells that mediate foreign tissue rejection. If the mixed lymphocyte culture shows no evidence of immune reactivity after seven days, compatibility between the donor and client is confirmed.

CONCEPT XVI:
As with any other organ transplant, the client's tissue rejection potential must be suppressed prior to a bone marrow transplant.

Rejection of foreign tissue is a function of cellular immunity mediated by T-lymphocytes, so suppression of cellular immunity is crucial for a successful bone marrow transplant. High-dose cyclophosphamide (Cytoxan) is the most commonly used agent for immunosuppression, and further immunosuppression can be achieved with whole-body irradiation.

The transplant procedure itself is a simple one. The donor is given general surgical anesthesia, and multiple bone marrow aspirations are taken from the anterior and posterior iliac crests. The risk to the donor is no greater than the risk of receiving general anesthesia. The aspirated donor marrow is then mixed with an anticoagulant and strained to remove fat and bony debris. The strained donor marrow is then infused intravenously into the recipient by a peripheral intravenous line. The cells of the donor bone marrow then migrate from the client's general circulation to the bone marrow spaces by a poorly understood mechanism.

CONCEPT XVII:
Evidence of a successful bone marrow transplant is the presence of leukocyte, erythrocyte, and platelet precursors in the client's bone marrow.

The earliest signs of a successful bone marrow transplant appear one to three weeks after the procedure, and peripheral blood counts do not begin to rise until about four weeks after the transplant. Failure of bone marrow transplantation is infrequent.

CONCEPT XVIII:
Alterations in immune status, vulnerability to infection, bleeding tendencies, and anemia are common sequelae that leave the client at risk until an adequate number of cells are released into the general circulation.

The most common complication is infection. Because of the client's inability to mount an inflammatory response, infections are usually not localized, and even normal flora may cause opportunistic infections because of the client's impaired immunity. Fever, which is a systemic rather than local sign of infection, must be treated aggressively and promptly. Daily infusions of leukocytes may be carried out for suspected infection.

Severe stomatitis may occur secondary to whole body irradiation and leukopenia. Prophylactic mouth care with mycostatin, an antifungal antibiotic, may prevent secondary infection of the mouth. Total parenteral nutrition may be necessary to prevent malnutrition.

Interstitial pneumonia characterized by diffuse pleural infiltrates, hypoxemia, tachypnea, and tachycardia, may cause death after a bone marrow transplant. *Cytomegalovirus* and *pneumocystis carinii* (a protozoan) are the most common pathogens. Many times, however, the disease is idiopathic with no demonstrable cause and so is treated with broad-spectrum antibiotics. Often, the pneumonia is fulminating, rapidly progressive, and fatal before treatment is effective.

Protective isolation with a private room and sterile supplies and equipment may be used to help prevent infection. A laminar air flow unit can provide a continuous flow of sterile air and can remove any airborne pathogens introduced by staff or visitors. All staff and visitors must wear caps, masks, shoe covers, sterile gowns, and gloves, and sterile technique is used for all procedures. A sterile diet is served, and a nonabsorbable oral antibiotic is administered to sterilize the gastrointestinal tract. An antimicrobial agent is used twice daily to bathe the skin and hair. A germ-free state is achieved when cultures of the skin, oropharynx, stool, and external environment are negative. The client must remain in the room unless a portable air-recycling system is available for use.

Minimal infection precautions may also be used after the bone marrow transplant. The client is placed in a private room but other people need not dress in a special manner before entering the room. Clean, rather than sterile, technique is used for procedures, and good handwashing is carried out by all people before contact with the client. A regular diet is served, and routine sterilization of the gastrointestinal tract is not done. Good oral care and body hygiene remains an important nursing consideration. Cultures are performed only when infection is suspected.

CONCEPT XIX:
Graft versus host disease (GVHD) is a common development within two months after the transplant procedure.

Graft versus host disease is a phenomenon that occurs when T-lymphocytes mount a cellular immune response because of the recognition of foreign tissue. GHVD often occurs despite apparent histocompatibility between the donor and recipient. Acute GHVD can range from a mild, self-limiting disease process involving only one organ system to a severe and fulminating multisystem disease that may result in death.

GVHD is characterized by infiltration of skin, liver, and gastrointestinal tract by T-lymphocytes. The skin becomes erythematous with a maculopapular rash on the extremities and/or trunk. Skin involvement may be minor and transient, or it may progress to generalized erythroderma and desquamation (scaling). Liver involvement is characterized by hepatitis-like symptoms with hepatomegaly and an increase in serum bilirubin levels. Gastrointestinal involvement is characterized by mucosal ulceration, nausea, vomiting, diarrhea, abdominal pain, and malabsorption. The disease process may become a chronic and debilitating condition characterized by progressive skin involvement, chronic anorexia, fatigue, episodic diarrhea, and an increased vulnerability to infection.

GVHD is usually treated pharmaceutically in an effort to suppress T-lymphocyte activity. Intravenous methotrexate is administered in scheduled doses after bone marrow transplantation to prevent severe GVHD. When the condition occurs, corticosteroids and antihuman thymocyteglobulin (ATG) are given.

CONCEPT XX:
Clients who are free from complications and who have adequate oral nutrition are discharged from the hospital when blood counts are stable and within normal ranges.

The total leukocyte count must be near normal, and platelet and hemoglobin levels must be self-sustaining. The client must be taught to avoid infections for at least three months. Full maturity of the client's immune system requires approximately one year.

REFERENCES

1. Bakemeier, R. F. Basic Principles of Tumor Immunology and Immunotherapy. In P. Rubin (Ed.). *Clinical Oncology for Medical Students and Physicians: A Multidisciplinary Approach* (5th Ed.). New York: American Cancer Society, 1978. Pp. 320–325.

2. Ben-Hur, E., Elking, M. M., and Burk, B. V. Thermally Enhanced Radio Response of Cultured Chinese Hamster Cells: Inhibition of Repair of Sublethal Damage and Enhancement of Lethal Damage. *Radiat Res* 58:38, 1974.

3. Bowman, W. P., Melvin, S. L., Aur, R. J. A., and Mauer, A. M. A Clinical Perspective on Cell Markers in Acute Lymphocytic Leukemia. *Cancer Res* 41:4794, 1981.

4. Carroll, R. M. BCG Immunotherapy by the Tine Technique: The Nurse's Role. *Cancer Nurs* 1:241, 1978.

5. Cavalierre, R., Ciocatto, E. G., Giovanella, B. C., et al. Selective Heat Senstivity of Cancer Cells: Biochemical and Clinical Studies. *Cancer* 20:1351, 1967.

6. Coley, W. B. The Treatment of Malignant Tumors by Repeated Innoculations of Erysipelas: With a Report of Ten Original Cases. *Am J Med Sci* 105:487, 1893.

7. Coley, W. B. The Therapeutic Value of the Mixed Toxins of the Streptococcus of Erysipelas and Bacillus Prodigeosus in the Treatment of Inoperable Malignant Tumors. *Am J Med Sci* 112:251, 1896.

8. Coral, F. S. A Perspective on Cancer Immunotherapy. In C. J. Kellogg and B. P. Sullivan (Eds.). *Current Perspectives in Oncologic Nursing*, Vol. 2. St. Louis: C. V. Mosby, 1978. Pp. 35–44.

9. Couch, W. D. Combined Effusion Tumor Marker Assay, Carcinoembryonic Antigen (CEA), and Human Chorionic Gonadotropin (HCG) in the Detection of Malignant Tumors. *Cancer* 48:2475, 1981.

10. Cox, K. O. and Ern, M. Immunotherapy II. In F. Pilapel and K. V. Studva (Eds.). *Programmed Instruction: Immunology.* New York: Masson, 1981. Pp. 7–16.

11. Crile, G. Jr. The Effects of Heat and Radiation on Cancers Implanted in the Feet of Mice. *Cancer Res* 23:372, 1963.

12. Ern, M. Immunity: Basic Concepts. In F. Pilapel and K. V. Studva (Eds.). *Programmed Instruction: Immunology.* New York: Masson, 1981. Pp. 7–16.

13. Ern, M. Immunology: Immunity and Cancer. In F. Pilapel and K. V. Studva (Eds.). *Programmed Instruction: Immunology.* New York: Masson, 1981. Pp. 17–25.

14. Ern, M. Immunotherapy I. In F. Pilapel and K. V. Studva (Eds.). *Programmed Instruction: Immunology.* New York: Masson, 1981. Pp. 27–36.

15. Ern, M. Bone Marrow Transplantation. In F. Pilapel and K. V. Studva (Eds.). *Programmed Instruction: Immunology.* New York: Masson, 1981. Pp. 53–66.

16. Hahn, G. M. Metabolic Aspects of the Role of Hyperthermia in Mammalian Cell Inactivation and Their Possible Relevance to Cancer Treatment. *Cancer Res* 34:3117, 1974.

17. Hoogstraten, B. Adjuvant Melanoma Protocol. Southwest Oncology Group Protocol #7521. San Antonio, TX: Southwest Oncology Group, 1976.

18. Kaplan, H. S. Basic Principles in Radiation Oncology. *Cancer* 39:689, 1977.

19. Kim, J., Hahn, E., and Tokita, N. Combination Hyperthermia and Radiation Therapy for Cutaneous Malignant Melanoma. *Cancer* 41:2143, 1978.

20. Leith, J. T., Miller, R. C., Gerner, E. W., and Boone, M. L. M. Hyperthermic Potentiation: Biological Aspects and Application to Radiation Therapy. *Cancer* 39:766, 1977.

21. Manning, M. R. Hyperthermia: Renewed Interest in an Old Treatment for Cancer. In L. C. Kruse, J. L. Reese, and L. K. Hart (Eds.). *Cancer: Pathophysiology, Etiology, and Management.* St. Louis: C. V. Mosby, 1979. Pp. 188–192.

22. McCalla, J. L. Immunotherapy: Concepts and Nursing Implications. *Nurs Clin North Am* 11(1):59, 1976.

23. McKhann, C. Cancer Immunotherapy: A Realistic Appraisal. *CA* 80:286, 1980.

24. McKhann, C. F. and Yarlott, M. A. *Tumor Immunology.* New York: American Cancer Society, 1975.

25. McNeally, M., Mauer, C., and Kausel, H. Regional Immunotherapy of Lung Cancer with Intrapleural BCG. *Lancet* 1:377, 1976.

26. Morton, D. L. Horizons in Tumor Immunology. *Surgery* 74:69, 1973.

27. Morton, D. L. Cancer Immunotherapy: An Overview. In L. C. Kruse, J. L. Reese, and L. K. Hart (Eds.). *Cancer: Pathophysiology, Etiology, and Management.* St. Louis: C. V. Mosby, 1979. Pp. 219–237.

28. Morton, D. L., Eilber, F. R., Holmes, E. C., et al. BCG Immunotherapy of Malignant Melanoma: Summary of a Seven-Year Experience. *Ann Surg* 180:635, 1974.

29. Oppenheimer, S. B. *Cancer: A Biological and Clinical Introduction.* Boston: Allyn and Bacon, 1982.

30. Order, S. E. The Effects of Therapeutic Irradiation on Lymphocytes and Immunity. *Cancer* 39:737, 1977.

31. Patterson, W. B. Principles of Surgical Oncology. In P. Rubin (Ed.). *Clinical Oncology for Medical Students and Physicians: A Multidisciplinary Approach* (5th Ed.). New York: American Cancer Society, 1978. P. 27.

32. Pettigrew, R. T., Galt, J. M., et al. Circulatory and Biochemical Effects of Whole Body Hyperthermia. *Br J Surg* 61:727, 1964.

33. Portlock, C. S. and Goffinet, D. R. *Manual of Clinical Problems in Oncology.* Boston: Little, Brown and Co., 1980.

34. Prehn, R. T. and Main, J. M. Immunity to Methylcholanthrene-induced Sarcomas. *J Natl Cancer Inst* 18:769, 1957.

35. Robinson, J. E., Wizenberg, M. J., and McCready, W. A. Radiation and Hyperthermal Response of Normal Tissue *in situ. Radiology* 113:195, 1974.

36. Stehlin, J. S., Giovanella, B. C., Ipolyi, P. P., Muenz, L. R., and Anderson, R. Results of Hyperthermic Perfusion for Melanoma of the Extremities. *Surg Gynecol Obstet* 140:339, 1975.

37. Warren, S. L. Preliminary Study of the Effect of Artificial Fever Upon Hopeless Tumor Cases. *Am J Roentgenol* 33:75, 1969.

PART III

TREATMENT AND NURSING CARE FOR THE CHILD WITH CANCER

Chapter 9

Cancer in Children

CONCEPT I:
Although cancer remains the number one disease killer among children in the United States, survival rates have increased so significantly that health professionals are beginning to cautiously use the word "cure" regarding certain childhood malignancies.

The outcome for the child with cancer just thirty years ago was abysmal. Every child diagnosed with acute leukemia was dead within a few weeks and the child who survived a solid tumor was rare. Now, however, more than 50 percent of children with leukemia survive five or more years, and survival rates in other pediatric tumors have increased dramatically (see Table 9.1). Thus, although pediatric malignancies still kill more children between the ages of three and fourteen than any other disease (see Figure 9.1), most childhood cancers are no longer considered to be necessarily terminal illnesses. Instead, these malignant diseases in children are considered to be chronic, life-threatening diseases.

CONCEPT II:
Epidemiological patterns of childhood cancer help to identify that part of the pediatric population at risk for developing a malignancy.

INCIDENCE OF CHILDHOOD CANCERS

Every year, approximately 121 white children and 93 black children per one million children in the United States are diagnosed with some form of cancer. Leukemias and lymphomas account for 45 percent of all malignancies in white

Table 9.1. Anticipated Biological Cure Rates of Common Childhood Cancers

Type of Cancer	Anticipated Cure Rate
Acute lymphocytic leukemia [39, 75, 94]	40%–50%
Hodgkin's Disease [17, 75]	70%–80%
Neuroblastoma [42, 78]	30%
Wilms' Tumor [13, 38, 78]	70%–80%
Osteosarcoma [22, 26, 74, 96]	40%
Ewing's Sarcoma [73]	40%
Rhabdomyosarcoma [8, 105]	40%
Retinoblastoma [92]	90%

Figure 9.1. Most Common Childhood Malignancies.
Leukemia
Central Nervous System Tumors
Lymphoma
Neuroblastoma
Wilms' tumor
Bone Tumors
Rhabdomyosarcoma
Retinoblastoma

children and 35 percent of all cancers in black children. Central nervous system tumors and neuroblastomas (tumors of the sympathetic nervous system) are responsible for 26 percent of cancers in white children and 29 percent of cancers in black children [33].

AGE [33]

Forty-one percent of pediatric malignancies occur between birth and age four. Many of the malignancies in this age group are embryonal cell tumors, thus strongly implying that prenatal determinants are involved in carcinogenesis. Examples of these cancers are acute lymphocytic leukemia, neuroblastoma, Wilms' tumor, retinoblastoma, and primary liver cancer—all of which peak in incidence before the age of five.

Other malignancies such as Hodgkin's disease, bone cancers, and acute myelogenous leukemia peak in incidence after the age of five. These data suggest a strong postnatal influence, probably environmental in origin.

The incidence of cancer among children younger than one year of age is 183.4 cases per million children of that age group in the United States. For newborns, cancer incidence is 36.5 cases per million American newborn children. In American children younger than one year of age, the primary malignancies are (in decreasing order) neuroblastoma, leukemia, Wilms' tumor, sarcomas, and tumors of the central nervous system. Two-thirds of these malignancies in this age group are diagnosed by the time the child is one week old.

SEX [33]

In general, cancer is more common among male children than among female children. In the United States, the overall ratio is 1.2 boys to 1 girl.

RACE

With some exceptions, most childhood cancers are equal in relative incidence between whites and nonwhites in the United States. The notable exceptions are acute lymphocytic leukemia, melanoma, and Ewing's sarcoma. White children have an increased overall incidence as compared to the incidence in black children. In addition, acute lymphocytic leukemia exhibits a mortality peak at age four in white children, but no such peak is observed in blacks [109], and black children exhibit a lower incidence of Ewing's sarcoma than do white children [88, 109]. These findings suggest that genetic differences between the two races may result in differences in the child's vulnerability to the development of cancer.

MORTALITY PEAKS

Peaks in mortality occur under the age of five for several of the common childhood tumors, including Wilms' tumor, neuroblastoma, and retinoblastoma, which strengthens the hypothesis that these tumors have a prenatal origin. Peaks in mortality for other childhood tumors occur at later ages, again suggesting post-natal influence [88]. For example, malignant tumors of the bone exhibit a progressive rise in mortality throughout childhood with a pattern closely resembling the age curve for bone growth, suggesting that bone growth rate may be a stimulus for the development of this type of cancer [62].

CONCEPT III:
In attempting to identify etiological factors in the development of childhood cancers, one must remain aware of both prenatal and postnatal influences that may have a carcinogenic effect on the child.

Although most childhood cancers seem to be genetically influenced, environmental agents have been increasingly implicated in causation of the malignancies of childhood. It seems likely that genetic factors interact with environmental stressors to produce cancer in the pediatric population since several cancers have short enough latency periods that diagnosis can be made during childhood, whereas others clinically manifest themselves in adulthood but originate prenatally or during childhood (for example, adult tumors consisting of embryonal cells).

GENETIC FACTORS INFLUENCING CHILDHOOD CARCINOGENESIS

The hypothesis of two mutational events has been proposed to explain both childhood and adult carcinogenesis. This theory postulates that there are two mutational events that are involved in the development of certain childhood cancers. The first mutational event may occur even before conception and "sets the stage" for the development of malignancy by increasing the baby's vulnerability to certain postconception carcinogenic influences. The second mutational event always takes place after conception and is necessary for actual development of the cancer [46]. For example, when retinoblastoma is unilateral and sporadic, it is thought that both mutational events occur after conception; but when the retino-blastoma is familial and/or bilateral, it is hypothesized that the first mutational event occurs before conception and the second mutational event occurs after conception. The two mutational event theory is thought to apply to retinoblastoma, Wilms' tumor [46], pheochromocytoma, and medullary thyroid carcinoma [7].

Genetic, familial, or congenital factors are conspicuous in many childhood malignancies. Genetic factors are secondary to chromosomal mutations. Familial factors refer to a disease or trait occurring in several members of the same family and may be related to environmental, genetic, or unknown stressors. Congenital factors refer to those abnormalities present at birth and may be secondary to environmental, genetic, or unknown stressors. Although there is a considerable body of data linking genetic factors with carcinogenesis in children, it is difficult to definitively separate the roles of the genetic and environmental factors.

Bilateral retinoblastoma is the malignancy of childhood that has most strongly been linked to the transmission of mutated genes. Bilateral retinoblastoma is more likely to be genetically induced than is unilateral disease [65]. If a long-term survivor of bilateral retinoblastoma has children, the tumor will develop in approximately 50 percent of the afflicted parent's children, indicating that the ''cancer gene'' is an autosomal dominant gene [88].

Childhood leukemia is another disease that may be linked to genetic and congenital factors. When an identical twin develops leukemia during infancy, the risk of leukemia to the other twin is nearly 100 percent. The risk to the other twin decreases progressively after one year of age. This age-dependent risk is thought to be attributed to the phenomenon of one twin developing leukemia in utero and subsequently ''passing'' leukemia cells to the other twin through placental vessels [61]. Other genetic links with the subsequent development of childhood leukemia have been proposed. Three classic syndromes, all of which occur because of autosomal recessive traits, have been found to predispose the afflicted child to acute leukemia: ataxia telangiectasia, Fanconi's anemia, and Bloom's syndrome [65]. In addition, Down's syndrome (trisomy-31) has been linked with an excessive risk of subsequent leukemia, with leukemia occurring in these children ten or more times more often than in children without trisomy-31 [88].

Neuroblastoma exhibits its prenatal hereditary origin by its high incidence among the very young (it is the most common tumor in neonates and infants) as well as by its pathology. Neuroblastoma arises from primitive ectoderm tissue that otherwise would differentiate into sympathetic nervous tissue. Although some evidence exists that neuroblastoma may be related to other congenital defects, no definite link between neuroblastoma and other congenital abnormalities has been established. Neuroblastoma is, however, considered to be a hereditary disease [79].

Cryptorchism, a congenital abnormality in which one or both of a male infant's testicles are undescended, affects approximately 2 percent of male babies. These male infants have a thirty-three times greater risk of developing testicular cancer later in life than normal male infants [88].

Wilms' tumor (nephroblastoma) is linked strongly with three congenital urogenital abnormalities: (1) pseudohermaphroditism coupled with a congenital nephron disorder, (2) hemihypertrophy that may affect just one extremity or the tongue and that may be contralateral to the tumor, and (3) visceral cytomegaly syndrome of Wiedeman and Beckwith, consisting of a large tongue, omphalocele, and large viscera secondary to an increase in the number and size of cells [65]. Thus, Wilms' tumor is strongly associated with the concurrent presence of one of three congenital urogenital abnormalities, but the linkage is not clearly understood.

IONIZING RADIATION INFLUENCING CHILDHOOD CARCINOGENESIS

Ionizing radiation is carcinogenic no matter how small the dose [63, 88]. One study illustrates the danger of even maternal medical X-rays on the developing fetus: the study demonstrates an increased incidence of childhood cancers in children born of mothers who had medical X-rays done while they were pregnant. Results of the study allowed the investigators to estimate that, among children who developed cancer, there was a 1.5-fold greater incidence of maternal prenatal X-rays than among the control group [5]. However, it must be pointed out that this effect was not observed among children whose mothers were survivors of the Japanese atomic bomb attack. A large sample of Japanese children who were prenatally exposed to radioactive fallout from the atomic bomb did not show an excess in cancer-related mortality [41]. It has thus been postulated that genetic and environmental influences (such as ionizing radiation) interact in children who have disease conditions characterized by defective repair of DNA, resulting in the development of malignancy.

VIRUSES INFLUENCING CHILDHOOD CARCINOGENESIS

Although viruses have been implicated in carcinogenesis in a number of studies, only one childhood malignancy has been definitely associated with a viral etiology: Burkitt's lymphoma. The Epstein-Barr virus has been positively identified as an etiological factor in the development of Burkitt's lymphoma, but it must be remembered that other environmental factors may also influence development of this childhood malignancy [63, 88]. The phenomenon of clusters of cancer seem to occur by chance, and there is no definitive evidence that any of the cancerous diseases are contagious in the usual sense of the word.

DRUGS INFLUENCING CHILDHOOD CARCINOGENESIS

The discovery that adenocarcinoma of the vagina and/or cervix could be induced by the child's mother's ingestion of diethylstilbestrol (DES) was the first concrete evidence of transplacental chemical carcinogenesis in humans, and DES still remains the only positively identified transplacental carcinogen in humans exposed to the drug in utero [63, 88], but phenytoin is suspected to be a carcinogenic agent with the ability to cross the placental barrier. Other prenatal carcinogenic drug exposures involve the anabolic androgenic steroids used to treat aplastic and Fanconi's anemia, with maternal ingestion of these drugs being associated with primary liver neoplasia [63].

Treatment of the child with immunosuppressive drugs, as in renal transplants, is also associated with an increased risk of development of cancer. The malignancy most commonly associated with immunosuppressive drugs is reticulum cell carcinoma, especially of the brain. Onset of symptoms may occur as soon as three months after the initiation of immunosuppressive therapy [63]. The incidence of reticulum cell carcinoma after immunosuppressive drug therapy is from 150 to 350 times greater than would be expected in the general population [63, 88].

Another class of drugs that are immunosuppressive and carcinogenic are antineoplastic drugs. Children who survive five years or longer after diagnosis and treatment with antineoplastic drugs have twenty times more multiple primary cancers than do the normal population of children [52].

MISCELLANEOUS FACTORS INFLUENCING CHILDHOOD CARCINOGENESIS

Exogenous chemicals, such as pollution and dietary additives, may accumulate throughout the life-span and may contribute to carcinogenesis. These factors may be transplacental and prenatal in nature, or they may be postnatal and exert carcinogenic effects on the child after birth. The exogenous carcinogenic factors now pose a greater threat to the child since chemical and dietary pollution continue to worsen.

THE OVERALL GOAL OF NURSING

Nurses must first minimize the impact of definite or possible carcinogens on the unborn child. Education of pregnant women and women who plan to have children regarding carcinogens that might predispose their child to cancer is a primary nursing function.

CONCEPT IV:
There are certain types of cancer that are peculiar to children and are rarely, if ever, seen in adults.

GRADING OF PEDIATRIC TUMORS [4]

There are many serious problems involved in achieving an effective grading system for pediatric tumors. First, tumors are often not of a uniform grade. Many pediatric solid tumors are complex, mixed, embryonal neoplasms in which there are wide varieties of cell and tissue types within a single tumor. Teratomas, Wilms' tumor, hepatoblastoma, and osteosarcomas are examples of such pediatric malignancies. Second, grading is generally based on very subjective criteria that may vary widely from pathologist to pathologist, and tumor grade cannot be reliably applied except in the context of other prognostic indicators. Finally, tumor structure, and thus its grade, may change over time.

CHILDHOOD LEUKEMIA

Acute leukemia is the most frequently encountered malignancy in children. Before the advent of chemotherapy, leukemic children rarely survived more than two or three months after diagnosis. Now, however, more than 50 percent of children with certain types of leukemia are free of both the disease and its symptoms five years after diagnosis [78], and the word "cure" is beginning to be cautiously used with these children.

Leukemia appears to originate in the bone marrow and is characterized by uncontrollable growth of one of the components of the blood, usually the leukocytes. This overproliferation of the white blood cells results in overcrowding of the bone marrow and inhibition of its normal functioning, causing subsequent anemia, increased vulnerability to infection, and risk of bleeding. Childhood leukemia can invade any organ and is always widespread at time of diagnosis.

Overall incidence of childhood leukemia in the United States is 4.2 white children per 100,000 and 2.4 black children per 100,000. Peak frequency of childhood leukemia occurs at age four. Boys develop acute leukemia more often than do girls, and the male:female ratio continues to increase through puberty [78].

Efforts to determine etiological factors causing leukemia are focused on four broad areas: (1) genetic susceptibility, (2) environmental factors, (3) the role of viruses, and (4) immunological considerations. The idea that some children are genetically predisposed to leukemia is based on four major observations: the occurrence of familial leukemias, the high incidence of leukemia in both individuals of identical twin sets, the apparent increased susceptibility to leukemia in children with certain chromosomal aberrations, and the presence of karyotypic abnormalities in children with leukemia. The focus on environmental factors is based on the increased incidence of leukemia in children exposed to ionizing irradiation and/or certain toxic chemicals (e.g., benzene; antineoplastic chemotherapy, especially the alkylating agents; and either the disease processes of Hodgkin's disease or Wilms' tumor or their treatments). Although there has been no absolute definitive linkage between human leukemia and oncogenic viruses, the role of a viral etiology in human leukemia is being intensively studied. The Epstein-Barr virus, a DNA-virus of the herpes virus group, has been strongly (although not absolutely) implicated in the etiology of human leukemia. There is also a large body of evidence linking leukemia and viruses in animals, although the majority of these leukemia-causing viruses are of the RNA-virus group. Finally, immunodeficiency may be an etiological factor in the development of leukemia. Children with congenital or drug-induced immunodeficiency exhibit an increased risk of leukemia development. It is hypothesized that a breakdown in normal host immunological surveillance may allow a malignancy, such as leukemia, to develop [78]. Defects in delayed hypersensitivity skin tests (which assess the cellular immune system) and decreased immunoglobulin levels (which assess the humoral immune system) have been observed in children newly diagnosed with a certain type of leukemia [36, 47]. However, it is not yet known if these immunological abnormalities precede the development of leukemia or result from malignant involvement of the immune system by leukemic cells.

Clustering of leukemia refers to the appearance of a number of cases of childhood leukemia greater than expected within a given geographic locale and time period. With the exception of the clustering of leukemic children who survived Hiroshima and Nagasaki, most studies have failed to demonstrate any statistically significant clustering of leukemic children [78].

Three major types of leukemia occur among children: acute lymphocytic or lymphoblastic leukemia (ALL), acute myelogenous or nonlymphocytic leukemia (AML or ANLL), and chronic myelogenous leukemia (CML). ALL accounts for 80 percent of childhood leukemias, whereas ANLL and CML are responsible for 18 percent and 2 percent of leukemias in children, respectively [93].

Acute Lymphocytic Leukemia (ALL)

ALL is the most common type of pediatric leukemia. Prognosis for the child with ALL has changed dramatically in just the last three decades. Before the advent of chemotherapy, the child with ALL was dead within a few weeks; but now, approximately 50 percent of these children are disease-free and asymptomatic for five years or more after initiation of medical therapy [93], and the word "cure" is beginning to be cautiously used with these long-term survivors. A method of staging children with ALL has been developed and is predictive of survival.

Signs and symptoms associated with ALL reflect myelosuppression secondary to bone marrow infiltration by leukemic cells as well as to the presence of extramedullary leukemic spread. Common findings include (1) fatigue, pallor, purpura, petechiae, bleeding, and fever secondary to anemia, thrombocytopenia, and dysfunctional white cells; (2) anorexia, malaise, and irritability probably secondary to a general sense of simply feeling unwell; (3) bone pain, especially in the long bones and perhaps accompanied by a limp or an outright refusal to walk, secondary to leukemic infiltration of the joints and/or bone marrow; and (4) lymphadenopathy secondary to extramedullary infiltration. It is rare for the child to present with signs of central nervous system involvement.

Extramedullary infiltration often heralds impending bone marrow relapse. This bone marrow relapse is often due to metastatic seeding of the marrow from the involved extramedullary sites. The most common sites of extramedullary infiltration are the central nervous system, testes, liver, kidney, and spleen. Extramedullary spread can result in lymphadenopathy, splenomegaly, hepatomegaly, and bone tenderness and pain.

Although there is no standard treatment for ALL, combination chemotherapy is the most common treatment modality currently being used. There are four phases of curative chemotherapy for acute leukemia: (1) remission-induction, (2) central nervous system prophylaxis, (3) consolidation therapy, and (4) maintenance therapy. Central nervous system prophylaxis is designed to eradicate leukemic cells that may sequester themselves behind the blood-brain barrier, thus out of reach for most systemically administered chemotherapeutic drugs. Prophylactic or curative treatment of the central nervous system involves the use of cranial irradiation and intrathecal chemotherapy. When cranial irradiation is combined with multiple-drug chemotherapy, approximately half of the treated children remain in remission for five or more years and are at little risk of relapse [75]. Supportive treatment may include any or all of the following: transfusion of red blood cells, leukocytes, or platelets; aggressive diagnosis and treatment of overt or suspected infection; metabolic and nutritional care; pain control; and comprehensive personal-social care. The major cause of treatment failure is bone marrow relapse.

Another aspect to medical treatment of ALL is bone marrow transplantation, usually reserved for those children whose leukemia has been refractory to the more traditional treatment methods. The procedure involves treatment with extremely high doses of chemotherapy plus total whole body irradiation in doses that are lethal to the child's own bone marrow. Subsequent bone marrow rescue is then achieved by the intravenous infusion of bone marrow obtained from a compatible donor. In one series of 110 clients with acute leukemia who were treated with bone marrow transplants, fourteen survived two to seven years postgraft. After two years, there were no leukemic relapses in the survivors, which led the investigators to suggest that bone marrow transplant might eventually lead to cure. The overall one-year survival rate for clients who received bone marrow transplant while in relapse was 25 percent, as compared to a one-year survival rate of 50 percent in clients receiving the transplant while in remission [95]. In another bone marrow transplant study involving 125 children with ALL, there were 28 long-term survivors who experienced no relapse after the transplant. Survival time ranged from ten to ninety-six months, and the median survival time was twenty months [98]. Causes of death in the children who had received bone marrow transplantation included recurrent leukemia, graft-versus-host disease, and infection. Further discussion of bone marrow transplant and appropriate nursing treatment may be found in Chapter 8.

By virtue of the phenomenal increase in survival in children with ALL, late sequelae have become increasingly important in the provision of health care to these children. Rehabilitation of the child with ALL must be focused on mainstreaming him or her into the larger society. Since the general prognosis for children with ALL points to survival rates of more than 50 percent, many leukemic children must reenter a society that still views cancer as a stigmatizing, loathsome disease that carries an automatic death sentence. Thus, incorporation of these children into the larger society has become an increasingly important issue, and acceptance of the child into normal community activities may be threatened by the old obstacles of fear and ignorance.

Acute Myelogenous or Nonlymphocytic Leukemia (AML or ANLL)

These childhood leukemias encompass various subtypes of acute myeloid leukemia, such as acute myelocytic leukemia, myelomonocytic leukemia, monocytic leukemia, progranulocytic leukemia, and acute erythroleukemia. The proliferating cells originate in the bone marrow, and acute myelocytic leukemia is the most common type of ANLL.

ANLL is a rare disease, affecting five children per one million under the age of fifteen. ANLL peaks in frequency during the first two years of life, has a greater incidence among whites than nonwhites, and is thought to be slightly more common in males [104].

Little is known about the etiology or pathology of ANLL. It is possible that genetic factors may interact with environmental factors to produce the disease, a hypothesis partially supported by the high frequency of ANLL in children with certain chromosomal disorders (e.g., Down's syndrome, Fanconi's anemia, and so on) as well as the increased frequency of ANLL in identical twins and other siblings of an afflicted child.

As with ALL, the presenting signs and symptoms of ANLL usually include those reflective of myelosuppression. However, ANLL characteristically exhibits an extremely high white blood cell count. When the serum blast count is greater than 200,000/mm^3, there is significant risk of fatal central nervous system bleeding resulting from plugging of intracerebral capillary lumens at the venous ends. The increased viscosity of the blood and the decreased blood flow may cause rupture of the capillary and subsequent bleeding into the brain. Extreme enlargement of the liver and/or spleen is common, as is extreme lymphadenopathy. Gingival hypertrophy, which occurs in ANLL but not in ALL, is helpful in determining the diagnosis. Meningeal leukemic infiltration is observed more often in ANLL, and bone pain is less common than in ALL.

With ANLL, there may be direct or indirect involvement of the skin. Leukemic infiltration of the cutaneous tissue produces nontender raised nodules. Nonspecific exfoliative dermatitis of an unknown etiology may be a treatment-induced phenomenon. Also of unknown etiology is a febrile neutrophilic dermatosis, characterized by painful indurated plaques on the skin and by fever. Development of this syndrome may be suggestive of systemic infection.

Ocular involvement in ANLL may take several forms. The child may develop retinal hemorrhages or fundal lesions secondary to leukemic infiltration. Fundal lesions are often associated with other central nervous system involvement. Additionally, the child may develop granulocytic sarcoma of the orbit, the dura mater, and/or other head-neck regions. Focal neurological signs accompany invasion of the dura mater, and the painless mass in the head-neck area may compromise the child's ability to breathe or chew.

Abdominal or gastrointestinal symptoms in the child with ANLL may include gastrointestinal bleeding secondary to thrombocytopenia or, rarely, leukemic infiltration. Benign, necrotizing enterocolitis of the terminal ileum or colon may occur, as may perirectal abscess.

Central nervous system signs and symptoms are similar to those seen in ALL, and the incidence of central nervous system involvement in ANLL approaches that observed in ALL. Bone pain accompanied by X-ray evidence of bony involvement is frequent in children with ANLL. Peridontal disease, which may partially be initiated by the gingival hypertrophy common in ANLL, may lead to sepsis if the child is also leukopenic.

Medical treatment for ANLL is, in principle, similar to that given for ALL, but the necessary increased intensity of chemotherapy for ANLL may be life-threatening in itself because of the severe and prolonged suppression of bone marrow function. Preventive cranial irradiation is effective in controlling meningeal infiltration in children with ANLL, but the radiotherapy's effectiveness does not affect overall survival because of the inadequacy of chemotherapy in controlling bone marrow disease [75]. Because of these treatment difficulties, increased supportive care is indicated for children with ANLL. Sooner or later, virtually all children with ANLL become resistant to all medical therapy and subsequently die [104].

Prognosis for the child with ANLL is measured in terms of months rather than years. Survival ranges from 0.9 to 38 months, depending upon the age of the child, clinical condition, and the child's response to treatment [11, 24, 25, 64, 71, 103].

Congenital leukemia is a subtype of ANLL that is present at birth or occurs within the first month. It is a relatively rare disease, and there have been no reports of congenital leukemia occurring in infants of mothers who had leukemia before or during their pregnancies. Congenital leukemia is associated with chromosomal and other congenital abnormalities, most often Down's syndrome [78].

Common presenting signs and symptoms of congenital leukemia are skin lesions of ecchymoses and purpura as well as leukemic infiltration of the skin. Profound hepatosplenomegaly is common, but lymphadenopathy is only infrequently observed. Anemia and leukocytosis are usually present, and respiratory distress is often evident and probably secondary to leukemic infiltration.

Without medical treatment, these infants experience an extremely short survival time, and there are *no* long-term survivors. Even with aggressive chemotherapy, remissions are short-lived and prognosis is extremely poor.

Chronic Myelogenous Leukemia (CML)

CML may occur in adults, older children, infants, or very young children. CML in older children is indistinguishable from that seen in adults. Juvenile CML, which is seen in infants and very young children, differs substantially from the adult type. The incidence of CML is 1 percent to 5 percent of all childhood leukemias [78].

The adult type of CML is the more common of the two among childhood leukemias. Its frequency peaks during adolescence with a male:female ratio of 6:1. A consistent chromosomal abnormality (the so-called "Philadelphia chromosome") has been observed in cells of granulocytic, megakaryocytic, and erythroid lines in clients with CML, adult type [78].

CML, adult type, has an insidious onset. Signs and symptoms may vary widely but the most common presenting manifestations have been identified. The initial leukocytosis commonly seen in all leukemias consists of predominately mature white blood cells in CML. The leukocytosis is profound with this type of leukemia, frequently exceeding 100,000/mm^3, with immature leukocytes taking up less than 10 percent of the circulating white cells. Fatigue and malaise resulting from mild, normocytic, normochromic anemia is common, as is splenomegaly and abdominal protrusion. Thrombocytopenia is uncommon, and some clients actually exhibit a significant increase in the serum platelet count. Hypercellular marrow with a predominance of myeloid cells is accompanied by bone pain owing to the marrow hyperplasia. Pallor, bone tenderness, lymphadenopathy, and hepatosplenomegaly are also common presenting signs and symptoms of CML, adult type.

This disease is characterized by an asymptomatic initial chronic period that is eventually marked by transition to a refractory state characterized by hematological dedifferentiation. This transitional event is frequently heralded by fever, night sweats, weight loss, and organomegaly. Clients with CML usually progress to what is called a "blast crisis" or "acute blastic transformation" [8]. During the blast crisis, there is a rapidly increasing peripheral blast count (immature leukocytes), profound pancytopenia, and rapid clinical deterioration. Blast crisis may occasionally be preceded by extramedullary disease development or by bone marrow evidence of myelofibrosis. The blast crisis is the most serious period of time for the client with CML. It is generally refractory to treatment and is associated with a subsequently poor prognosis. Studies to date indicate that chemotherapy during CML's chronic phase does not alter the seemingly inevitable transformation to the blast crisis [119]. Thus, although CML is treated with intensive chemotherapy, treatment failure resulting from acute blastic transformation (which may not be preventable) is the usual cause of death.

Juvenile CML is substantially different from adult CML in that the former usually involves myelomonocytic cells whereas adult CML is associated with granulocytic cells. The peak incidence occurs during infancy, with almost all cases diagnosed before age five. The male:female ratio for CML, juvenile type, is 2:1. Another significant difference between adult and juvenile CML is that, unlike adult CML, juvenile CML is not associated with the Philadelphia chromosome abnormality [78].

Common presenting signs and symptoms in juvenile CML again reflect bone marrow dysfunction: fatigue, pallor, recurrent infections, eczematoid facial rash, and prominent suppurative lymphadenopathy. Leukocytosis is almost always present, usually at a level less than $100,000/mm^3$. Thrombocytopenia and subsequent recurrent bleeding is also present, and there is an unexplained myeloid and erythroid bone marrow hyperplasia. Splenomegaly is also common, although less frequently observed than in adult CML. Additionally, there is also an unexplained immunological abnormality present in juvenile CML, manifested by an increased level of serum immunoglobulins [119].

Despite the name of the disease, the clinical course is not usually chronic in the common sense but instead is characterized by progressive deterioration. Medical treatment is similar to other types of leukemia, although treatment seems to have minimal effects on the course and severity of the disease. Treatment failure and resulting death is due to erythroid hyperplasia of the bone marrow rather than the terminal blast crisis associated with adult CML. Median survival time of children with juvenile CML is less than nine months [78].

SOLID TUMORS OF THE CENTRAL NERVOUS SYSTEM

Primary tumors of the central nervous system are the most common solid tumors and the second most common malignancy in children, with leukemia being twice as frequent and lymphoma half as frequent. The most common types of primary central nervous system tumors in children are astrocytoma, other gliomas, medulloblastoma, and ependymoma. In all four types, males outnumber females in disease frequency. There is a wide variety of histological, anatomical, and biological aspects within the spectrum of central nervous system solid tumors. In brain neoplasms—whether benign or malignant—even relatively small masses constitute a lethal tumor burden. Although children and especially infants have an amazing capacity to adapt to space-occupying intracranial lesions because of the relative flexibility of the cranium and nonunion of the sutures [49], a supratentorial lesion of 10^{11} cells (approximately 100 grams) is lethal and approximately one to three times 10^{11} cells is a deadly posterior fossa mass. If, however, a tumor impinges upon important areas of the brain, a tumor as small as 10^9 cells may be a fatal tumor burden. Diagnosis of a central nervous system tumor is accomplished by a neurological examination and a CT scan. The incidence of primary brain tumors in children is 6.5 per 100,000 children up to the age of fourteen, or about 21 percent of all childhood cancers [102].

Because of the child's greater flexibility in cranial bony structure, focal signs and symptoms are often preceded by the general neurological symptoms of malaise, failure to thrive, irritability, vomiting, ataxia, and clumsiness [107, 108]. Focal signs and/or a significant increase in head size will not appear until there is a sudden partial or complete blockage of cerebrospinal fluid flow through the ventricles or subarachnoid spaces [56].

Medical treatment of primary brain tumors includes all three traditional treatment modalities: surgery, radiotherapy, and chemotherapy. Surgical goals are threefold: (1) to establish the diagnosis by brain biopsy, if possible, (2) to totally remove those tumors that are accessible and that have good operative prognoses, and (3) decompression of the brain. It is virtually impossible to achieve total surgical removal of astrocytomas and gliomas, and even debulking operations leave behind enough cells for tumor regrowth. Thus, surgical goals for these tumor types are (1) control of intracranial pressure, (2) reduction of the child's tumor burden, and (3) maintenance of the child's neurological functioning for as long as possible.

The use of ventricular shunts in children with brain tumors has generated much controversy in the literature. Proponents of ventricular shunts state that they are useful in the control of most cases of obstructive hydrocephalus resulting from tumor pressure and that shunts allow the child to achieve proper fluid and electrolyte balance and nutritional stabilization, especially before extensive neurosurgery. Opponents state that permanent shunts are not indicated except in cases of postoperative increased intracranial pressure or hydrocephalus, basing their opposition on the evidence that the use of shunts to control cerebrospinal fluid pressure may result in seeding of the peritoneal cavity with tumor cells.

Medical treatment also includes fractionated radiotherapy, the site and dosage varying with the type, location, and size of the tumor. Chemotherapy is only sporadically used because of the number of problems that are encountered. Because of the blood-brain barrier, most systemic chemotherapy cannot reach the tumor in appropriate concentrations. Even when given intrathecally, unacceptable toxicities of the chemotherapeutic drug frequently occur not far from the dose where slight therapeutic effects are seen. Corticosteroids are much safer to use for the child with a brain tumor and may have a direct oncolytic effect as well as having a definite effect in controlling cerebral edema.

Prognosis for the child with a primary brain tumor varies according to the type of tumor, size, and location, but the overall prognosis is not good. With brain tumors, there has not been the dramatic increase in survival rates that has been seen with other childhood cancers.

LYMPHOMA IN CHILDREN

Lymphoma, or cancer of the lymphoreticular system, has a narrow range of types in children. Childhood lymphoma is never of the nodular type that may be seen in adults. The primary lymph organs, which are the bone marrow and thymus, are responsible for differentiation of stem cells, thus replenishing the cells of the immune system. Secondary lymph organs, which are the spleen and lymph nodes, provide sites for the augmentation of the immune response. Because all bodily tissues require surveillance by lymphocytes, there is considerable blurring of the relationship between the type of lymphoma and the anatomical origin of the involved overproliferating cell. The bone marrow is an extremely complex organ containing both lymphoid and hematopoietic stem cells. Thus, the primary difference between childhood leukemia and lymphoma is the type of cell that is overproliferating rather than the exact intravascular or extravascular location of the disease.

There are a variety of different types of lymphoma, depending on the type of cell involved. Hodgkin's disease is the most common type seen in the pediatric population. Childhood lymphoma, far from having an indolent clinical course, is almost always rapidly progressive. Incidence of the disease is markedly age-dependent, with a peak generally under twenty years of age. Lymphoma in general is much more common in adults. Lymphoma probably results from either an increased proliferation or increased life-span of lymphocytes, and immunodeficiency appears to have a major role in lymphoma's etiology [53].

Malignant lymphoma cells will initially cluster in the same anatomical location as would the equivalent normal cell type, thus presenting signs and symptoms are variable. The predominant malignant cells are almost always immature.

Hodgkin's Disease

Hodgkin's disease is relatively uncommon among children in America, although it is the most common type of childhood lymphoma. Males outnumber females between ages five and eleven by a ratio of 3:1. There is a progressive decline in the sex ratio until the age of seventeen, when the adult ratio of 1.5 males:1 female is reached and maintained [60]. In the Hodgkin's disease of childhood, radiotherapy may effect a cure for clients with Stages I-A, II-A, and III-A disease, and radiotherapy contributes to the chemotherapeutic treatment of more advanced disease.

Non-Hodgkin's Lymphoma

Non-Hodgkin's lymphoma is vastly different in children than in adults. In children, this disease is almost always diffuse and poorly differentiated with a much higher rate of bone marrow spread than is seen in adults. Primary anatomical sites in children are usually the mediastinum and abdomen [106].

With intensive chemotherapy, the majority of afflicted children can have the disease eradicated and achieve long-term remission. Thus, the prognosis for non-Hodgkin's lymphoma in the pediatric population is good.

There are several subtypes of non-Hodgkin's lymphoma, primarily undifferentiated Burkitt's lymphoma (see the next section of this chapter), undifferentiated lymphoblastic lymphoma, histiocytic or immunoblastic lymphoma, and diffuse poorly differentiated lymphoma. The first subtype, undifferentiated Burkitt's lymphoma, involves malignant cells of B-cell derivation and is highly malignant with a generally poor prognosis. It accounts for about 3 percent of non-Hodgkin's lymphoma in the United States, making it a relatively rare neoplasm. In undifferentiated lymphoblastic lymphoma, the malignant cell is of T-cell derivation and is commonly associated with the development of a mediastinal mass, especially in adolescent males. This subtype has early and frequent spread to the bone marrow and central nervous system. Diffuse poorly differentiated lymphoma demonstrates a larger incidence among the pediatric population than any of the other subtypes of non-Hodgkin's lymphoma.

Burkitt's Lymphoma

Burkitt's lymphoma, a type of non-Hodgkin's lymphoma, represents the proliferation of clones of immunocytes that underwent malignant transformation at a particular stage of differentiation or activation [90], and is a malignancy involving B-lymphocytes. The Epstein-Barr virus, which causes mononucleosis, is highly suspected as an etiological agent in the development of Burkitt's lymphoma [23, 110]. It is thought that the Epstein-Barr virus selectively infects B-cells and is associated with nasopharyngeal carcinoma in humans and Burkitt's lymphoma in older children. Normally, suppressor T-lymphocytes control B-cell proliferation and neoplasia does not develop. Burkitt's lymphoma is thought to occur when a B-cell clone escapes immunological surveillance by suppressor T-cells. The relationship between the Epstein-Barr virus and Burkitt's lymphoma provides compelling evidence for a link between viral infection and human cancer.

Classic symptomatology of Burkitt's lymphoma includes a distinct syndrome of large, extranodal tumors affecting the bones of the jaw and the abdominal viscera, primarily the ovaries, kidneys, and retroperitoneal structures. Involvement of the bone marrow, lymph nodes, lungs, mediastinum, liver, and spleen is rare. Paraplegia may result from retroperitoneal or extradural tumors either because of vascular compromise or direct spinal cord involvement. Involvement of the central nervous system is rarely the presenting sign of Burkitt's lymphoma but becomes an increasingly common manifestation characteristic of relapse [111]. Cranial neuropathy and malignant involvement with cancerous cells in the central nervous system are usually the presenting signs of central nervous system involvement.

The mean age for Burkitt's lymphoma was eleven years in one study. The majority of children in the study had intra-abdominal tumors, and the most frequent presentation was either intestinal obstruction or abdominal mass [2].

Burkitt's lymphoma is the fastest growing human tumor with a potential cell doubling time of twenty-four hours. Because of this rapid growth, persons with Burkitt's lymphoma often present with an emergency situation with the fast-growing tumor obstructing the airway, intestines, or ureters. The emergency situation may also be one of increased serum uric acid and subsequent urate nephropathy resulting from the excessive tumor growth.

Because of the fast tumor growth that is characteristic of Burkitt's lymphoma, there is little time for a leisurely medical workup, and the staging workup should be completed within twenty-four to forty-eight hours. Medical treatment is focused on (1) debulking surgery to rid the child, even if temporarily, of the mass of rapidly proliferating tumor cells and (2) early achievement of metabolic stability, especially control of serum uric acid. Medical treatment of choice for Burkitt's lymphoma consists of surgical debulking followed by aggressive systemic chemotherapy. Precise identification of every tumor site is not necessary, since that may take an inordinate amount of time. Radiotherapy is not usually used as a primary or sole treatment modality, and even its role as an adjuvant treatment is unclear. Lack of success of radiotherapy is attributed to the rapidity of tumor growth.

Aggressive prophylactic intrathecal chemotherapy with or without high-dose methotrexate is used to prevent central nervous system relapse. The same therapy is also successful if there is actual involvement of the central nervous system.

Burkitt's lymphoma has an unusual relapse pattern with both early and late peaks of relapse. Early relapse occurs within three months of diagnosis and is characterized by tumor regrowth in the original sites. There is a high incidence of central nervous system involvement in early relapse, and prognosis is poor with a usually relentless downhill course. Early relapse represents clones of inadequately treated or drug-resistant tumor cells from the original tumor mass.

Late relapse occurs between three months and ten years after initial treatment and is characterized by tumors in new, previously uninvolved sites. Central nervous system involvement is infrequent, and children respond readily to reinduction chemotherapy. The second remission is frequently prolonged, and thus the prognosis is better. Late relapses are usually observed with Epstein-Barr-positive tumors.

Maintenance chemotherapy for Burkitt's lymphoma is a subject of much controversy. The general opinion is that chemotherapy can be safely terminated after one year if remission has been achieved [110].

Tumor-directed host immunity may be partially responsible for prolonged remissions. However, two early trials of BCG immunotherapy have shown no clinical evidence of significant effect on duration of remission or on survival [31, 54].

Overall prognosis for children with Burkitt's lymphoma is fairly good, with an overall survival rate of 70 percent. The disease rarely recurs after complete remission lasts beyond one year. Children who fail to respond to prompt diagnosis, careful medical/nursing management, and aggressive chemotherapy usually die within the first several months despite continued chemotherapy. Early death may also be attributed to fatal sequelae of rapidly growing or very large tumors, such as acute airway obstruction, bilateral ureteral obstruction, or intestinal obstruction. Metabolic abnormalities, especially hyperuricemia, may also contribute to early death [110].

NEUROBLASTOMA

Neuroblastoma is the most frequently diagnosed malignant tumor in children under one year of age, and more than 80 percent of cases occur in children less than five years old [33]. Neuroblastoma is a tumor of the sympathetic nervous system, arising from primitive neurectoderm that otherwise would have become normal sympathetic nervous tissue. This, plus the early age of incidence, points to its probable prenatal origin. The tumor is slightly more frequent in males than in females, and nonwhite children develop neuroblastoma less frequently than do white children. Approximately two-thirds of children have demonstrable metastases at diagnosis, most commonly in the liver, long bones, and skull. The annual death rate from neuroblastoma in the United States is about ten per million for children up to four years of age, four per million for children aged five to nine, and one per million for children aged ten to fourteen, showing a broad mortality peak before age five and a progressive decline thereafter [79].

Three cell types of neuroblastoma have been identified: neuroblastoma, ganglioneuroblastoma, and ganglioneuroma. Neuroblastomas are the most malignant of the three types and consist of very primitive cancerous cells. They may be encapsulated or, when very invasive, soft with poorly defined edges. Neuroblastomas are often characterized by hemorrhage, cyst formation, and necrosis. Ganglioneuroblastomas may have extremely primitive cells and more differentiated cells within the same tumor. Ganglioneuroblastomas have the potential for invasion and are capable of metastasis. Ganglioneuromas are the most benign of all three types of neuroblastoma. Ganglioneuromas are composed primarily of mature ganglion cells and nerve fibers, and this tumor usually does not metastasize. Instead, ganglioneuromas may cause symptoms merely by compression of surrounding structures.

The etiology of neuroblastoma is uncertain. Although some evidence exists, there is no definite relationship with other congenital defects, and it is not considered to be a hereditary disease.

Signs and symptoms vary widely since the tumor may arise at any point along the course of the sympathetic nervous system. The most common presenting sign is an abdominal mass, appearing in about 65 percent of cases. Primary abdominal disease is usually retroperitoneal, involving the adrenal glands, although the abdominal mass may be due to liver metastases from a primary tumor at another site. Extrinsic compression of intra-abdominal structures, such as the bowel and bladder, may cause other abdominal signs and symptoms. Intractable diarrhea is thought to result from the production of vasoactive intestinal peptides by neuroblastoma cells and may resolve with the removal of the tumor. If the primary tumor is in the chest, it is usually located in the posterior-superior mediastinum, and clinical manifestations are secondary to the compression of vital structures (trachea, bronchi, lymphatics, or mediastinal vessels). The tumor may also involve areas of the central nervous system, producing signs and symptoms. Paravertebral tumors may result in nerve root and plexi compression, whereas invasive vertebral tumors may cause spinal cord compression and subsequent paraplegia. Bone pain is generally negligible; if present, it is often secondary to pathological fractures. An enlarging head in infants indicates skull involvement with widening of the cranial sutures. Bone marrow metastases occur in approximately 50 percent of children with neuroblastoma, producing anemia and either thrombocythemia or thrombocytopenia. Generalized common symptoms are weight loss, fatigue, irritability, and lymphadenopathy.

Signs and symptoms of metastatic neuroblastoma may be observed in tumor involvement of the skin and soft tissues. Cutaneous manifestations of neuroblastoma include firm and nontender subcutaneous nodules that are bluish in color. Compression of these nodules results in an erythematous flush followed by localized blanching, probably secondary to catecholamine release into surrounding tissues. Soft-tissue involvement is usually manifested by periorbital edema and ecchymoses. See Table 9.2 for one method of staging neuroblastoma.

Of all malignant tumors, neuroblastoma has the highest rate of spontaneous remission. This phenomenon is usually seen in children under two years of age with

Stages I and II disease. This remission constitutes an actual spontaneous disappearance of the tumor, not merely a change in cell type or shrinkage of the tumor mass. Needless to say, the mechanism for this phenomenon is unknown.

Neuroblastomas synthesize and metabolize catecholamines, which explains the high frequency of catecholamines and their precursors in the urine of children with this tumor [79]. Tumor regression, whether spontaneous or treatment-induced, can thus easily be monitored by the measurement of catecholamine precursors or products of catecholamine degradation (VMA, HVA) in the child's urine.

Medical treatment of neuroblastoma utilizes a variety of methods. Surgery has five major goals: (1) establishment of diagnosis by biopsy, (2) exploration for an occult primary tumor, (3) staging, (4) placement of silver clips for the design of radiotherapy ports and for following treatment response, and (5) debulking or complete tumor resection. With Stages I and II disease, tumor resection produces two-year survivals of 95 percent [79].

Radiotherapy is useful because neuroblastoma is a relatively radiosensitive tumor. Radiotherapy, however, is not the primary treatment modality for neuroblastoma because of its relatively high incidence of distant dissemination at the time of diagnosis. Radiotherapy has a useful place in the treatment of emergency situations such as spinal cord compression or respiratory distress secondary to mediastinal disease.

Chemotherapy may also be used in the treatment of neuroblastoma. As with other childhood cancers, combination chemotherapy is more effective than the use of a single agent. In children with resectable Stage I-III tumors, chemotherapy seems to provide no additional benefit. However, in Stage IV disease, there is some palliative benefit from chemotherapy, although there is no change in survival statistics [79].

Immunotherapy with BCG and MER is being investigated. However, immunotherapy is not currently a widespread treatment modality for neuroblastoma.

Prognosis for neuroblastoma is highly dependent upon the age of the child. Infants have almost 100 percent survival following therapy, even if metastases are present, and children under one year of age have a 60 percent to 65 percent chance of cure. On the other hand, children older than two years have only a 15 percent survival rate, partly owing to the larger proportion of Stage IV disease at the time of diagnosis in this age group [81].

Wilms' Tumor

Wilms' tumor is a malignant childhood tumor of the kidney, sometimes called nephroblastoma. The tumor is usually unilateral, and bilateral tumors are rare. Median age at diagnosis is between three and four years [14, 33], with an incidence of 10 to 15 cases for every 100,000 children younger than age fifteen [14]. Black children are more likely to develop Wilms' tumor than are white children.

The etiology of Wilms' tumor is uncertain, although it is seen excessively in children with one of three other congenital urogenital malformations: (1) pseudohermaphroditism and a congenital nephron disorder; (2) hemihypertrophy, which may affect just one extremity or the tongue and is often contralateral to the tumor; and (3) visceral cytomegaly syndrome of Wiedemann and Beckwith, consisting of a large tongue, omphalocele, and a large viscera secondary to cells that are increased both in size and in number.

The most common manifestation of Wilms' tumor is an abdominal mass that is smooth to palpation and confined to one side of the abdomen. Most children have few, if any, other signs or symptoms besides the abdominal mass itself. Distortion of the kidney's collecting system may occur; and, if extreme, this may cause a flank mass, anemia, fever, and hypertension. Abdominal pain and hematuria may occur. Bone metastases are almost never seen at the time of diagnosis.

Surgery is the primary medical treatment for the primary tumor. It is crucial that the surgeon litigate the renal veins before resecting the tumor in order to avoid spread of microscopic malignant cells. It is also important during surgery to avoid tumor rupture and intraperitoneal spillage.

Surgery is often followed by radiotherapy to the area of the primary tumor as well as to any areas of metastasis. In one five-year study of thirty-two children with Wilms' tumor, radiotherapy was shown to be uniformly effective in the prevention of local relapse in unilateral disease [10]. Chemotherapy is primarily used for metastatic disease or for preventing recurrence.

Late sequelae of medical treatment for Wilms' tumor can be attributed to the use of radiotherapy [14]. The most pronounced late effect of treatment involves the hematopoietic system, with hematopoietic toxicity seen between the first and sixth week. Hematological adverse effects are more common in infants and are worsened by the treatment combination of radiotherapy and chemotherapy. Although the most common effect consists of leukopenia and thrombocytopenia, major drops in levels of white blood cells and platelets are not frequently seen. Secondary malignancies and other dysfunctions secondary to radiotherapy may occur in the liver and lungs and is relative to the volume of tissue that is irradiated and the dose delivered. Scoliosis, which is usually subclinical, may develop secondary to the effects of radiotherapy on growing tissues. Infertility, teratogenesis, and genetic abnormalities may occur secondary to gonadal irradiation.

The prognosis in Wilms' tumor is excellent. A death rate of 90 percent in 1920 has changed to a survival rate of 90 percent in 1980 [14]. Even with children whose primary tumor has spread beyond the original site (but with no distant metastases), there is a 90 percent survival rate at two years if optimal medical and nursing therapies have been administered [99].

BONE SARCOMA

The two most common childhood sarcomas of the bone are osteosarcoma and Ewing's sarcoma. Prognosis for both types of bone sarcomas is good, with a two-year disease-free survival rate of over 80 percent for osteosarcoma and over 75 percent for Ewing's sarcoma [86]. Mortality rates for both osteosarcoma and Ewing's sarcoma rise progressively until age fifteen to eighteen, after which there is a sharp drop [33]. Medical treatment for both types of bone sarcomas commonly consists of preoperative chemotherapy (high-dose methotrexate with leucovorin

Table 9.2.   A Staging Format for Neuroblastoma [66]

Pretreatment Clinical Staging—TNM System	
TX	Inadequate Information
T0	Primary Site Not Detected
T1	Primary Site Less Than 5 Cm. in Diameter
T2	Primary Site 5–10 Cm. in Diameter
T3	Primary Site More Than 10 Cm. in Diameter
T4	Multicentric Tumors
Corresponding Traditional Staging of Pretreatment Disease	
CS I	Primary Tumor Less Than 5 Cm. in Diameter, Normal Nodes $(T_1N_xN_0M_0)$
CS II	Primary Tumor 5–10 Cm. in Diameter, Normal Nodes $(T_2N_xN_0M_0)$
CS III	Primary Tumor More Than 10 Cm. in Diameter or Tumor with Suspected Nodal Involvement $(T_3N_xN_0M_0$ or $T_1T_2N_1M_0)$
CS IV	Metastatic Disease $(T_xT_0T_1T_2T_3N_xN_0N_1M_1)$
CS V	Multicentric Tumors $(T_5$ any NM)
Postsurgical-Histopathological Staging—TNM System	
PTX	Inadequate Information
PT0	Primary Site Not Established
PT1	Complete Excision, Histologically Confirmed
PT3A	Microscopic Residual Tumor Left After Excision
PT3B	Macroscopic Residual Tumor Left After Excision
PT5	Multicentric Tumors
PNX	Inadequate Information
PN0	Sampled Lymph Nodes Negative
PN1	Lymph Nodes Positive, Complete Resected
PN2	Lymph Nodes Positive, Incompletely Resected
PMX	Inadequate Information
PM0	No Metastases Demonstrated At Time of Surgery
PM1	Metastatic Disease Confirmed or Found at Surgery
Corresponding Traditional Staging, Postsurgical-Histopathological	
PS I	Primary Tumor Completely Resected, Lymph Nodes Negative $(PT_1PN_xPN_1PM_0)$
PS II	Primary Tumor Completely Resected, Lymph Nodes Positive $(PT_1PN_1PM_0)$
PS IIIA	Incomplete Resection of Primary Tumor with Microscopic Residual Tumor Left Behind $(PT_{3A}PN_xPN_0PN_1)$
PS IIIB	Incomplete Resection of Primary Tumor with Macroscopic Residual Tumor Left Behind $(PT_{3B}PN_xPN_0PN_1)$
PS IV	Metastatic Disease (Any PT $PN_1PM_1)$
PS V	Multicentric Tumors $(PT_3$Any PN, PM)

rescue plus Adriamycin) followed by local therapy, which may be an en bloc surgical resection, amputation, and/or radiotherapy.

Osteosarcoma

Another name for this bone cancer is osteogenic sarcoma. It is a malignant neoplasm characterized by osteoid formation from malignant stromal cells in the bone. It is the sixth most common malignancy in children under age fifteen, and the third most common tumor in adolescence. The growth spurt of adolescence is a peak time for the development of osteosarcoma. Males are slightly more affected than females [6].

There are three primary etiological factors related to the development of osteosarcoma: rate of bone growth, genetic and congenital factors, and environmental factors. First, there is an apparent relationship between the development of osteosarcoma and the child's rate of bone growth. The most frequent sites for osteosarcoma are the most rapidly growing ends of the most rapidly growing bones—sites of increased cellular activity—with increased incidence of the disease during the adolescent growth spurt. Second, genetic and congenital factors seem to have etiological significance. The disease seems to be familial. Also, there is a definite relationship between the presence of retinoblastoma and the subsequent development of osteosarcoma. Children with retinoblastoma have a 500-times greater risk for the development of osteosarcoma than do children without bilateral retinoblastoma. Additionally, the child who receives radiotherapy for retinoblastoma carries a high risk for the subsequent development of orbital osteosarcoma. Relationship among these genetic and congenital factors is not clear. Finally, environmental factors appear to be of etiological significance in this disease. Although no RNA- or DNA-virus has been reproducibly isolated from human osteosarcoma, evidence does point toward a viral etiology. Ionizing radiation may be another environmental factor in the development of osteosarcoma, as the tumor may arise in previously irradiated bone [6].

Half of all osteosarcomas are located in the upper leg above the knee. The child may complain of pain and swelling may appear, but neither manifestation can be linked to an obvious traumatic cause. Occasionally, erythema, tenderness, warmth, and limitation of movement in the adjacent joint may occur, and pathological fractures may precede diagnosis. Systemic manifestations of osteosarcoma are rare, and laboratory findings are usually unremarkable except for an occasional rise in serum alkaline phosphatase.

Osteosarcoma classically arises in the central portion of the bone, destroying the cortex and invading surrounding tissues. The lungs, other areas of bone, pleura, lymph nodes, pericardium, kidney, brain, and adrenal glands are frequent sites of metastatic disease. The average duration of symptoms before diagnosis is three months, and 10 percent to 20 percent of the afflicted children have metastatic disease at the time of diagnosis [6].

Medical treatment currently focuses on preoperative chemotherapy with high-dose methotrexate with leucovorin rescue plus Adriamycin. This preoperative chemotherapeutic regimen may, however, be replaced by radiotherapy followed by intra-arterial chemotherapy. This preoperative therapy is then followed by en bloc tumor resection and replacement of the bone with a prosthesis. Long-term results of the latter treatment method are not yet known.

Ablation of the tumor by amputation is still widely used for osteosarcoma, usually with those children who have no demonstrable metastases at the time of diagnosis. However, in approximately 50 percent of those children with no detectable metastases who had their tumor totally removed by amputation, pulmonary metastases appeared within six to ten months after amputation and death occurred within twelve to fifteen months [6]. Since amputation has not proven to be a highly successful mode of treatment and since it causes considerable rehabilitation problems, the "bone-sparing" treatment of preoperative chemotherapy or radio-therapy followed by en bloc resection and bone prosthesis is being looked upon with increasing favor.

The role of radiotherapy alone as a medical treatment for osteosarcoma is limited to those children whose tumor is inoperable because of site (skull, pelvis, ribs) and who demonstrate metastatic disease at the time of diagnosis. Osteosarcoma is a relatively radioresistant tumor, and a tumoricidal dose ranges from 6,000 to 12,000 rad. Thus, much damage can be done by this high dose of irradiation to surround-ing vital structures [6, 97].

Chemotherapy may also be used as an adjuvant treatment for micrometastases. There have been disappointing results when chemotherapy has been utilized as the sole treatment modality. Immunotherapy has also been disappointing in the treat-ment of this disease.

Prognosis is generally fairly poor for children with osteosarcoma. The five-year disease-free survival in children without initial overt metastases is less than 20 per-cent, and survival is rare when nodal involvement is present [6].

Ewing's Sarcoma [28]

Ewing's sarcoma is a relatively rare neoplasm, accounting for 10 percent of all childhood bone cancers. The tumor usually occurs in bone tissue, although a variant of Ewing's sarcoma arises in soft tissue. Ewing's sarcoma, unlike osteosar-coma, is not characterized by osteoid formation. The tumor frequently has areas of blood vessels, hemorrhage, and necrosis. Ewing's sarcoma characteristically arises in the midshaft region of long bones and in flat bone rather than the growing ends of long bones where osteosarcoma usually develops. Ewing's sarcoma produces large amounts of bone destruction and may spread through the periosteum into surrounding soft tissue, creating a mass. Ewing's sarcoma has a peak incidence in the second decade of life and is extremely rare in blacks. The male to female ratio is 1.6:1, and females exhibit a slightly better prognosis. The most common sites for Ewing's sarcoma are the femur and pelvic bones.

The most common manifestations of Ewing's sarcoma are local pain and swelling at the site of the tumor, as well as leukocytosis and an increased erythrocyte sedi-mentation rate (ESR) reflective of the concurrent inflammatory process. There may also be neurological symptoms secondary to nerve entrapment by the tumor. Com-mon metastatic sites are the lung and bone. Metastasis to visceral organs usually occurs late in the disease process. Metastatic involvement of the central nervous system, also occurring late in the course of Ewing's sarcoma, is not common and so central nervous system prophylaxis is not generally carried out. If, however, central nervous system involvement does occur, it is postulated to be a result of the sanctuary provided for malignant cells by the blood-brain barrier similar to that seen in leukemia.

Primary medical treatment for Ewing's sarcoma consists of radiotherapy plus aggressive systemic chemotherapy. Surgery is not of great value in this disease because of the relative inaccessibility of the usual tumor sites to surgical pro-cedures.

One late sequelae of treatment for Ewing's sarcoma is particularly notable. Children with Ewing's sarcoma demonstrate a significantly increased incidence of osteosarcoma, and the incidence increases with time since the treatment of the Ewing's sarcoma. This late sequelae is probably radiation-induced. There are few other complications related to the currently utilized protocols.

Prognosis for children with Ewing's sarcoma is highly dependent upon whether or not metastatic disease is present at the time of diagnosis. Of those individuals without metastases at the time of diagnosis, 45 percent will enjoy a long-term, disease-free survival if adequate medical treatment with radiotherapy and chemotherapy has been administered. However, survival statistics for those children presenting with metastatic disease are very poor.

SOFT-TISSUE SARCOMA

Soft-tissue sarcomas include malignancies of both smooth and striated muscle, both fibrous and adipose connective tissues, connective tissue (fascia and synovia), and both blood and lymphatic vascular tissue [77]. Thus, while soft-tissue sarcomas most commonly arise in the extremities, the head and neck area, and the genitourinary tract, this type of tumor can occur in virtually any part of the body. Soft-tissue sarcomas have an incidence of 8.4 per million white children and 3.9 per million black children in the United States, and are more common in males than females. Histogenesis of soft-tissue sarcomas is detailed in Figure 9.2.

Rhabdomyosarcoma

Approximately 50 percent of soft-tissue sarcomas are rhabdomyosarcomas, and rhabdomyosarcoma is the prototype for medical and nursing treatments of all soft-tissue sarcomas. This type of tumor is usually a firm, fleshy, gray-white mass and is a locally invasive tumor with a pseudo-capsule. The pseudo-capsule makes surgical resection of rhabdomyosarcoma difficult. There are three subtypes of rhabdomyosarcoma: embryonal, alveolar, and pleomorphic. Embryonal rhabdomyosarcoma is the subtype most commonly seen in children, responsible for 50 percent to 65 percent of childhood rhabdomyosarcomas. The alveolar subtype is most commonly seen during the ages of ten to twenty years. This type of tumor generally arises in the extremities or the perineal/perirectal area. Pleomorphic rhabdomyosarcoma is rarely found in children, its peak occurrence being ages thirty to fifty [109].

Childhood rhabdomyosarcoma has an incidence of 4.4. per million white children and 1.3 per million black children with a slight male predominance. Peak occurrence of the disease is between the ages of two and six [77].

Rhabdomyosarcoma can be induced in animals by inoculation with viruses. Although this evidence suggests a viral etiology, human studies are still inconclusive. It is also possible that genetic factors and immunodeficiency increase the child's vulnerability to the development of rhabdomyosarcoma.

Manifestations of rhabdomyosarcoma may vary, since the tumor may arise in any body site containing striated muscle. The most frequent sites are the head and

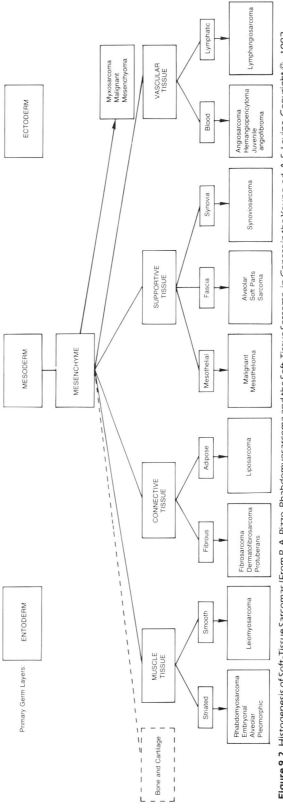

Figure 9.2. Histogenesis of Soft-Tissue Sarcomas (From P. A. Pizzo, Rhabdomyosarcoma and the Soft-Tissue Sarcoma, in *Cancer in the Young*, ed. A. S. Levine. Copyright © 1982, Masson Publishing USA, Inc., New York. Reprinted by permission of the publisher and the author.)

neck region (41 percent), genitourinary and intra-abdominal areas (34 percent), and the trunk or extremities (25 percent). The primary tumor mass is generally painless and has a variable growth rate. The mode of spread is commonly a combination of local infiltration plus metastatic dissemination by blood and lymphatic vessels. Common metastatic sites are the lungs, lymph nodes, bone marrow, bone, liver, brain, and breast; and 20 percent to 40 percent of afflicted children have metastatic disease at the time of diagnosis [12].

Medical treatment for rhabdomyosarcoma includes all three major treatment modalities. Surgery and radiotherapy are used to treat the primary tumor, and chemotherapy is utilized for the treatment of distant metastases.

Prognosis is strongly related to the stage of tumor at the time of diagnosis. Two-year survival rates with multimodal medical treatment is 85 percent for Stage I disease, 72 percent for Stage II, 60 percent for Stage III, and only 25 percent for Stage IV [77].

RETINOBLASTOMA

Retinoblastoma is a relatively rare, highly malignant tumor of the retina in young children. Although it is not generally recognized at birth, it is considered to be a congenital, inheritable tumor. The incidence of retinoblastoma is eleven new cases per million children less than five years old per year, or approximately one in 18,000 live births. Most cases are unilateral disease, and there is no racial or sexual preference [16].

Retinoblastoma often infiltrates the optic nerve, traveling through the subarachnoid space to invade the central nervous system. The tumor may also extend into the orbit and cause secondary glaucoma. Pulmonary metastases are rare. Spontaneous regression of the retinoblastoma has been observed and is attributed to the tumor outgrowing its blood supply.

Approximately 40 percent of retinoblastoma cases are bilateral and 60 percent are unilateral. Bilateral retinoblastoma is the malignancy of childhood most strongly linked to genetic etiological factors. All children with bilateral retinoblastoma have the autosomal dominant mutant gene thought to cause the disease. This mutant gene reflects a germinal mutation, and even 15 percent of the children with unilateral disease carry the retinoblastoma gene [1, 16].

Sixty-six percent to 75 percent of children with retinoblastoma present with a classic syndrome of leukokoria, strabismus, and red and painful eye with or without glaucoma, and poor vision. Leukokoria is the most frequently observed sign of retinoblastoma, consisting of a white pupillary reflection ("cat's eye reflex") indicative of a mass behind the lens. Strabismus is due to the macular involvement of the tumor; and the red and painful eye reflects intraocular inflammation, uveitis secondary to tumor necrosis, or vitreous hemorrhage. Poor vision is secondary to macular involvement, a cloudy vitreous, or detachment of the retina.

There is no standardized staging system for retinoblastoma. There is a need to correlate the stage of the disease with respect to the extent of the intraocular tumor, optic nerve involvement, orbital extension of the tumor, and/or distant metastases.

Medical treatment must be correlated to the stage of the disease, vague as the distinctions may be.

Medical treatment for retinoblastoma consists of a wide variety of treatment modalities. The traditional rule of thumb for determining medical treatment has been that, if there is no chance to save vision, enucleation of the eye is done whereas if vision might be preserved, other treatment modalities must be considered before surgical removal of the eye is carried out.

Enucleation is the primary surgical procedure used for treatment of retinoblastoma. It is advocated for advanced disease when there is no hope for the preservation of vision and also in the follow-up phase if the tumor recurs. During enucleation, approximately ten millimeters of the optic nerve is also resected to ensure complete removal of the malignancy and to reduce the risk of orbital recurrence. Enucleation may be followed by radiotherapy to the surgical site.

If orbital or intracranial extension of the retinoblastoma has occurred, radiotherapy plus systemic chemotherapy is advocated rather than enucleation. If radiotherapy is utilized in treatment, the use of the linear accelerator is recommended since the high voltage rays produce better clinical results. Retinoblastoma is a very radiosensitive tumor; thus irradiation is an extremely effective curative medical treatment for the diseased eye(s) if there is any chance at all to save the vision. Radiotherapy is also very effective for palliation of large masses, central nervous system disease, or symptomatic distant metastases. For radiotherapy, the child is anesthetized and immobilized to prevent unnecessary and dangerous scattering of the radiation to the brain and other vital areas within the region of the head.

Chemotherapy has a limited use in the medical treatment of retinoblastoma. It is primarily used for the treatment of distant metastatic disease.

Photocoagulation may be utilized for small tumors, and it is done under general anesthesia with the exenon-arc photocoagulator. The tumor itself is not treated but instead photocoagulation is applied to retinal blood vessels. With only one or sometimes more photocoagulation sessions, more than 75 percent of small retinoblastomas can be eradicated and cured [1].

Cryotherapy is a simple, safe, and effective treatment modality used in conjunction with photocoagulation. Cryotherapy plus photocoagulation may be curative for small tumors and is also useful as an adjuvant therapy in conjunction with irradiation for more advanced disease or tumor recurrence. Cryotherapy requires a primary tumor that is small, distinct from the optic nerve head and macula, without large blood vessels for nutrient supply, and without involvement of the choroid. The freezing probe is applied under direct visualization until an ice-ball completely covers the tumor. A freeze-thaw cycle is repeated three times, utilizing both photocoagulation and cryotherapy. Therapy is repeated at intervals of six to eight weeks until a flat scar is formed at the primary tumor site. Potential adverse effects of cryotherapy are retinal detachment and hemorrhage [1, 16].

Localized radioactive applicators that emit either gamma or beta radiation have been used successfully in the treatment of small retinoblastomas. Cobalt-60 plaques have been utilized most frequently. The plaque is surgically attached to the sclera and then surgically removed after four to seven days [1].

The most important late sequelae of retinoblastoma and its treatment is the development of secondary nonocular malignancies. Osteosarcoma of the skull, for example, occurs two thousand times more often in the survivors of bilateral reti-noblastoma than in the general population, and osteogenic sarcoma of the femur occurs five hundred times more often. The latency period for these sarcomas may be as long as ten to eleven years, and there seems to be no relationship between the secondary tumor development and whether or not the client had received ra-diation treatment. Mortality rates for these secondary tumors are still very high. More children with retinoblastoma die from the second tumor than from the reti-noblastoma itself [1].

Prognosis for retinoblastoma is excellent, with successful treatment now being measured in terms of disease eradication and cure without vision loss. For the last two decades, the five-year survival rate in the United States has been more than 90 percent [16].

Both nurses and physicians should ensure that genetic counseling is done at some point in time for the survivors of retinoblastoma. A parent who has survived bilateral retinoblastoma will have a 50 percent chance of passing the disease on to a child. If the disease is unilateral and truly multifocal, there is again a 50 percent chance of transmitting the dominant mutant gene for retinoblastoma on to a child. If the disease is unilateral and not multifocal, then the risk of the client's children developing retinoblastoma is much lower—15 percent.

Additionally, a normal child without the disease who is born to a parent who has had bilateral retinoblastoma has a 1 percent chance of carrying the gene and thus a 0.5 percent chance of passing the disease on to his or her children, the grandchildren of the original client [1].

UNCOMMON MALIGNANCIES OF CHILDHOOD

Testicular Carcinoma

The most common type of testicular carcinoma is embryonal carcinoma. There is an early peak in incidence and mortality at age two. This malignancy is rarely found in blacks and black males generally develop the disease later in life [33].

An etiological factor of significance is cryptorchidism (unilateral or bilateral fail-ure of the testes to descend), and male children with this congenital defect have a 33-times greater incidence of testicular carcinoma. If surgical repair of the defect is performed by age six, the child's risk for testicular carcinoma returns to normal. If surgical repair is not accomplished by age six, the child's risk remains high. An-other etiological factor is that the disease has some familial aspects. If one child in the family has testicular carcinoma, his male siblings have three times the expected risk for the disease [65].

Clear Cell Adenocarcinoma of the Vagina [27]

Before 1970, carcinoma of the vagina was considered to be primarily a disease of postmenopausal women and was usually a squamous cell adenocarci-noma. However, since 1970, the discovery of clear cell carcinoma of the vagina in young, premenopausal women has been linked to their exposure in utero to non-steroidal estrogens, the primary agent being diethylstilbestrol (DES). Mothers of these young women had taken diethylstilbestrol to prevent threatened spontaneous abortion. It is estimated that more than one million young women in the United States have been exposed in utero to diethylstilbestrol since 1940, and 50 percent to 90 percent of young women who were exposed to the agent during the eighth to eighteenth weeks of their gestation will have detectable abnormality in the vagina and/or cervix.

Although the risk of developing overt clear cell adenocarcinoma of the vagina is quite low (about fifty cases are diagnosed each year), any female child with vaginal bleeding or discharge in whom the possibility of DES exposure exists should be examined for malignancy. In exposed female children who are asymptomatic, this physical examination can be safely delayed until menarche or age fourteen because the occurrence of clear cell vaginal carcinoma is rare before that time. Cytology specimens alone will detect about 80 percent of these malignancies.

The age of the client ranges from seven to twenty-nine years with 90 percent of the cases developing after age fourteen. Peak incidence occurs at age nineteen. About 66 percent of young women with this disease have a documented history of in utero exposure to diethylstilbestrol, and the exposure generally occurred between the eighth and eighteenth weeks of gestation. This period of time is the time of fetal genital development.

Eighty percent of these young women present with vaginal bleeding or discharge. Less than 20 percent are asymptomatic at the time of diagnosis. Approximately half of the cancers are well differentiated. Spread to the pelvic lymph nodes seems to be associated with both increasing tumor size and depth of invasion.

Medical treatment depends on the primary site of the tumor (cervix or vaginal vault) as well as the extent of the disease. For Stages I and II of cervical disease, medical treatment of choice is radical hysterectomy with pelvic lymph node dissection and preservation of one or both ovaries. For Stages I and II of vaginal disease, medical treatment is the same as for cervical disease plus radical vaginectomy. For more advanced disease, regardless of the primary site, radiotherapy is added to the medical treatment regimen. If metastases have occurred, radiotherapy and systemic chemotherapy are both used to supplement surgery. Vaginal reconstruction is done early, perhaps even immediately, for young women receiving a vaginectomy.

Prognosis regarding physiological aspects of clear cell adenocarcinoma of the vagina is highly dependent upon the presence or absence of metastases at the time of diagnosis. If the diagnostic workup reveals metastatic disease in the pelvic lymph nodes, survival is less than 50 percent. Personal and social aspects of prognosis are less well defined. Intensive counseling *must* be a part of the routine medical and nursing treatment regimens to assist the young woman to attain optimal personal, sexual, and social levels of functioning.

Another aspect of nursing and medical intervention has been the aspect of the client's mother's response to the diagnosis, treatment, and perhaps death of her daughter. Because the causative stressor for the development of this malignancy was the mother's decision to take diethylstilbestrol in order to prevent a threatened miscarriage, the client's mother is apt to feel an enormous sense of guilt [15]. Intensive counselng and consistent support, or "emotional hyperalimentation," is indicated for the client's mother as well as for the client herself.

Hepatoblastoma

Primary carcinoma of the liver is one of the least common malignancies in children, with an annual incidence of 0.6 cases per million white children [33]. Although the significance is unclear, there seems to be an etiological relationship between hepatoblastoma and the hemihypertrophy and visceral cytomegaly syndrome of Wiedemann and Beckwith (which is also etiologically assoiated with Wilms' tumor) [65]. Primary liver cancer in children originates in utero and may attain considerable size prior to birth [40].

Teratoma

The pathogenesis of teratoma probably arises from embryonal germ cell carcinogenic transformation in utero. Teratomas are more frequently diagnosed in females. There is an early peak in both incidence and mortality before age three, and a second rise in mortality begins at age six and peaks at fifteen to eighteen years of age [33]. Sacrococcygeal teratomas are more common in females, and are often associated with major defects of the lower spine and perhaps duplication of the lower intestine and organs of the urogenital regions [65].

CONCEPT V:
Disease- and treatment-related complications have a profound biological impact on the child with cancer.

THE PHYSICAL COSTS OF DISEASE AND TREATMENT

Overall, the physical costs to the child with cancer exact a tremendous price. Pain, morbidity related to either disease or treatment, changes in body appearance, infection, complications related to supportive therapy, malaise, fatigue, a general syndrome of "just not feeling well," late sequelae of treatment, secondary malignancies, and even physical death are but a few of the physical costs that the child must experience and endure. An incomplete list of the physical costs would include (1) significant physical deformity secondary to surgery, such as amputation, orchiectomy, vaginectomy, unsightly scars, or an Ommaya reservoir, (2) physical deformities secondary to radiotherapy or chemotherapy, such as weight gain, drug extravasation, allergic reactions, nausea and vomiting, diarrhea, mucositis, or alopecia, (3) adverse effects of the malignancy itself, including weight loss, pain, decreased mobility, or pathological fractures, and (4) other oncologic emergencies shared with adults.

In order to minimize or prevent these predictable complications of cancer and its treatment, nurses and physicians must carefully attend to subtle signs and symptoms of disease progression or treatment complications. If this is done, prophylactic or curative nursing and medical treatments can be instituted early, thus averting or at least minimizing potential physical catastrophes.

Pain

A child's response to pain is different from that of an adult, and children's reports of pain are often ignored by their caregivers. Control of acute pain should provide complete relief, whereas control of chronic pain must achieve a balance between pain control and drug toxicity so that the child's functioning is maintained. Uncontrolled chronic pain in the child may cause behavioral and/or school-related problems which, in the final analysis, may be the child's only way of asking for help in controlling the pain. To assess the impairment caused by chronic pain in the child, the nurse and physician must evaluate (1) the child's suffering, (2) social restrictions imposed by pain, (3) pain's interference with developmental tasks, and (4) the effect of the child's pain on others in the environment [21].

A child's chronic pain secondary to cancer may be effectively controlled by use of potent narcotic analgesics. As with adults, routine use of potent narcotics will produce tolerance and physical dependence in the child but rarely addiction. Dosage and intervals between drug administration should be manipulated until the child can maintain pain relief at a steady level without loss of awareness of the external environment [67]. Again, as with adults, the nursing and medical goal is to provide freedom from chronic pain so that the child can participate and enjoy the pleasurable activities available to him or her.

Another intervention that has been demonstrated to be effective in the control of the child's chronic pain is neuroaugmentation through transcutaneous electrical nerve stimulation (TENS). In one study, 60 percent of children with chronic pain obtained sufficient relief with TENS and needed no further medical therapy [21].

For further discussion of pain control, refer to Chapter 11.

Nausea and Vomiting

Nausea and vomiting is usually iatrogenic in children, being induced by surgical anesthesia, radiotherapy, chemotherapy, and/or immunotherapy. This distressing physical burden for the child should be treated prophylactically (or at least with *prompt* curative treatment) by phenothiazines. For further discussion of nursing and medical management of nausea and vomiting, refer to Chapters 6 and 7.

Drug Toxicity [82]

The toxicities of the drugs that are commonly used in children are discussed in the following section. For further in-depth discussion of the toxicities associated with these and other chemotherapeutic agents, refer to Chapter 7.

L-asparaginase.   L-asparaginase is primarily used in the medical treatment of acute lymphocytic or lymphoblastic leukemia. Manifestations of toxicity include drug fever, anorexia, nausea and vomiting, aberrations of the central nervous system, azotemia, liver dysfunction, pancreatitis, hyperglycemia, and anaphylaxis. Children are less likely to require discontinuance of the drug because of dangerous side effects than are adults. If the drug must be discontinued in a child, it is primarily because of hypersensitivity and anaphylaxis.

Doxorubicin and Daunorubicin. These two chemotherapeutic drugs are primarily used in children for the medical treatment of leukemia, and doxorubicin (Adriamycin) is also utilized for the treatment of solid tumors. The number of treatment courses is limited by the cardiotoxicity of these two drugs, which may appear in children as life-threatening congestive heart failure. Children have an equal or perhaps even increased vulnerability to the development of drug-induced cardiac damage as do adults, although some controversy about this exists in the literature. If the child also receives mediastinal radiotherapy, there is an increased risk of cardiac damage secondary to doxorubicin and daunorubicin.

Methotrexate. Intrathecal administration of methotrexate is commonly used in preventing or treating leukemic central nervous system infiltration in children. Three dangerous toxic syndromes may result: (1) arachnoiditis, (2) demyelination of spinal root nerves, and (3) demyelinating encephalopathy. When peripheral systemic methotrexate is given to children, the major toxicity is pulmonary dysfunction with cough, fever, and dyspnea.

Cis-platinum. Cis-platinum's primary use in children is in treatment of osteosarcoma and neuroblastoma. Toxicities in children are similar to those observed in adults: severe vomiting and dangerous renal damage. Children, however, are more likely to develop hypomagnesemia secondary to cis-platinum administration than are adults.

Teniposide (VM-26). This is an investigational drug used for the medical treatment of neuroblastoma and primary brain tumors in children. Major toxicities include vomiting, diarrhea, and myelosuppression.

Infection [76]

Precise diagnosis of a febrile child who is granulocytopenic is difficult since the classic signs and symptoms of infection are likely to be absent. Types of infections common to the granulocytopenic child with cancer include oral mucositis, otitis media, pulmonary infection, esophagitis, perianal infections, and cutaneous (skin) infections. Nevertheless, simply because the child has a fever does not necessarily mean that he or she has an infection since the incidence of drug fever is significantly high. On the other hand, an afebrile child does not rule out serious infection since the granulocytic child with sepsis may exhibit no fever at all and may even have a subnormal temperature.

Fever of undetermined origin (FUO) with or without initial neutropenia that resolves within seven days after the initiation of antibiotic therapy indicates that the child has low risk for the development of sepsis. Resolution of the condition is defined as absence of fever and a serum neutrophil level of more than $500/mm^3$. If the child has a fever of undetermined origin and neutropenia that last for more than seven days after antibiotics have been started, the child is considered to be at high risk for the development of sepsis. If any neutropenic child is suspected of infection (occult or overt), culture and sensitivity tests should be carried out on nasal secretions, throat secretions, urine, and stool. Two additional blood samples should be drawn from different venipuncture sites for culture and sensitivity tests. If the child has an intravenous line, it should be removed and the intravenous catheter cultured. All culture samples must be taken before antibiotic therapy is initiated. In addition, a chest X-ray should be done. Even with this extensive diagnostic workup, however, only 55 percent to 70 percent of febrile neutropenic children clearly demonstrate an infection. Negative culture results do not rule out infection, and morbidity and mortality secondary to infectious complications are decreased if broad-spectrum antibiotics are started immediately after cultures are taken but before culture results are back.

Septicemia accounts for approximately 20 percent of febrile episodes in neutropenic children. The primary bacteria involved in sepsis are gram-negative bacilli, such as *E. coli, Pseudomonas aeruginosa,* and *Klebsiella pneumoniae.* Mortality rates for gram-negative sepsis ranges form 25 percent to 40 percent. If the septicemia is polymycrobial in etiology, the mortality rate is approximately 70 percent. For further discussion of nursing and medical management of infectious complications, refer to Chapters 7 and 13.

Complications of Blood Component Therapy

The advantages, disadvantages, and potential complications of blood component therapy are outlined in Table 9.3. For further discussion of nursing and medical management, refer to Chapter 13.

Late Side Effects of Antineoplastic Therapy

Both chemotherapy and radiotherapy may cause a wide variety of adverse effects on normal body tissues, becoming clinically apparent months or even years after termination of the therapy. These late effects may affect any bodily system and vary in severity from simple laboratory abnormalities to life-threatening complications. Long-term deleterious results of chemotherapy and irradiation can be divided into two broad categories: disruption of function and the development of secondary neoplasms (see Figure 9.3).

Disruption of Function

Impaired Growth and Development.   This late sequelae may manifest itself by temporary delays in bone and soft-tissue growth resulting from a deficiency in the secretion of growth hormones, especially noted in children who received treatment for brain tumors. Major structural deformities are uncommon.

Central Nervous System Damage.   Neuropsychological and intellectual damage may occur as a late consequence of chemotherapy and/or radiotherapy, but this adverse effect is difficult to definitively diagnose because of the long latency

Table 9.3. Advantages, Disadvantages, and Potential Complications of Blood Component Therapy

Blood Component	Advantages	Disadvantages and Complications
Packed Red Blood Cells	Correct anemia Increase capacity for oxygen transport Reduced risk of circulatory overload (able to give a large amount of erythrocytes in a small volume)	Residual leukocytes and platelets immunize client Potential anaphylactic response
Leukocyte-poor Red Blood Cells	Virtually free of white blood cells, platelets and plasma Excellent oxygen transport capacity Consists of erythrocytes only	Outdates in 24 hours Blood must be less than seven days Potential anaphylactic response
Frozen-Thawed Red Blood Cells	Same advantages as leukocyte-poor red blood cells	Very expensive Potential anaphylactic response
Platelets	Correct thrombocytopenia and decrease risk of bleeding Increases chance of client survival With platelet pheresis method, donor can give 8–10 units of platelets without significant blood loss Few adverse side effects	If platelets are not HLA-matched, will produce eventual immunization to future platelet transfusions (refractory thrombocytopenia)
Granulocytes	Protects client against infection Increases client's chance for survival	Short life-span of white blood cells requires many transfusions Donor and recipient must be HLA-matched Transfusion-induced fever and chills may be severe Transfusion reaction may be life-threatening

period between the time of antineoplastic therapy and the clinical onset of abnormalities. Another factor confusing definitive diagnosis is that one or more factors may be responsible, such as the treatment, the disease itself, or the personal stress response associated with prolonged disease and treatment. Neuropsychological or intellectual dysfunction may take the form of physical or mental handicaps, including subnormal intelligence and/or abnormal psychological tests revealing aberrations in perceptual behavior, language development, and learning disabilities [3, 58, 59, 69]. Intellectual dysfunction may be associated with moderate to high doses of radiotherapy administered to the developing brain, and actual dementia may result from treatment with high-dose methotrexate. Incidence and severity of both the aforementioned side effects are increased significantly when cranial irradiation and systemic chemotherapy are used together [12]. A small pilot study of leukemic children revealed a significant decrease in relative intelligence after the children had

Figure 9.3 Adverse Late Effects of Antineoplastic Treatment

I. DISRUPTION OF FUNCTION
    A. Impaired Growth and Development
    B. Central Nervous System Damage
        1. Neuropsychological and intellectual problems
        2. Generalized neurological problems
        3. Chronic encephalopathy
        4. Postintrathecal chemotherapy syndrome
        5. Peripheral neuropathy
    C. Gonadal Dysfunction
        1. Reproductive
        2. Genetic and teratogenic
    D. Dysfunction of Other Organs and Systems
        1. Liver
        2. Cardiovascular system
        3. Pulmonary system
        4. Gastrointestinal system
        5. Renal system
        6. Endocrine system
        7. Skeletal system
        8. Immune system
II. DEVELOPMENT OF SECONDARY MALIGNANCIES

received central nervous system irradiation [19]. It has also been demonstrated that there is a definite reduction in quantitative memory and motor skills among some young leukemic children after antineoplastic treatment [20]. Thus far, it has not been possible to determine the relative effects of contributions from the disease process, complications, treatment modalities, and the child's relative stress response (including the emotional regression commonly observed in chronically ill children) to the development of these neuropsychological and intellectual changes. The actual prevalence of postcancer learning disorders is unknown [55].

Generalized neurological problems may result from chemotherapy, radiotherapy, or both. A variety of generalized neurological dysfunctions are associated with survivors of acute lymphocytic leukemia and may range from slight slowing of electroencephalographic (EEG) activity to seizure disorders or paraplegia. In the case of brain tumors that have been treated by a combination of surgery, radiotherapy, and chemotherapy, many central nervous system abnormalities have appeared as late sequelae. These include deficiencies in growth hormone and subsequent retarded bone growth, residual visual and hearing losses, motor abnormalities, decreased intellectual capacity, and cranial and peripheral nerve damage [43].

Chronic encephalopathy constitutes a neurotoxicity that often causes permanent neurological deficits or death. This condition is frequently not clinically detectable for months or years after antineoplastic treatment has been discontinued. Most cases of chronic encephalopathy arise in children whose acute leukemia required prophylactic or curative chemotherapy for cerebral infiltration and/or cranial irradiation [69]. It is thought that as many as 55 percent of asymptomatic children who had received central nervous system prophylaxis (cranial irradiation plus intrathecal chemotherapy) for acute lymphocytic leukemia developed abnormal CT brain scans [74]. Upon autopsy, chronic encephalopathy manifests the following abnormalities: multiple noninflammatory necrotic foci in the central white matter of the brain, extensive areas of demyelinization, and vascular changes such as sclerotic microangiopathy and thickened capillary walls [69]. Symptomatology of chronic encephalopathy includes lethargy, sleepiness, dementia, seizure activity, visual disturbances, spastic paraplegia or quadriplegia, coma, and/or death. Symptoms of meningeal irritation—nuchal rigidity, fever, and photophobia—may also occur. Medical and nursing treatments are primarily supportive since the neurological damage is irreversible. Prognosis is variable. If it is possible to modify or discontinue any ongoing antineoplastic treatment, the client may completely recover. However, only partial recovery with permanent neurological defects or progression to coma and death may also occur, even if any ongoing treatment has been discontinued [18, 57, 59, 69].

After intrathecal chemotherapy, temporary or permanent central nervous system abnormalities may occur. These include: (1) cranial nerve palsies, (2) paraplegia, (3) encephalopathy, (4) motor disturbances, (5) dementia, (6) dysfunction in perceptual, behavioral, or language development, (7) fever, and (8) even sudden and unexpected death [43].

Sensory or motor peripheral neuropathies may occur as late sequelae to treatment of intracranial tumors with surgery, radiotherapy, and chemotherapy or may be drug-induced by the administration of vinca alkaloids. Damage to a peripheral nerve by radiotherapy usually requires months to years to manifest itself, and adverse effects are generally observed in the cranial nerves and brachial plexus [69]. Peripheral nerve toxicities associated with the vinca alkaloids, especially vincristine, are usually manifested by muscle weakness and/or parasthesias. The vinca alkaloids produce mixed sensory-motor peripheral neuropathies that are common and usually reversible by either decreasing drug dosage or by completely discontinuing the drug. Incidence of vinca alkaloid-induced neuropathies is highly dose-related. Up to 67 percent of clients develop symptoms of parasthesia or peripheral pain, and 100 percent of clients exhibit depressed or absent deep tendon reflexes at doses of fifty micrograms per kilogram of body weight per week. Fewer clients develop anesthesia, foot or wrist drop, muscle atrophy, or paralysis [37, 89]. However, these manifestations occur in a large enough proportion of patients that assessment, preventive measures, and, if necessary, curative treatment are indeed appropriate. Vincristine can also affect the autonomic nervous system, resulting in bladder atony, ileus, and/or orthostatic hypotension. In addition, the vinca alkaloids can cause cranial nerve palsies [9, 29, 37].

Gonadal Dysfunction

Gonadal dysfunction may occur as the result of either chemotherapy or irradiation and has tremendous implications for the child or adolescent who survives their cancer. Either chemotherapy or irradiation may result in infertility, gynecomastia in males, premature menopause in females, and a decrease in libido. Of particular significance to young survivors of cancer is the effect of antineoplastic treatment on their sexual maturation since it is dependent upon normal gonadal function.

Permanent gonadal failure has been observed in children who are long-term survivors of infant and childhood malignancies. Of particular risk are those young females who received pelvic and/or abdominal irradiation and those young males who received chemotherapeutic treatment with alkylating agents [43].

Reproductive dysfunction. Reproductive capacity in both males and females is adversely affected by chemotherapy and radiotherapy to the gonads. Infertility may be reversible but also may persist for three to four years after antineoplastic therapy is terminated. However, this induced infertility may be permanent [69].

In sexually mature adolescent males, antineoplastic therapy affects the complex cell division responsible for spermatogenesis and causes testicular atrophy, both of which result in the production of less than normal amounts of sperm or no sperm at all. Oligospermia or azospermia are more common after the young man receives treatment with cyclophosphamide (Cytoxan) or chlorambucil. Return of spermatogenesis may occur after discontinuance of the drug. If the production of sperm is adversely affected by radiotherapy, it appears that younger adolescents are less vulnerable than are older adolescents. Serum testosterone levels may drop in adolescent males after combined chemotherapy of nitrogen mustard, vincristine, procarbazine, and prednisone (often used to treat Hodgkin's disease), although the reduction of testosterone levels is not necessarily permanent [43]. If there is a possibility that a young man will be irreversibly sterile after antineoplastic therapy, pretreatment sperm storage is strongly advocated.

Ovarian failure in females is usually characterized by amenorrhea and may occur after treatment with cyclophosphamide (Cytoxan). Menses may return after the drug has been discontinued [43]. Additionally, gonadal irradiation in female children and adolescents may result in oocyte depletion [12].

Total or near-total eradication of reproductive capacity in both males and females can result from highly aggressive chemotherapy using multiple drugs. The alkylating agents are the most likely to cause this complication, and males are more vulnerable than are females. Females, however, are relatively more vulnerable if the treatment is administered after puberty [12].

Genetic Abnormalities and Teratogenesis. Both chemotherapy and radiotherapy are teratogenetic in man, primarily in the first trimester of pregnancy. Although actual chromosomal (genetic) damage associated with antineoplastic therapy has probably been overestimated in the past, development of the fetus has been demonstrated to be adversely affected in a number of studies if the mother receives antineoplastic chemotherapy or irradiation during the first trimester [12, 43]. Many anticancer drugs are demonstrably teratogenic in animals; for example, the administration of aminopterin and 6-mercaptopurine to laboratory animals during the first trimester of pregnancy results in approximately 80 percent of the offspring being spontaneously aborted. Although human studies are as yet inconclusive, it appears that the vast majority of the offspring of female cancer clients will be carried to term and will be normal with normal chromosomal patterns [43]. Birth defects are apparently not any more common in children born of parents who were previously treated and cured of various pediatric cancers than children born to parents within the general population. Parents who have been cured of cancer exhibit an 11 percent spontaneous abortion rate, which is approximately the same as that within the general population. Progeny of parents with cancer or who have been cured of cancer have not demonstrated congenital malignancy, with only few and certain exceptions such as retinoblastoma [51].

The issue of whether or not to treat pregnant young women who have a malignancy is rarely encountered. The severity of the effect of antineoplastic treatment on the fetus depends upon the gestational age of the baby, the drug concentration in maternal blood, the ability of the drug to cross the placental barrier, the anatomical area of the mother that is being irradiated, the radiation dose, and the vulnerability of developing organs and structures to fetal blood levels of specific drugs and/or irradiation. Toxic doses of chemotherapy or irradiation given during the sensitive first trimester are generally embryolethal, and a spontaneous abortion will almost always occur.

The earlier in gestation that the developing embryo is exposed to radiation, the more likely it is to develop serious damage secondary to irradiation. There is, however, an initial resistant period of time very early in the pregnancy—approximately the first two and one-half weeks after conception—which is the phase of embryonal development prior to cell differentiation and organogenesis when radiation effects are minimal. After that initial phase of resistance, the effects of radiation on the fetus for the remainder of the first trimester are profound, ranging from death to major developmental abnormalities even if radiotherapy doses are as low as 10 rad. The central nervous system of the fetus is especially vulnerable during the first trimester, with pronounced ocular and central nervous system aberrations (including varying degrees of mental retardation) ensuing after 100 rad. After the first trimester, however, adverse fatal reactions to radiotherapy are progressively more uncommon. Thus, the developing embryo, especially if exposed during the sensitive first trimester, can be expected to sustain substantial damage after either maternal pelvic radiotherapy or intensive chemotherapy, especially with alkylating agents [43]. The probable result is spontaneous abortion or stillbirth.

The likelihood of severe malformation is dependent upon the gestational age of the baby, as well as upon the dose, time, and frequency of irradiation. The human fetus is most vulnerable to the damaging effects of radiation during gestational weeks 3 to 10, the period of differentiation and organogenesis. Damaging effects are dose-dependent and more pronounced with multiple treatments. During the last half of the pregnancy, the mother requiring antineoplastic treatment may be allowed to go to term if the radiotherapy is kept to the minimum necessary for effective treatment of the mother. In this situation, severe deformities in the baby are unlikely to occur [12].

Dysfunction of Other Organs and Structures

Hepatic Dysfunction [43]. Liver toxicity is primarily seen as a secondary adverse effect of chemotherapy. Methotrexate is associated with hepatic fibrosis, as are aminopterin, chlorambucil, cytosine arabinoside, and the anthracyclines. The incidence of hepatic fibrosis is increased if the treatment regimen is low in dosage, daily, and given orally; whereas hepatic fibrosis occurs less often if the treatment is given in higher dosages and on an intermittent schedule. The fibrotic changes in the liver tend to worsen as the duration of the treatment is lengthier. Some cases of hepatic fibrosis will progress to frank cirrhosis which may develop insidiously over a period of months to years after treatment. This type of cirrhosis is not detectable by laboratory studies but requires a liver biopsy for definitive diagnosis. Other chemotherapeutic agents implicated in hepatic toxicity in children include 6-mercaptopurine with or without concurrent use of Adriamycin (hepatic damage) and 6-mercaptopurine given concurrently with methotrexate (hepatic cirrhosis and portal hypertension). Additionally, actinomycin-D or radiotherapy can inhibit liver cell regeneration and thus enhance development of hepatic fibrosis. For further discussion of nursing care appropriate for hepatic dysfunciton, refers to Chapters 7 and 13.

Cardiovascular Dysfunction.   Cardiovascular dysfunction is among the most serious of late complications of antineoplastic therapy. Severe congestive cardiomyopathy and radiation-induced constrictive pericarditis are the late sequelae of chemotherapy and/or radiotherapy that are potentially fatal. For further discussion of nursing care appropriate for cardiovascular dysfunction, refer to Chapters 7 and 13.

Severe congestive cardiomyopathy is almost always secondary to the administration of the anthracyclines doxorubicin (Adriamycin) and daunorubicin (daunomycin). Anthracyclines have a lifetime cumulative dosage limit that must not be exceeded, and both children under the age of fifteen and elderly individuals over the age of seventy are particularly vulnerable to the development of this complication. Manifestations of congestive cardiomyopathy include the abrupt onset of biventricular congestive heart failure, tachypnea, tachycardia, edema, hepatomegaly, cardiomegaly, gallop rhythms, and pleural effusions. Medical treatment is generally supportive and usually not very effective. Prognosis for those children who develop severe congestive cardiomyopathy is poor, and 60 percent to 80 percent die within a few months of diagnosis [100, 101].

Radiation-induced pericarditis is another late sequelae of antineoplastic therapy affecting the cardiovascular system and is usually associated with mediastinal irradiation. Incidence and severity of this complication is dose-dependent and develops from a few months to forty-five years after the radiation therapy has been discontinued [32, 91]. Signs and symptoms of radiation-induced pericarditis are similar to other forms of pericarditis: chest pain and dyspnea, fever, pulse irregularities, and friction rubs upon auscultation. Electrocardiogram changes include inversion of the T-wave and elevation of the S-T segment. The pericarditis may be self-limiting and resolve spontaneously without nursing or medical intervention. Older children with radiation-induced pericarditis may require medical therapy with steroids or pericardectomy [69].

Pulmonary Dysfunction.   Both chemotherapy and radiotherapy have been implicated in the development of late complications affecting the child's pulmonary system. Interstitial pneumonitis, diffuse pulmonary fibrosis, and diffuse generalized pulmonary damage are the most commonly observed late complications of antineoplastic therapy.

Interstitial pneumonitis may develop as a result of either radiation or treatment with such chemotherapeutic agents as cyclophosphamide (Cytoxan), chlorambucil, and bleomycin. Radiation-induced pneumonitis generally occurs two to six months after radiotherapy. Signs and symptoms associated with radiation-induced pneumonitis include dyspnea, fever, and a nonproductive cough.

Interstitial pneumonitis associated with cyclophosphamide and bleomycin is heralded by the subtle sign of fine rales upon auscultation. Signs and symptoms are otherwise similar to those seen with radiation-induced pneumonitis. Bleomycin-induced disease has the additional symptoms of reduced diffusion capacity and restrictive ventilation with subsequent arterial hypoxemia [43]. Most cases of interstitial pneumonitis resolve spontaneously without medical intervention. However, administration of high-dose steroids may reduce the child's pulmonary inflammation.

Diffuse pulmonary fibrosis is particularly associated with the anticancer drugs busulfan and chlorambucil, and interstitial pneumonitis secondary to cyclophosphamide, bleomycin, and radiation therapy may progress to pulmonary fibrosis. Busulfan-induced pulmonary fibrosis has an insidious onset of symptoms, usually appearing three to four years after treatment with the drug [43]. Progressive radiation-induced pulmonary fibrosis may initially appear as long as nine to twelve months after irradiation has been discontinued. Signs and symptoms indicative of pulmonary fibrosis include increased dyspnea and restrictive ventilatory function [69].

Diffuse generalized pulmonary disease is usually a self-limiting process requiring little or no intervention. It is most often seen after intermittent administration of methotrexate or radiotherapy. For further discussion of appropriate nursing care for pulmonary dysfunction, refer to Chapters 6, 7, and 13.

Gastrointestinal Dysfunction.   A late complication of radiotherapy is chronic enteritis in which the pathological changes are similar throughout the gastrointestinal system. The most common pathological changes are characterized by areas of fibrosis throughout the gastrointestinal tract leading to either stricture formation or mucosal ulcerations with bleeding. Gastric lesions secondary to radiotherapy may result in intractable epigastric pain, stomach bleeding, and vomiting. Lesions in the small intestine may cause colicky abdominal pain, recurrent vomiting, and bloody or mucous-containing diarrhea followed by constipation. Large bowel and rectal lesions cause crampy lower abdominal pain, alternating constipation and diarrhea, tenesmus, and recurrent bleeding. Medical treatment for these problems is primarily supportive. Surgical intervention may be necessary if an intestinal obstruction develops, although the procedure is often a difficult and dangerous one. A colostomy may be necessary if radiation damage is so extensive that anastamosis is impossible [69].

Chemotherapy rarely causes late gastrointestinal sequelae. One exception is the potentially fatal pancreatitis secondary to previous administration of L-asparaginase [12]. For further discussion of nursing care appropriate for gastrointestinal dysfunction, refer to Chapter 6, 7, and 13.

Renal Dysfunction.   Late development of renal dysfunction in the child previously treated for cancer may take the form of radiation nephritis. Radiation nephritis is a complex pathophysiological syndrome that may occur as an acute or chronic phenomenon. Acute radiation nephritis usually develops within six to twelve months after radiation treatment and is characterized by a rapid decrease in renal function with elevated serum blood urea nitrogen (BUN), proteinuria, anemia, hypertension, and symptoms of congestive heart failure. The chronic form of the disease occurs several months to several years after radiotherapy. In either case, the renal damage may be progressive, resulting in renal failure, uremia, and death. Medical and nursing treatments are generally supportive with emphasis on dietary changes as for renal failure. If only one kidney is involved and the damage is serious enough to cause hypertension, nephrectomy may be performed.

Chronic hemorrhagic cystitis may be induced in the child who has received either pelvic irradiation or treatment with cyclophosphamide (Cytoxan). The onset of this syndrome may be very rapid (one day after initiation of therapy) or may take several years to develop. The syndrome is more likely to occur if the child receives both cyclophosphamide and pelvic irradiation. The severity of the cystitis is highly variable, ranging from chronic microscopic hematuria to life-threatening hemorrhage. Symptoms include microscopic or frank hematuria and urinary frequency. The best treatment for chronic hemorrhagic cystitis is prophylactic: minimizing exposure of the bladder to ionizing radiation during pelvic radiotherapy and adequate hydration of the child before and during cyclophosphamide treatment. If the disease is overt, medical and nursing treatments are primarily supportive.

Renal failure may be the end result of both radiation nephritis and chronic hemorrhagic nephritis. Potentially fatal renal failure may also be a late complication of high-dose radiation administered to the kidney.

Other renal aberrations may occur as a late complication of treatment with 6-mercaptopurine [43]. Manifestations may include any or all of the following: tubular defects, chronic glomerulonephritis, and a nephrotic syndrome. For further discussion of the nursing care appropriate for renal dysfunction, refer to Chapters 6, 7, and 13.

Dysfunction of the Endocrine System [29].   Endocrine system abnormalities are usually a late complication of radiotherapy. The primary glands affected are the pituitary and thyroid glands.

Hypopituitarism may be a late complication in the child if the radiotherapy field includes the hypothalamus and/or pituitary. Incidence and severity of the dysfunction is dependent upon the radiation dose delivered to those sensitive areas. Since the pituitary gland affects many hormonal systems, signs and symptoms vary widely according to the hormonal systems that are affected. Manifestations of radiation-induced hypopituitarism may range from simple growth hormone deficiency to panhypopituitarism with short stature, hypothyroidism, hypofunction of the gonads, and Addison's disease. Medical treatment consisting of the replacement of the deficient hormones has been consistently successful.

Radiation-induced hypothyroidism is probably secondary to atrophy or fibrosis of thyroid tissue. Severity of the condition ranges from asymptomatic depletion of thyroid hormone reserve to life-threatening myxedematous coma. Medical treatment consists of hormone replacement.

Abnormalities of the Skeletal System. Various skeletal abnormalities may result as late complications of antineoplastic treatment. Long-term administration of methotrexate may cause osteoporosis, growth arrest, and dental abnormalities. The administration of steroids such as prednisone may result in the late development of osteoporosis. Vertebral deformities may result from radiotherapy administered to the vertebral column and is more likely to occur if the child is less than six years old when radiotherapy is given or if the irradiation is delivered at the time of puberty.

Dysfunction of the Immune System. Long-term suppression of the immune system and of bone marrow function may be seen after extensive radiotherapy or prolonged chemotherapy with alkylating agents, especially busulfan. The extent of damage to the bone marrow and the immune system depends upon the amount of marrow that has been irradiated and whether radiotherapy has been combined with marrow-toxic chemotherapy [43, 70, 87].

Late Development of Secondary Malignancies

Most data regarding the late development of secondary malignancies have been gathered from the survivors of pediatric solid tumors and acute childhood leukemia. Results of these studies strongly indicate that the risks of a later cancer must be balanced against the severity of the first malignancy and the potential benefits of antineoplastic therapy.

Incidence of Secondary Malignancies. It has been postulated that the overall incidence of secondary cancers among twenty-year survivors of childhood malignancies may be as high as 12 percent. The overall risk for secondary malignancies following radiotherapy appears to be 17 percent with a peak occurrence at fifteen to nineteen years after the initial diagnosis [50]. Thus, an average of six children per one thousand children with cancer develop a secondary malignancy in each year of medical follow-up [65].

The risk among survivors of Hodgkin's disease is estimated to be 3 percent at five years after treatment and 4 percent at seven years. Risk among survivors of non-Hodgkin's lymphoma who have received both chemotherapy and radiotherapy is thought to be 4.5 percent at ten years [48].

Causative Stressors: General Information. Although the relative carcinogenic potential of radiotherapy and chemotherapy are unclear, both modalities of antineoplastic therapy—as well as immunosuppression and increased susceptibility of the child—are thought to be the primary causative stressors associated with the development of secondary malignancies. Most forms of antineoplastic treatment carry the risk of inducing neoplasia, and the combination of both radiotherapy and chemotherapy seems to be more oncogenic than either modality alone. Besides the carcinogenic effects of radiotherapy and chemotherapy, they are also immunosuppressive, which adds to the risk of developing a second malignancy since immunosuppression has been shown to enhance the growth of malignant cells in man.

Carcinogenic activity of antineoplastic treatment in man may also be modified by other host factors such as the child's age at time of treatment and variations in drug metabolism. Chemotherapeutic agents most clearly associated with the development of secondary malignancies are alkylating agents [44, 50]; the antineoplastic antibiotics doxorubicin (Adriamycin), procarbazine, and actinomycin-D [83, 84]; methotrexate; and the combination of vincristine, procarbazine, nitrogen mustard, and prednisone [43]. Possible mechanisms of drug-induced carcinogenesis include chromosomal damage, immunosuppression, and activation of dormant oncogenic viruses [35]. Most secondary malignancies have been associated with the use of orthovoltage radiation rather than the newer megavoltage treatments [69]. Some chemotherapeutic drugs such as doxorubicin and actinomycin-D may potentiate the carcinogenicity of radiotherapy.

Causative Stressors: Chemotherapeutic Agents. The alkylating agents are apparently strongly carcinogenic. Follow-up studies of children successfully treated with these drugs have demonstrated increased carcinogenic effects probably resulting from the use of alkylating agents [8, 34]. Acute nonlymphocytic leukemia has been shown to occur in high frequency after the administration of alkylating agents for cancers of the breast, lung, brain, and ovary [83, 85]. Individuals treated with alkylating agents for ovarian carcinoma and who survive for at least two years, for example, have a relative risk for later development of acute nonlymphocytic leukemia more than 170 percent greater than that of the general population. Thus, approximately 5 percent to 10 percent of ten-year survivors of ovarian carcinoma will develop acute nonlymphocytic leukemia [72, 85], and the five-year cumulative risk is postulated to be 7.6 percent. Neither concurrent radiotherapy nor total drug dosage seems to be a major influencing factor [72].

Among the antineoplastic antibiotics, actinomycin-D, procarbazine, and doxorubicin have shown to be carcinogenic in animal studies, with procarbazine showing the strongest oncogenic activity [83]. In one study, for example, 100 percent of rats that received procarbazine developed breast carcinoma as a late sequelae to the drug [45]. In another investigation, a high incidence of acute leukemia developed in nonhuman primates (Rhesus monkeys) after prolonged treatment with procarbazine [68]. Additionally, both doxorubicin and antinomycin-D are capable of enhancing the oncogenic effects of radiotherapy [30, 84].

Antimetabolites are not as carcinogenic as the other two classes of drugs mentioned, and there is controversy in the literature regarding the carcinogenicity of methotrexate in particular. Some researchers have demonstrated that methotrexate does indeed have carcinogenic effects [43], whereas other studies have not shown methotrexate-induced malignancy to develop in laboratory animals [83].

Causative Stressor: Radiotherapy. Therapeutic radiation in the treatment of childhood cancers is potentially carcinogenic. As previously mentioned, the development of secondary malignancies is more likely to occur if the child receives treatment with the older orthovoltage equipment than from the newer megavoltage radiation equipment. Treatment with megavoltage equipment causes less skin and bone absorption of radiation as well as less scattering of the radiation beam, and thus may be less carcinogenic. There have been, however, many reports of malignancies arising in previously irradiated areas [43].

REFERENCES

1. Abramson, D. II. Retinoblastoma: Diagnosis and Management. *CA* 32:120, 1982.
2. Arseneau, J. C., Canellos, G. P., Banks, P. M., et al. American Burkitt's Lymphoma: A Clinicopathologic Study of 30 Cases: I. Clinical Factors Relating to Prolonged Survival. *Am J Med* 58:514, 1975.
3. Bamford, F. N., Morris-Jones, P., Pearson, D., Ribeiro, G. G., Shalet, S. M., and Beardwell, C. G. Residual Disabilities in Children Treated for Intracranial Space-Occupying Lesions. *Cancer* 37:1149, 1976.
4. Beckwith, J. B. Grading of Pediatric Tumors. In American Cancer Society. *Proceedings of the National Conference on the Care of the Child with Cancer.* New York: American Cancer Society, 1979. Pp. 39–44.
5. Bithell, J. F. and Steward, A. M. Prenatal Irradiation and Childhood Malignancy: A Review of British Data From the Oxford Survey. *Br. J Cancer* 31:271, 1975.
6. Bode, U. and Levine, A. S. The Biology and Management of Osteosarcoma. In A. S. Levine (Ed.). *Cancer in the Young.* New York: Masson Publishing, 1982. Chapter 20.
7. Borstein, I. J. and Klein, A. Parents of Fatally Ill Children in a Parent's Group. In B. Schoenberg, A. C. Carr, A. H. Kutscher, D. Peretz, and I. Goldberg (Eds.). *Anticipatory Grief.* New York: Columbia University Press, 1974. Chapter 19.
8. Canellos, G. P. Reconstitution or Resurrection of Normal Stem Cells in Chronic Granulocytic Leukemia. *N Engl J Med* 300:360, 1979.
9. Carmichael, S. M., Eagleton, L., Ayers, C. R., and Mohler, D. Orthostatic Hypotension During Vincristine Therapy. *Arch Intern Med* 126:290, 1970.
10. Cassady, J. R., Jaffe, N., Paed, D., and Fuller, R. M. The Increasing Importance of Radiation Therapy in the Improved Prognosis of Children with Wilms' Tumor. *Cancer* 39:825, 1977.
11. Chard, R. L. Jr., Finklestein, J. Z., Sonley, M. J., et al. Increased Survival in Childhood Nonlymphocytic Leukemia After Treatment with Prednisone, Cytosine Arabinoside, 6-Thioguanine, Cyclophosphamide, and Oncovin (PATCO) Combination Chemotherapy. *Med Pediatr Oncol* 4:263, 1978.
12. D'Angio, G. J. Late Adversities of Treatment in Long-Term Survivors of Childhood Cancer. In American Cancer Society. *Proceedings of the American Cancer Society Second National Conference on Human Values and Cancer.* New York: American Cancer Society, 1978. Pp. 59–72.
13. D'Angio, G. J., Evans, A. E., Breslow, N., et al. The Treatment of Wilms' Tumor. *Cancer* 38:633, 1976.
14. D'Angio, G. J. and the National Wilms' Tumor Study Writing Committee. Biology and Management of Wilms' Tumor. In A. S. Levine (Ed.). *Cancer in the Young.* New York: Masson Publishing, 1982. Chapter 23.
15. Donahue, D. DES: A Case Study. *Cancer Nurs* 1:207, 1978.
16. Donaldson, S. S. Retinoblastoma. In A. S. Levine (Ed.). *Cancer in the Young.* New York: Masson Publishing, 1982. Chapter 25.
17. Donaldson, S. S., Glatstein, E., Rosenberg, S. A., and Kaplan, H. S. Pediatric Hodgkin's Disease: II. Results of Therapy. *Cancer* 37:2436, 1976.

18. Duttera, M. J., Bleyer, W. A., Pomeroy, T. C., Leventhal, C. M., and Levanthal, B. G. Irradiation, Methotrexate Toxicity, and the Treatment of Meningeal Leukemia. *Lancet* 2:703, 1973.

19. Eiser, C. Intellectual Abilities Among Survivors of Childhood Leukemia as a Function of CNS Radiation. *Arch Dis Child* 53:391, 1978.

20. Eiser, C. and Landsdown, R. Retrospective Study of Intellectual Development in Children with Acute Lymphoblastic Leukemia. *Arch Dis Child* 52:525, 1977.

21. Epstein, M. H. and Harris, J. Jr. Children with Chronic Pain—Can They Be Helped? *Pediatr Nurs* 4(1):42, 1978.

22. Ethcubanas, E. and Wilbur, J. R. Adjuvant Chemotherapy for Osteogenic Sarcoma. *Cancer Treat Rep* 62:283, 1978.

23. Evans, A. S., Niederman, J. C., and McCollum, A. T. Seroepidemiologic Studies of Infectious Mononucleosis with EB Virus. *N Engl J Med* 279:1121, 1968.

24. Evans, D. I. K., Jones, P. H. M., and Morley, C. J. Treatment of Acute Myeloid Leukemia of Childhood with Cytosine Arabinoside, Daunorubicin, Prednisone, and Mercaptopurine of Thioguanine. *Cancer* 36:1547, 1975.

25. Fleming, I., Simone, J., Jackson, R., Johnson, W., Walters, T., and Mason, C. Splenectomy and Chemotherapy in Acute Myelocytic Leukemia of Childhood. *Cancer* 33:427, 1974.

26. Frei, E. III, Jaffe, N., Paed, D., Gero, M., Skipper, H., and Watts, H. Guest Editorial— Adjuvant Chemotherapy of Osteogenic Sarcoma: Progress and Perspectives. *J Natl Cancer Inst* 60:3, 1978.

27. Fuller, A. F. The DES Syndrome and Clear Cell Adenocarcinoma in Young Women. *Cancer Nurs* 1:201, 1978.

28. Glaubiger, D. L., Tepper, J., and Makuch, R. Ewing's Sarcoma. In A. S. Levine (Ed.). *Cancer in the Young.* New York: Masson Publishing, 1982. Chapter 21.

29. Gottlieb, R. J. and Cuttner, J. Vincristine-Induced Bladder Atony. *Cancer* 30:674, 1971.

30. Greco, F. A., Brereton, H. D., Kent, H., Zimbler, H., Merrill, J., and Johnson, R. E. Adriamycin and Enhanced Radiation Reaction in Normal Esophagus and Skin. *Ann Intern Med* 85:294, 1976.

31. Gunven, P., Klein, G., Onyango, J., et al. Antibodies Associated with Epstein-Barr Virus in Burkitt's Lymphoma During Injection of BCG of Irradiated Autologous Tumor Cells. *J Natl Cancer Inst* 51:45, 1973.

32. Haas, J. M. Symptomatic Constrictive Pericarditis Developing 45 Years After Radiation to Mediastinum: A Review of Radiation Pericarditis: Case Reports. *Am Heart J* 77:89, 1969.

33. Hanson, M. R. and Mulvihill, J. J. Epidemiology of Cancer in the Young. In A. S. Levine (Ed.). *Cancer in the Young.* New York: Masson Publishing, 1982. Chapter 1.

34. Harris, C. C. Immunosuppressive Anticancer Drugs in Man: Their Oncogenic Potential. *Radiology* 114:163, 1975.

35. Harris, C. C. The Carcinogenicity of Anticancer Drugs: A Hazard in Man. *Cancer* 37:1014, 1976.

36. Hearsh, E. M., Whitcar, J. P., McCredie, K. B., Bodey, G. P., and Freireich, E. J. Chemotherapy, Immunocompetence, Immunosuppression and Prognosis in Acute Leukemia. *N Engl J Med* 285:1211, 1971.

37. Holland, J. F., Scharlau, C., Gailani, S., et al. Vincristine Treatment of Advanced Cancer: A Cooperative Study of 392 Cases. *Cancer Res* 33:1258, 1973.

38. Hussey, D. H., Castro, J. R., Sullivan, M. P., and Sutow, W. W. Radiation Therapy in Management of Wilms' Tumor. *Radiology* 101:633, 1971.

39. Husto, H. O., Pinkel, D., and Pratt, C. B. Treatment of Clinically Localized Ewing's Sarcoma with Radiotherapy and Combination Chemotherapy. *Cancer* 30:1522, 1972.

40. Ishak, K. G. and Glunz, P. R. Hepatoblastoma and Hepatocarcinoma in Infancy and Childhood: Report of 47 Cases. *Cancer* 20:396, 1967.

41. Jablon, S. and Kato, H. Childhood Cancer in Relation to Prenatal Exposure to Atomic Bomb Radiation. *Lancet* 2:1000, 1970.

42. Jaffe, N. Neuroblastoma: Review of the Literature and an Examination of Factors Contributing to Its Enigmatic Character. *Cancer Treat Rev* 3:61, 1976.

43. Jaffe, N. Pediatric Cancer—Delayed Sequelae of Treatment. In American Cancer Society. *Proceedings of the National Conference on the Care of the Child with Cancer.* New York: American Cancer Society, 1979. Pp. 118–130.

44. Karchmer, R. K., Amare, M., Larsen, W. E., et al. Alkylating Agents as Leukemogens in Mutiple Myeloma. *Cancer* 33:1103, 1974.

45. Kelly, M. G., O'Gara, R. W., Yancey, S. T., and Botkin, C. Introduction of Tumors in Rats with Procarbazine Hydrochloride. *J Natl Cancer Inst* 40:1027, 1968.

46. Knudson, A. G. Jr. and Strong, L. C. Mutation and Cancer: A Model for Wilms' Tumor of the Kidney. *J Natl Cancer Inst* 48:313, 1972.

47. Konior, G. S. and Leventhall, B. G. Immunocompetence and Prognosis in Acute Leukemia. *Semin Oncol* 3:283, 1976.

48. Krikorian, J. C., Burke, J. S., Rosenberg, S. A., and Kaplan, H. S. Occurrence of Non-Hodgkin's Lymphoma After Therapy for Hodgkin's Disease. *N Engl J Med* 300:452, 1979.

49. Kyle, R. H., Susen, A. F., and Napolitano, L. Brain Tumors in Children: A Clinical and Ultrastructural Study. *Surgery* 56:734, 1964.

50. Li, F. P., Cassady, R., and Jaffe, N. Risk of Second Tumors in Survivors of Childhood Cancer. *Cancer* 35:1230, 1975.

51. Li, F. P. and Jaffe, N. Progeny of Childhood Cancer Survivors. *Lancet* 2:707, 1974.

52. Li, F. P., Myers, M. H., Heise, H. W., and Jaffe, N. The Course of Five-Year Survivors of Cancer of Childhood. *J Pediatr* 93:185, 1978.

53. Magrath, I. Malignant Lymphomas (Including Hodgkin's Disease). In R. S. Levine (Ed.). *Cancer in the Young.* New York: Masson Publishing, 1982. Chapter 19.

54. Magrath, I. T. and Ziegler, J. L. Failure of BCG Immunostimulation to Affect the Clinical Course of Burkitt's Lymphoma. *Br Med J* 1:615, 1976.

55. Marten, G. W., Goff, J. R., Powazek, M., and Payne, J. S. Psychosocial Evaluation of Children with Cancer. In American Cancer Society. *Proceedings of the National Conference on the Care of the Child with Cancer.* New York: American Cancer Society, 1979. Pp. 45–49.

56. Matson, D. D. Benign Intracranial Tumors of Childhood. *N Engl J Med* 259:330, 1958.

57. McIntosh, S. and Aspnes, G. T. Encephalopathy Following CNS Prophylaxis in Childhood Lymphoblastic Leukemia. *Pediatrics* 52:612, 1973.

58. McIntosh, S., Klatskin, E. H., O'Brien, R. T., et al. Chronic Neurologic Disturbance in Childhood Leukemia. *Cancer* 37:853, 1976.

59. Meadows, A. T. and Evans, A. E. Effects of Chemotherapy on the Central Nervous System. *Cancer* 37:1079, 1976.

60. Miller, R. W. Mortality in Childhood Hodgkin's Disease: An Etiologic Clue. *JAMA* 198:1216, 1966.

61. Miller, R. W. Persons with Exceptionally High Risk of Leukemia. *Cancer Res* 27:2420, 1967.

62. Miller, R. W. Relation Between Cancer and Congenital Defects: An Epidemiological Evaluation. *J Natl Cancer Inst* 40:1079, 1968.

63. Miller, R. W. Etiology of Cancer During Childhood: Recent Advances. In American Cancer Society. *Proceedings of the National Conference on the Care of the Child with Cancer.* New York: American Cancer Society, 1979. Pp. 7–12.

64. Moreno, H., Castleberry, R. P., and McCann, N. P. Cytosine Arabinoside and 6-Thioguanine in the Treatment of Childhood Acute Myeloblastic Leukemia. *Cancer* 40:998, 1977.

65. Mulvihill, J. J. Ecogenetic Origins of Cancer in the Young: Environmental and Genetic Determinants. In A. S. Levine (Ed.). *Cancer in the Young.* New York: Masson Publishing, 1982. Chapter 2.

66. Nesbit, M. E., Coccia, P. F., Sather, H. N., et al. Staging in Pediatric Malignancies. In American Cancer Society. *Proceedings of the National Conference on the Care of the Child with Cancer.* New York: American Cancer Society, 1979. Pp. 31–38.

67. Newburger, P. E. and Sallen, S. E. Symptom Control in Childhood Malignancy: Pain and Vomiting. In American Cancer Society. *Proceedings of the National Conference on the Care of the Child with Cancer.* New York: American Cancer Society, 1979. Pp. 106–117.

68. O'Gara, R. W., Adamson, R. H., Kelly, M. G., and Dalgard, D. W. Neoplasms of the Hematopoietic System in Nonhuman Primates: Report of One Spontaneous Tumor and Two Leukemias Induced by Procarbazine. *J Natl Cancer Inst* 46:1121, 1971.

69. Oliff, A. and Levine, A. S. Late Effects of Anti-Neoplastic Therapy. In A. S. Levine (Ed.). *Cancer in the Young.* New York: Masson Publishing, 1982. Chapter 28.

70. Parker, R. G. and Bery, H. C. Late Effects of Therapeutic Irradiation on the Skeleton and Bone Marrow. *Cancer* 37:1162, 1976.

71. Pavlovsky, S., Penalver, J., Eppinger-Helft, M., et al. Induction and Maintenance of Remission in Acute Leukemia. *Cancer* 31:273, 1973.

72. Pederson-Bjergaard, J., Nissen, N. E., Sorensen, H. M., et al. Acute Nonlymphocytic Leukemia in Patients with Ovarian Carcinoma Following Long-Term Treatment with Tresulfan (Dihydroxybusulfan). *Cancer* 45:19, 1980.

73. Perez, C. A., Razek, A., Tefft, M., et al. Analysis of Local Tumor Control in Ewing's Sarcoma: Preliminary Results of a Cooperative Intergroup Study. *Cancer* 40:2864, 1977.

74. Peylan-Ramu, N., Poplack, D. G., Pizzo, P. A., et al. Abnormal CT Scans of the Brain in Asymptomatic Children with Acute Lymphocytic Leukemia After Prophylactic Treatment of the CNS with Radiation and Intrathecal Chemotherapy. *N Engl J Med* 298:8, 1972.

75. Pinkel, D., Husto, H. O., Rhomes, J. A. A., et al. Radiotherapy in Leukemia and Lymphoma of Children. *Cancer* 39:817, 1977.

76. Pizzo, P. A. Infectious Complications in the Young Patient with Cancer: Etiology, Pathogenesis, Diagnosis, Management, and Prevention. In A. S. Levine (Ed.). *Cancer in the Young.* New York: Masson Publishing, 1982. Chapter 13.

77. Pizzo, P. A. Rhabdomyosarcoma and the Soft-Tissue Sarcomas. In A. S. Levine (Ed.). *Cancer in the Young.* New York: Masson Publishing, 1982. Chapter 22.

78. Poplack, D. G. Acute Lymphoblastic Leukemia and Less Frequently Occurring Leukemias in the Young. in A. S. Levine (Ed.). *Cancer in the Young.* New York: Masson Publishing, 1982. Chapter 17.

79. Poplack, D. G. and Blatt, J. Neuroblastoma. In A. S. Levine (Ed.). *Cancer in the Young.* New York: Masson Publishing, 1982. Chapter 24.

80. Pratt, C. B., Husto, H. O., and Pinkel, D. Coordinated Treatment of Childhood Rhabdomyosarcoma. *Prog Clin Cancer* 6:87, 1975.

81. Putnam, T. C., Nelson, D. F., and Klemperer, M. Pediatric Solid Tumors. In P. Rubin (Ed.). *Clinical Oncology for Medical Students and Physicians: A Multidisciplinary Approach* (5th Ed.). New York: American Cancer Society, 1978. Chapter 23.

82. Reich, S. D. Toxicity of Anticancer Drugs Used in Children. *Cancer Nurs* 3:385, 1980.

83. Reimer, R. R. Risk of a Second Malignancy Related to the Use of Cytotoxic Chemotherapy. *CA* 32:286, 1982.

84. Reimer, R. R. and Groppe, C. W. Jr. Acute Nonlymphocytic Leukemia Following Treatment with Radiomimetic Drugs. *Ann Intern Med* 90:989, 1979.

85. Reimer, R. R., Hoover, R., Fraumenia, F. F. Jr., and Young, R. C. Acute Leukemia After Alkylating Agent Therapy of Ovarian Cancer. *N Engl J Med* 292:177, 1977.

86. Rosen, G. Malignant Musculoskeletal Tumors: The Clinical Investigative Approach to Combined Therapy. In American Cancer Society. *Proceedings of the National Conference on the Care of the Child with Cancer.* New York: American Cancer Society, 1979. Pp. 71–82.

87. Rubin, P., Landman, S., Mayer, E., Keller, B., and Ciccio, S. Bone Marrow Regeneration After Extended Field Irradiation in Hodgkin's Disease. *Cancer* 32:699, 1973.

88. Safyer, A. W. and Miller, R. W. Childhood Cancer: Etiologic Clues From Epidemiology. *J Sch Health* 47(3):158, 1977.

89. Sandler, S. G., Tobin, W., and Henderson, E. S. Vincristine-induced Neuropathy: A Clinical Study of Fifty Patients. *Neurology* 19:397, 1969.

90. Schwartz, D. B. The Teenager and Cancer: I. Treatment. In United States Department of Health and Human Services. *Proceedings of the First National Conference for Parents of Children with Cancer,* NIH Publication No. 80–2176. Bethesda, MD: United States Department of Health and Human Services, 1980. Pp. 29–40.

91. Scott, D. L. and Thomas, R. D. Late Onset Constrictive Pericarditis After Thoracic Radiotherapy. *Br Med J* 1:341, 1978.

92. Shidnia, H., Hornback, N. B., Helveston, E. M., Gettlefinger, T., and Biglan, A. W. Treatment Results of Retinoblastoma at Indiana University Hospitals. *Cancer* 40:2917, 1977.

93. Simone, J. G. Leukemia. In American Cancer Society. *Proceedings of the National Conference on the Care of the Child with Cancer.* New York: American Cancer Society, 1979. Pp. 50–55.

94. Simone, J. V., Aur, R. J. A., Husto, H. O., VerZosa, M. S., and Pinkell, D. Three to Ten Years after Cessation of Therapy in Children with Leukemia. *Cancer* 42:839, 1978.

95. Stream, P., Harrington, E., and Clark, M. Bone Marrow Transplantation: An Option for Children with Acute Leukemia. *Cancer Nurs* 3:195, 1980.

96. Sutow, W. W., Gehan, E. A., et al. Multidrug Adjuvant Chemotherapy for Osteosarcoma: Interim Report of the Southwest Oncology Group Studies. *Cancer Treat Rep* 62:265, 1978.

97. Tefft, M., Chabora, B., and Rosen, G. Radiation in Bone Sarcomas: A Re-Evaluation in the Era of Intensive Systemic Chemotherapy. *Cancer* 39:806, 1977.

98. Thomas, E. D., Sanders, J. E., and Johnson, F. L. Marrow Transplantation in the Therapy of Children with Acute Leukemia. In American Cancer Society. *Proceedings of the National Conference on the Care of the Child with Cancer.* New York: American Cancer Society, 1979. Pp. 172–175.

99. VanEys, J. The Outlook for the Child with Cancer. *J Sch Health* 47:165, 1977.

100. VonHoff, D. D., Layard, M. W., Basa, P., et al. Risk Factors of Doxorubicin-induced Congestive Heart Failure. *Ann Intern Med* 91:710, 1979.

101. VonHoff, D. D., Rozencweig, M., Layard, M., Slavik, M., and Muggia, F. M. Daunomycin-induced Cardiotoxicity in Children and Adults. *Am J Med* 62:200, 1977.

102. Walker, M. D. Tumors of the Central Nervous System. In A. S. Levine (Ed.). *Cancer in the Young.* New York: Masson Publishing, 1982. Chapter 26.

103. Weinstein, H. H., Mayer, R. J., Rosenthal, D. S., et al. Treatment of Acute Myelogenous Leukemia in Children and Adults. *N Engl J Med* 303:473, 1980.

104. Wiernik, P. H. Acute Nonlymphocytic Leukemia in Young People. In A. S. Levine (Ed.). *Cancer in the Young.* New York: Masson Publishing, 1982. Chapter 18.

105. Wilbur, J. R. Combination Chemotherapy for Embryonal Rhabdomyosarcoma. *Cancer Chemother Rep* 58:281, 1974.

106. Wilbur, J. R. and Mott, M. G. Non-Hodgkin's Lymphoma in Children. In American

Cancer Society. *Proceedings of the National Conference on the Care of the Child with Cancer.* New York: American Cancer Society, 1979. Pp. 56–61.

107. Wilson, C. B. Medulloblastoma: Current Views Regarding the Tumor and Its Treatment. *Oncology* 24:273, 1970.

108. Yates, P. O. Tumors of the Central Nervous System in Children. *J Clin Pathol* 17:418, 1964.

109. Young, J. L. Jr. and Miller, R. W. Incidence of Malignant Tumors in U. S. Children. *J Pediatr* 86:254, 1975.

110. Ziegler, J. L. Burkitt's Lymphoma. *CA* 32:144, 1982.

111. Ziegler, J. L. and Bluming, A. Z. Intrathecal Chemotherapy in Burkitt's Lymphoma. *Br Med J* 3:508, 1971.

Chapter 10

Nursing Care of the Child With Cancer

INTRODUCTION

CONCEPT I:
Cancer and its treatment impede the child's normal growth and development.

Since childhood cancers pose major obstacles to the normal growth and development of the afflicted child, it may be said that the child with cancer is a handicapped child. The extent and severity of the handicap depends upon the magnitude of the obstacles to the child's fulfillment of his or her optimal functioning. The obstacles impeding normal growth and development in the child with cancer may be related to the disease itself or to the environmental alterations that occur because of the disease (e.g., hospitalization, isolation, disruption of school attendance, and side effects of treatment).

CONCEPT II:
The overall task of childhood is to prepare to be an independent, productive, and responsible adult.

AGE PROFILES

Infancy

The infant is totally dependent upon others for survival, as well as for the stimulation necessary for the development of personality, language, mobility, and so on. As bonding between the infant and parents strengthens, the baby's task of learning to trust is accomplished. Since nurses do not usually respond as quickly as the parents would to the infant's cry of pain or cry for food, it is not surprising that there are significant changes in the baby's eating, sleeping, and elimination habits if the infant is hospitalized [17].

Toddler

The toddler is busy exploring the world and increasing and refining language, social, and motor skills. If hospitalization is required, nurses should encourage the toddler's small steps toward independence and autonomy while simultaneously providing a safe environment for the child. The toddler needs his parents and attending health professionals to set and maintain behavioral limits, since unrestricted freedom of behavior and unwarranted permissiveness is a tremendous threat to the toddler's sense of safety and security [27].

Preschool age

The preschool child likes to be actively involved in group play. Organized group play allows the child to learn (1) to interact with and relate to other children and adults, (2) appropriate sex role behavior, (3) appropriate social behavior, and (4) the rewards and punishment associated with various behaviors and actions. The preschooler has little sense of time, living only in the present. A child of this age is also very egocentric and has great difficulty realizing that other people may have different viewpoints about a specific issue. Yet, this very egocentricity that is characteristic of preschool children allows them to attain some measure of control over what happens in their world. A primary characteristic of preschoolers is the phenomenon of precausal thinking, in which the child believes that there is a cause-and-effect relationship between his or her thoughts and subsequent events in the external environment. With precausal thinking, the child will assume responsibility for unpleasant occurrences which may result in a tremendous sense of self-blame and guilt if the unpleasant occurrence happens to be serious illness with its attendant painful procedures.

When nursing the hospitalized preschool child, it is both important and appropriate to encourage the child to make things, to color and draw, and to participate in playing with groups of other children in the playroom. Because of the child's lack of a sense of time, it is helpful to make a calendar that marks the days in terms of specific events, preferably events that are not treatment-related. An example of such a calendar might be "This day is Monday when your brothers and sisters will come to visit. Here is Tuesday, and that is the day when Mary the occupational therapist will come to play with you. The next day is Wednesday, when I will sit with you and we will read a book together," etc. By allowing the child to mark off the days on the calendar and by identifying the passage of time with concrete and pleasant events, the child will feel an increased sense of control and is less likely to fear that hospitalization will continue forever.

School-age

The school-age child's tasks include refinement of physical skills, building a positive self-image, the development of fundamental intellectual skills, developing a sense of values and morality, and achieving personal independence. If these tasks are not accomplished, a permanent sense of inferiority and inadequacy may result.

If a school-age child must be hospitalized, it is crucial for the nurse to facilitate the child's continued growth and development by enhancing his or her ability to progress toward achievement of these tasks. School-age children are characterized by industry and "busyness," so they may easily become bored and frustrated with the long hours in a hospital room with little to do. Again, encouragement of participation in playroom group activities is of value, as is the availability of materials necessary for art or craft projects. Nurses should display the things made by the school-age child in a prominent place where the child can see that "their" nurses value their art projects.

Continuation of school even while the child is hospitalized is important. Utilization of the hospital-based teacher will help ensure that the child does not fall behind in school work and face subsequent embarrassment upon return to the regular school. In addition, continuation of school work as much as possible will enhance the child's sense of security and normalcy, lessening fear, providing distraction, and reducing the child's feeling of "being different" from other children.

Adolescence

The tasks of the adolescent are to create a clear, positive self-concept and to initiate and maintain intimate relationships with others. If these tasks are not achieved during adolescence, then role confusion, cynicism, and apathy will result and may be irreparable. A more detailed description of the special needs and struggles of the adolescent may be found later in this chapter.

CHILDREN WITH CANCER

Though the child may be acutely ill at the time of diagnosis, few families or their sick children suspect a diagnosis as dire as cancer. Depending on how physically debilitated he or she is at the time of diagnostic workup, the child will experience emotions ranging from mild bewilderment to utter confusion and terror, and there is an aura of unreality about the situation in the hospital because everything happens so fast. In addition, for many children, the time of diagnosis is their first experience with hospitalization and thus is fraught with fear, separation from parents and loved ones, strange faces, bizarre and painful experiences, and foreign routines.

At the time of diagnosis, parents characteristically begin to blame themselves for not detecting symptoms sooner or for supposed errors in judgment. One of the primary tasks of parenting is to protect children from harm. Parents generally feel an extraordinary amount of guilt and self-blame when they suddenly are faced with the ultimate threat: the loss of their child. It is brutal for parents to realize that they are virtually helpless to protect their beloved child from pain and death. Parents commonly begin to seek ways to undo the past and to expiate their own tremendous guilt. They often become overprotective, permissive, and leap at opportunities to "do for" their child.

If, however, the overall task of childhood is preparation for responsible and independent adulthood, nothing can be more threatening to the child than to take this task away and to remove what autonomy and self-determination he or she has already achieved. The disease process of cancer, as well as its treatment, results in constantly changing external and internal environments. The disease itself may impose sudden and unexpected changes, and adverse side effects of antineoplastic treatment add even more stressors to an already highly stressful situation. It is important that health professionals realize that even positive changes or a sudden clinical improvement require as much adjustment as a deterioration of the child's condition [33]. As the child and parents begin to realize that treatment almost always requires years instead of days or weeks and that childhood cancer is characterized by an uncertain pattern of remission and relapse, their stress levels increase even more in anxious anticipation of what may come. As more effective medical treatments and increased survival rates have transformed childhood cancer from a rapidly fatal illness to a chronic yet life-threatening disease, the distress accompanying the illness has risen to enormous levels. Consequently, childhood cancer now exacts tremendous biological, personal, and social costs from both the ill child and the family.

COSTS OF CHILDHOOD CANCER

The costs of childhood malignancy include the biological, personal, and social aspects of (1) the morbidity accompanying the disease and its medical/nursing treatment, (2) the morbidity of late sequelae of antineoplastic treatment, which has only come under scrutiny as a result of more effective treatment and thus long-term survivors, and (3) the concerns and stressors experienced by long-term survivors that are not experienced by young people without a history of cancer.

Biological, personal, and social aspects of the morbidity associated with childhood malignancy and its treatment may cause serious disruption in the child's growth, development, and ability to form trusting, long-lasting relationships. Biological aspects of disease- or treatment-induced morbidity include changes in appearance because of surgery, radiotherapy, or drugs; pain; weight changes; and fatigue, bleeding, and infection secondary to myelosuppression. Some of the personal aspects of morbidity resulting from cancer and its treatment are fear, despair, helplessness, and hopelessness, as well as a wide range of other maladaptive coping mechanisms. Sudden enforced dependency upon others, whether at home or in the hospital, is incongruent with whatever level of autonomy and self-determination the child has achieved, and the child frequently is unable to perform well in school. Social aspects of cancer-related morbidity include drastic alterations in family life style and isolation from and changes in relationships with family members, friends, and peers.

Long-term survivors of childhood cancer must also deal with the morbidity associated with late sequelae of antineoplastic treatment and of the cancer experience, some of which may not manifest themselves for years after definitive treatment has been stopped. Costs for these children may include serious or even life-threatening physical dysfunction; the development of secondary malignancies; psychological, cognitive, or sexual disorders; and/or difficulties in establishing and maintaining an intimate, healthy relationship with a potential or actual marriage partner.

Long-term survivors of childhood cancer have other concerns and stressors not shared by young people who have not experienced cancer. These concerns include (1) obtaining adequate health and life insurance, (2) genetic counseling regarding the effects of antineoplastic treatment on future offspring, (3) vocational rehabilitation, (4) job security, and (5) living daily with the uncertainty and fear that the malignancy will recur [14].

MILITARY IMAGERY AND CANCER

The conversation of caregivers and the professional literature is replete with military imagery regarding cancer, and the verbiage itself subtly adds to the tension and fear surrounding childhood malignancy. Cancer is called the *enemy*, and both professional and lay groups have *declared war* on childhood cancer. The *killing* radiotherapy beam is focused on the *foreign* and *bad* cells. New drugs are added to the *arsenal* of *weapons*. Malignancy is described as a state of cellular *anarchy*, and antineoplastic treatment hopes to *eradicate* the cancer. Especially with children, the malignancy is to be *cut out, destroyed, burned,* or *killed* regardless of the physical, personal, or social costs involved. Chemotherapeutic drugs are referred to as the *toxins*, the *poisons*, and the *anti*neoplastics. In such a war, the end point is the total and permanent destruction of the enemy, with the child's body and psyche as the battleground [1].

The cancer cells, however, reside and exist within the children themselves. Perhaps the fear, despair, helplessness, and other stressors commonly accompanying childhood malignancies could be reduced by an awareness of and decrease in such military imagery. Increased survival time makes it mandatory that both the afflicted child and the parents must live continuously with the additional tension imposed by such destructive verbiage. Perhaps there needs to be a change in attitude in which cancer is not viewed as a *foreign killer* but instead as normal cells gone awry and not functioning as they ought. By reinforcing the militaristic attitude, both health professionals and lay people add to the negative stressors, fear, and tension of childhood cancer, and we *must* consider the cost of the "battle" to the child.

> **CONCEPT III:**
> **The definition of a "truly cured" child cannot be limited to the eradication of malignant cells from the body or to the absence of biological dysfunction; the definition of "true cure" must also include wellness in the personal and social aspects of the child's life [34, 39].**

Children with cancer must never be defined by their diagnoses. Regardless of the specific diagnosis, each child has unique and basic biological, personal, and social needs and rights that must be met in order to assure achievement of maximum development of total potential [40]. A true cure implies that, during the period of time between diagnosis and death, the child must be biologically, personally, and socially happy and well. Hope is focused on the child's eventual death from old age owing to causes unrelated to the former cancer. This is easier to achieve with a seventy-year-old person with cancer who dies five years later from a myocardial infarction. To achieve that same result with a five-year-old child, she or he must live for another seventy years. Thus, by this definition, cures of childhood cancer have not been frequently achieved [39].

BIOLOGICAL ASPECTS OF CURE

The above-stated example of a child living for seventy years after definitive antineoplastic treatment has been stopped and eventually dying from causes unrelated to cancer is part of the definition of biological cure. Another portion of the definition of biological cure is the proportion of children surviving with no indications of cancer or cancer-related symptoms, not receiving any antineoplastic medical therapy, and considered to have little or no risk of relapse [34]. However, it must be remembered that disease which is in remission is not clinically evident and without symptomatology. Although remission can last for periods of years, remission is *not* the same as cure. It is thus difficult to differentiate between biological cure and remission, and the word "cure" must be used with extreme caution since false and unrealistic hopes may be raised inappropriately.

PERSONAL ASPECTS OF CURE

The "psyche" and the "soma" cannot be separated. What affects one has an echo effect on the other. Personal aspects of the truly cured child include (1) the ability to think, grow, behave, and adapt in a healthy manner within the context of the child's own priorities, expectations, and values, and (2) the continual experience of feeling well and self-contented. Unfortunately, attention to the emotional implications of prolonged survival has not kept pace with attention to the rapid increase in the technological sophistication responsible for the increase in biological cures. The technical aspects of biological cure are most often the singular focus, and the more subjective aspects of personal and social cures are neglected.

SOCIAL ASPECTS OF CURE

The primary characteristic of social cure of the child with cancer is the ability to form intimate and satisfactory interpersonal relationships. Much of the potential for social cure depends upon the parental and staff relationships with and response to the child with cancer. For example, if a two-year-old is automatically expected to die—and so is indulged and spoiled—and then is declared biologically cured at age six, the child is not socially normal and may have a serious or even incurable handicap in adjusting to school, other people, and society.

BIOLOGICAL/PERSONAL/SOCIAL CURE

To achieve true cure in the child with cancer, holistic care is mandatory. The emphasis is not on care *rather than* cure, but on care *plus* cure. Cure has to be expected in order to be achieved. If one does not anticipate a biological cure and yet achieves it, a truly cured child will not be the result, for the aspects of personal and social cure will not have been attended to.

Thus, parents and staff must treat the child as normally as possible, including appropriate discipline, in order to achieve maximal biological/personal/social cure. After all, a child with cancer is just that—a normal child who happens to have cancer.

PERSONAL ASPECTS OF THE CHILDHOOD CANCER EXPERIENCE

CONCEPT IV:
The personal costs of the childhood cancer experience include disruptions in growth and development, psychological functioning, and cognitive abilities.

The child with cancer is suddenly thrust into a new role: that of being sick and "different" from healthy peers. For this child, tomorrow may not be of primary importance; rather the quality of life both now and during the period of time between now and tomorrow is of primary importance. Approximately 50 percent of children with cancer will survive for long periods of time and many will even be cured. Just a few decades ago, psychological issues and interventions surrounding children with cancer dealt with the aspect of death occurring at a young age. Now, however, with increased survival and even cures, new issues surrounding personal care of the child with cancer are raised. These children must deal with pain, disability, hospitalization, and the demands of diagnostic procedures and treatment that may extend over many years. The many remissions, relapses, and intermittent acute physical problems cause personal stress and anxiety, as does the separation between children with cancer and their families, peers, and communities. The necessity of developing positive relationships with new nurses and physicians is a further personal stress with which these children must deal.

All children, even very young toddlers and preschoolers, have varying levels of awareness of themselves and of others and variable degrees of the capacity to interpret and express their responses to experiences. The degree to which they express themselves depends upon their developmental stage, biological age, the degree to which their central nervous system is intact, and encountered experiences that facilitate or impede their introspective and expressive abilities [15].

Thus, the cancer experience presents major obstacles to normal psychological/emotional adjustment. Childhood cancer carries with it the risks that the disease process itself, disease-imposed restrictions, and/or severe anxiety will result in significant psychological crippling of the child. This, in turn, may result in the inability to form a healthy sense of self-esteem, may interfere with successful mastery of normal developmental tasks of childhood and adolescence, and may impede the development of cognitive skills and abilities [41].

CLINICAL COURSES OF CHILDHOOD CANCER

There are five possible clinical courses of childhood cancer, and each has both separate and overlapping personal and social implications (see Figure 10.1).

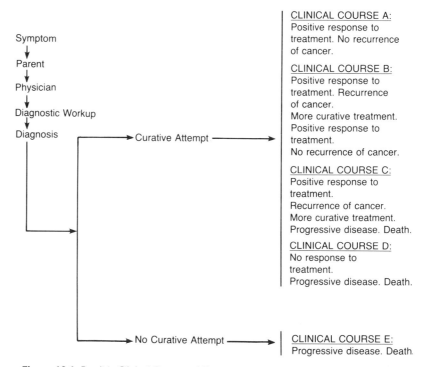

Figure 10.1. Possible Clinical Courses of Cancer.

Clinical course A represents early cancer that is eradicated by antineoplastic treatment. The child or adolescent is both elated and very fearful of a recurrence of symptoms and disease. As time and experience proves that the disease has not recurred, the young person is declared cured. Gradually, the child incorporates the frightening cancer experience into his or her life and, although left with a residual nagging fear regarding his or her vulnerability to cancer, the child basically resumes his or her former life style.

Clinical course B represents early cancer that may or may not be completely eradicated by antineoplastic therapy. Symptom recurrence eventually happens, and the child requires at least one more series of antineoplastic treatments. The antineoplastic therapy is finally successful in eradicating the disease, and cure is eventually achieved.

Clinical course C is the most common and conspicuous among children with cancer. Definitive curative treatment is given in an attempt to at least put the disease into remission. The remission may last months to years, and the child appears to be healthy and may even resume normal activities. However, both the child and the parents are frightened of disease recurrence. After long-term remission allows them to be more optimistic regarding the prognosis, they tend to relax. Yet this is only a period of grace, and metastatic or progressive disease eventually becomes evident. The first recurrence is particularly devastating because it abruptly indicates that the child's prognosis is poorer than the child and family had initially hoped. Newer treatments, perhaps including experimental drug protocols, are tried. Although some positive results occur, progressive disease is still apparent. Few children, especially adolescents, give up the fight altogether at this point, and it is not unusual for parents to request any treatment at all that may offer even a slim chance of cure.

Clinical course D is characterized by no clinical response at all to attempts at curative therapy. Regardless of the antineoplastic treatment that is administered, the disease progresses and death eventually ensues.

Clinical course E obviously has the worst prognosis. Curative treatment is not even attempted, and only palliation is possible. Disease progression is relentless and always culminates in death.

PSYCHOLOGICAL/EMOTIONAL DYSFUNCTION

Psychological/emotional dysfunction and problems with growth and development in the child with cancer are so intertwined that they will be dealt with simultaneously in this section.

A conscious, reflective awareness of self, others, and events does indeed exist in even very young children. Three stages of reaction to hospitalization have been identified: protest, despair, and denial, in that order [17]. The protest stage usually lasts less than twenty-four hours, and the child loudly and vocally protests examinations and procedures. During the despair phase, nursing and medical staff see the child "settling down and behaving" and being more cooperative with necessary procedures. This is a temporary stage and a period of extreme separation anxiety. Instead of insisting that the parent leave the hospital room during examinations and procedures, the staff's anxiety regarding presence of the parent must be weighed against the child's psychic pain of separation anxiety. Severe separation anxiety will decrease the child's cooperation as well as increase fear and the pain experience. During the denial stage, the child expresses no desire to go home. In fact, dismissal from the hospital may be a time of psychological crisis for the child, and parents may be overtly rebuffed.

The personal costs to the child with cancer are very real. The child has to cope with real threats to his or her mental/emotional stability secondary to low self-esteem, poor self-image, the experience of being "different" from normal healthy peers, and delayed physical and mental development. The developing child has a relatively short time to master specific skills and developmental tasks. Once these time opportunities are lost, subsequent development may be delayed or simply arrested. Older children and adolescents may have developed tentative career plans and life goals which, with cancer diagnosis and treatment, may become unrealistic and even impossible. Such children need extensive guidance and support in order to reprioritize and rearrange plans and goals. The costs of cancer and cancer treatment include the worry about possible sterility and/or defective children of their own. The latter is now known to be of minimal concern but it is still perceived by the children and parents as very real. Another personal cost of great magnitude is the issue of cure versus death, and the statistics don't mean much to the children or parents when it is themselves or their child who has a malignant disease. Finally, a significant mental cost is worry over the possible development of a secondary cancer.

Normal growth and development must be sustained in order to (1) preserve the child's emotional stability and sense of control, (2) develop an accurate perception of self, (3) nurture the child's self-esteem, (4) preserve relationships with family and friends, and (5) deal with an uncertain future [25]. Even though the child has a chronic, life-threatening disease, she or he will still continue to grow and develop. Extensive, overly intense, or persistent fears interfere with the child's normal mastery of developmental tasks and enjoyment of life.

Very young children may view hospitalization as punishment for real or imagined misdeeds, and they may react with separation anxiety and anger. Common responses from these young children include either clinging to or ignoring parents, refusal to eat or sleep, great fear of treatments, silence and withdrawal, and hostile reactions to friendly overtures.

School-age children with cancer are especially vulnerable to developing a sense of inferiority [40]. Loss of time from school has a negative effect on the child's peer relationships. Pain, weakness, and other symptoms decrease the child's energy and interferes with his or her sense of achievement. The strange and often painful world of the hospital or clinic forces the school-age child to be increasingly dependent upon adults, leading to a variety of responses from the child such as regression, anger, withdrawal, clinging, manipulative behavior, depression, and crying. Older children may keenly feel that they are burdensome to their parents and may react with pseudoindependence. The school-age child's growing awareness of the seriousness and chronicity of his or her condition is, however, balanced by an increased cognitive understanding and by the capacity to use language and activity to cope with the cancer experience.

Adolescence is the most demanding stage in life in which to have to deal with malignant disease. Although adolescents are old enough to fully understand the implications of their disease, they have not yet completed the personality integration or developed the adult defense mechanisms needed to effectively cope with the cancer experience. The transition from childhood to adulthood is a time of enormous physical, personal, and social growth and development. Adolescence is marked by sexual maturation, increased capacity for abstract thought, and changing relationships with family and peers. A primary task of adolescence is to assert independence constructively, yet the cancer experience increases dependence in every area. Hospital routines virtually eradicate any privacy for the adolescent, something which is especially valued as a symbol of independence. Forced into unwanted dependence, the adolescent may rebel by acting out, taking risks, or failing to comply with treatment regimens.

Once remission is induced, adolescents begin to be acutely aware of being different from their peers. Specific symptoms such as alopecia, amputation, and so on are the focal points around which the feelings of the adolescent revolve. At this point, the symptoms themselves are what the adolescent must adjust to. Some symptoms impinge more insistently upon the adolescent's awareness, some imply a greater threat of death, and some pose a larger threat to self-esteem [35]. Major problems for the adolescent are weakness, fatigue, and the hovering protectiveness of parents, all of which are embarrassing to the adolescent. To be different from peers causes distress at any age; but during adolescence, "being different" becomes a crisis of major significance. A major psychological turning point occurs when adolescents are able to demonstrate to themselves that they can still function like their peers.

Expression of Feelings

Often the child perceives that it is not acceptable to express feelings. If, for example, the child tries to talk to parents about the fearful and painful experiences only to have the parents cry, change the subject, or turn away, the child will be further burdened with the task of protecting his or her parents from distress. Allowing the child to express feelings of apprehension, pain, loneliness, and so on implies that adult caregivers and parents must allow the child to ask questions with the assurance of receiving honest answers. Health professionals must gently assist parents to maintain a relationship with their child that is as normal and healthy as possible. Honesty cannot be overemphasized, for the child will know when lies or partial truths are given. If the adults lie, the trust between the sick child and the adults will be destroyed, resulting in even greater fear in the child.

It is crucial for parents and staff to have accurate information about the child's disease process, treatment plans, and prognosis. It is as harmful to overemphasize discussion of death with a child who has a good prognosis as it is to ignore the subject of death with a child who will most probably die. If death is emphasized to the child with a good prognosis, the result may be psychological euthanasia. To assume a fatal outcome often results in a self-fulfilling prophecy. No promise of cure or death should be given, but all children with cancer should be viewed as children who are living and yet might die.

As the first remission continues for lengthening periods of time, the life of the child and family usually returns to near normal. With each well day and with each good medical report, the hoped-for cure seems more likely to be achieved. After all, the child has paid a high price for survival: pain, treatment side effects, possibly an amputated limb, and so on. Thus, the time of the first relapse is often the most difficult time for both the child and the family, for the fragile hope that the first remission would lead to cure is vaporized. Times of relapse are often times of great anger, and the child often expresses this anger toward himself or herself, parents, staff, and other children. By this time, most of these children have become good friends with other children who have cancer, and if some of these friends have died, it shakes the child badly. Very young children react to relapse with despair because of the repetition of the entire painful experience of hospitalization, treatments, and so on. Older children often respond with denial, anger, depression, and withdrawal. The adolescent frequently experiences a sense of growing entrapment during relapse, feeling terrible frustration because of the inability to make plans or to be normal. Times of relapse make the child even more acutely aware of the uncertainty with which he or she must live. Although the uncertainty allows for hope, it is in itself highly stressful. Parents may especially need help in understanding that their child, although seriously ill, is still growing up physically and emotionally and needs to continue to establish growing independence. Enhancement of the child's self-esteem is of crucial importance during times of relapse or progressive disease. Self-esteem is strengthened by parental acceptance, clearly defined and enforced behavioral limits, and the opportunity for the child to act independently within those defined limits [36].

Therapeutic Intervention Into Psychological/Emotional Problems

When assessing areas for intervention, the nurse must consider the child's cognitive level as well as his or her emotional needs. Two assessment methods particularly valuable with younger children are drawing pictures and play therapy, and these two methods are also useful for intervention into anxiety. Playing and drawing pictures provide pleasure for the child, serve as a safe method to express feelings, and can help the child master anxiety [9, 37].

Because of their greater cognitive abilities and larger capacity for abstract thinking, older children and adolescents will benefit by being given some degree of responsibility in their treatment. This will decrease the possibility of maladaptive rebellion and will increase the child's sense of independence. For example, the older child or adolescent might arrange the hospital scheduling of baths, physical therapy, and so on, and it may be necessary to give antineoplastic treatments in the evening for outpatients in order to minimize disruptions of school and social activities.

Conferences between nurses, physicians, and parents must include the child in order to avoid projectng a sense of conspiracy, and this intervention becomes increasingly important with the increasing age of the child. Discussions of death must be tempered with realistic hope in order to avoid the psychological euthanasia mentioned earlier. The child should clearly understand that problems such as disruptions in family finances are not his or her fault, any more than the disease is the child's fault. Finally, as a general rule, consistency and honesty from the adult caregivers will decrease the child's anxiety, but rigidity will only increase the child's sense of helplessness and loss of control.

COGNITIVE DISRUPTIONS

School is a child's work, and school-age children with cancer should return to their regular school and school activities as soon as possible. Cessation of the child's schooling strongly carries the implicit message that there is no hope. Disruptions in education have major negative effects on the child and the family, and there are major obstacles for the child with cancer to overcome in order to continue his education. These include parental, child, teacher, and medical obstacles [20].

Parental Obstacles

Parents may be reluctant to send their child back to school, reasoning that keeping the child at home will reduce the chance of infection or bleeding or that allowing the child to stay out of school will protect him or her from teasing and ridicule by the child's schoolmates. However, these reasons are not valid when compared with the more major threats to self-esteem and hope that are engendered by the cessation of school activities. Parental obstacles usually exist when the parents are unable to deal realistically with their child's disease process and prognosis. Thus, parental reluctance to return the child to school is generally symptomatic of deeper parental psychological problems.

Child Obstacles

Child-related obstacles are usually more minor than parental obstacles. A child's reluctance to return to school is most often secondary to changes in body image and is usually fairly easily managed by support from parents and teachers.

Teacher Obstacles

Teachers and school administrators must resist the idea that school life and home life are distinctly separate entities. When the student happens to be a child with cancer, school and home lives may even overlap more than usual. Teachers rarely receive any input at all from the health care team, which leaves the teachers in a most unfavorable position. The teacher may greatly overprotect the child with cancer because of the fear that the child may become seriously ill or even die during class. Teachers may also be fearful that the sick child or other students will ask questions that the teacher feels unprepared to answer, and they may also feel unprepared to deal with well students who tease the ill child. Teachers must be given adequate and appropriate information on a continuing basis about the child's disease, treatment side effects, and prognosis.

Medical Obstacles

The disease process itself, especially brain tumors or leukemic infiltration of the central nervous system, can impede cognitive development. The process of antineoplastic treatment certainly causes major disruptions in the child's school attendance. Medical obstacles can be minimized if the treatment team considers the child's return to regular school as an important rehabilitative goal. Treatments should be scheduled so as to reduce unnecessary or excessive school absences, and school nurses and teachers must receive appropriate and adequate information in order to facilitate the child's successful return to school.

Mainstreaming

Public Law 94–142, enacted in 1975, mandates that children who meet certain criteria have the right to an individualized educational program appropriate to both medical and educational needs [32]. Children with cancer need mainstreaming in school, just as other "different" children do under this public law. Since the child's disease outcome is uncertain, both health and educational professionals should assume that the child will be cured unless and until it is known that cure is impossible. School is appropriate even for the fatally ill child, since it can distract the child from pain and other symptoms by focusing attention on school and peer group activities at any level of which the child is capable.

SOCIAL ASPECTS OF THE CHILDHOOD CANCER EXPERIENCE

CONCEPT V:
If we are to effectively deal with the *child*, not with just the cancer, health professionals must realize that cancer is a powerful and negative social stigma.

Thirty years ago, children with cancer were relatively invisible to the larger community because the disease caused death in a matter of just a few weeks. Now, however, with extended survival times and even cures in children with cancer, childhood malignancy has become a chronic disease and thus the child with cancer is increasingly visible to the larger society. Still, most people interpret the statement, "This child has cancer," to mean "This child will die soon." Only a very small percentage of our population realizes that cancer, especially in children, is no longer synonymous with death. Most people believe that cure is a miracle to be prayed for, and they don't realize that approximately 50 percent of children with leukemia can expect to be alive and free of disease in five years. Although cancer is the leading cause of death from disease in children after the first year of life, it is still sufficiently rare that most people contact a child with cancer only occasionally. Thus, the social stigma of cancer disappears only slowly.

CONCEPT VI:
Since the family functions as a unit, regardless of which family member has cancer, each person within the family is significantly affected by the disease and will in turn affect the adjustment of other family members.

Most families have fairly predictable defense and coping strategies that are used if a child in the family develops cancer. If the family has marital or psychological problems before the child is diagnosed with cancer, the childhood cancer experience will exacerbate these problems because of the added stress and anxiety that accompany childhood malignancy. Each family member needs personal support, and each needs to realize that individual family members cope with the cancer experience in different ways.

PARENTS OF THE CHILD WITH CANCER

Parents play the predominant role in support of the child with cancer and thus require assistance from the health team so they may deliver this support effectively. Because of the rapid progression of childhood cancer, the parents, as well as the child, must cope with the rigors of treatment before the implications of the whole cancer experience are assimilated. Common immediate reactions of the parents to the diagnosis of cancer in their child are guilt, anger, frustration, helplessness, and despair. Parents, too, must cope with their child's pain, hospitalization, frequent clinic visits, disruption of normal family routines, sudden changes in family priorities, the needs of their other children, and possible catastrophic financial problems. Since the family unit as a whole is the target of nursing care—with the sick child receiving priority attention—nurses must attempt to promote adaptive coping responses from the family by viewing the parents as part of the treatment team.

Parental Tasks

The overall tasks of parents during the childhood cancer experience are threefold: (1) to help their sick child to respond to medical treatment, (2) to maintain intimacy, trust, and open communication within their marital relationship, and (3) to keep the entire family together and functioning during a period of great stress. Of primary importance to the achievement of these tasks is for the parents to learn to maintain as much family normalcy as possible even though they must face a life-threatening disease in one of their children.

Parents must not only deal with the physical health of the ill child but also with his personal and social health. This means that they must help the child fit comfortably and happily into the family and to cope with the ordinary tasks of childhood as well as the demands of the disease and treatment process. Increased survival means long-term distress for the parents instead of the short-term stress of childhood cancer and the almost universal early death of the child just a few years ago. Enhancing personal and social health of the sick child also implies attending to the needs of each other as spouses and of their other children; for if the family unit is broken, the sick child is further burdened by feelings of guilt, grief, and loss.

Parental Responses to Childhood Cancer

Parents, being individual people, vary in the ways in which they perceive and respond to the threat of childhood cancer. With each parent, coping and defense mechanisms will vary. Parents are usually the first in the family to know the diagnosis of cancer in one of the children. Frequent responses at this time are concurrent disbelief, anger, guilt, confusion, and grief. In the first few weeks after diagnosis, parents may also experience significant physical distress, inability to function in their usual roles, and notable depression with frequent bouts of crying. For the most part, the psychological distress at the time of diagnosis is more severe for the parents than for the child since the parents usually have a more realistic knowledge of the implications of their child's diagnosis. Recollections of other deaths that they have witnessed in their lifetimes come crowding into the parents' awareness. There are peak times when emotional responses such as disbelief, anger, and grieving are more intense: the time of diagnosis, the first relapse, and the time of death. Denial and disbelief during these times are adaptive, not maladaptive, responses unless they become overwhelming and significantly interfere with the parents' ability to function or make decisions. During these times, denial and disbelief decrease intolerable anxiety by providing emotional distance between the parent and unbearable psychic pain.

One of the first issues that the parents must face is whether or not to tell the child of the diagnosis. An important nursing intervention is to assist parents to realize that the real issue is *not* whether to tell, but *how* to tell and *how much* information to give to the child at first—both of which depend upon the child's developmental stage and cognitive abilities. If a parent wants to hide the diagnosis of cancer from the sick child, it most often reflects the parents' inability to face the diagnosis. Parents must be helped to realize that it is virtually impossible for their child not to realize the seriousness of his or her condition, for even infants respond to changes in their parents' tone of voice, touch, and mood. For both adults and children, incomplete information or evasion from the truth will result in the person filling in the void with fantasy, which is often more frightening and bizarre than even the grimmest truth. Silence or evasive chatter from the parents creates distrust and distance between them and their child. On the other hand, honest answers tempered with realistic hope and assurance of support will help to dispel the child's unwarranted fears and to solidify closeness and trust between parent and child. Few parents are really comfortable with deceit, and it is rarely in the best interests of the child to conceal the truth about his diagnosis, treatment plans, and even prognosis. Instead of protecting the child by concealing the truth, parents simply leave him or her alone with bizarre and fearful fantasies, partial truths, and the gut-level knowledge that something terrible is wrong.

Anger is a common parental response and may be directed toward the disease, the care team, God, fate, or each other. In one of its most destructive forms, parental anger may be turned toward the child for being sick, different, or dying. Anger is often an adaptive coping mechanism if it is used as a source of creative energy and is expressed in positive, nondestructive ways. Anger is a maladaptive response if parents direct their anger toward the child or do not express the anger at all. Anger that is not expressed is turned inward and results in guilt, deep depression, or somatic disease. Nurses can assist parents to express their anger by helping them to realistically identify the source of their anger—which in actuality is the situation—and to acknowledge anger in nondestructive verbal or physical ways. Helping parents to express their anger by venting their feelings to the treatment team or counselor will decrease the destructive result of directing anger toward the child, each other, or themselves.

Guilt, or anger turned inward, may be a significant stressor for the parents. Parents may feel guilty for several reasons, such as (1) their failure to seek medical care sooner, (2) suspected or real genetic defects that may have contributed to the malignancy, (3) worry over the emotional and financial resources that are being diverted away from the rest of the family, or (4) anger that they may feel toward the sick child. Some of the parents' guilt may be irrational and some rational, but it will always be present whether it is "deserved" or not. The parents may not even be aware that they are feeling guilty, and this subconscious guilt may manifest itself in discipline problems with the child, self-destructive or self-defeating behavior, or prolonged mourning. There are any number of ways that the human mind can find to punish itself, and guilt is anger turned inward toward the self. Nurses can best assist parents who feel guilty simply by listening, by allowing parents to express their feelings. Then, the nurse must reinforce the idea that, except for violent abuse, no parent has the power to wreak such havoc on a child.

Fear and worry seem to be the constant companions of parents who have a child with cancer, and they worry about and are frightened of many things. During remission, parents commonly worry about the uncertain promises offered by remission. They fear relapse, often becoming overprotective of their children and subjecting them to continual close scrutiny for a sign that something is wrong. Yet other parents deny their worry and thus deny the disease itself because of the absence of symptoms during remission. Most families exhibit a combination of both fear and denial during remission [25].

During times of relapse, parents are no longer able to deny the seriousness of the disease. The fear that their child might die becomes paramount once more, making relapse an event of tremendous significance. During both remission and relapse, parents often feel an enormous sense of loss of control as they turn over a major portion of their child's care to health professionals. Parents both want and fear the treatment team, finding it extremely difficult to fully trust those persons who are also responsible for some of their child's pain and suffering. Nurses can help parents keep fear and worry in optimal perspective by including them as part of the treatment team, offering full information with both candor and realistic hope, and giving the parents adequate instructions regarding home care of their sick child prior to the termination of hospitalization or office visit. Each hospitalization and office visit should conclude with a set of clearly understandable, written instructions plus the telephone number of the hospital nursing unit or physician. Parents should be encouraged to call the nursing unit or physician if they have any questions, no matter how trivial they might seem.

Underlying most, if not all, of the parents' responses are the aspects of grief and loss. Grief and mourning are continuous and intense processes in parents who have children with cancer. Health professionals must remember that the grief accompanying the actual loss of the child's health and the anticipatory grief experienced by parents in the face of potential death of their child are both normal, expected responses. Grief and mourning are maladaptive only in extreme cases. Parental grief must be expressed and supported by humane nursing and humane listening, and psychiatric consultation is most often premature.

Maladaptive Parent-Child Dyad

In most families when a child is ill, one parent (usually the mother) assumes the role of primary caretaker. This arrangement works well in short-term illnesses. However, in long-term chronic diseases like cancer, it usually has catastrophic effects on the well-being of the sick child, the marital relationship, and the entire family system. An inseparable dyad consisting of mother and child may develop in which both individuals withdraw together from external social contacts as well as from other members of the nuclear family. The child regresses to an earlier level of development and becomes progressively more dependent upon the mother. Although there may be significant hostility between the mother and the sick child in this situation, any attempt to separate them causes intense anxiety in both individuals. Thus, the mother-child dyad becomes hostile to any interference from others and even to therapeutic interventions from the health team. This type of mother-child dyad—or in some cases, father-child dyad—has far-reaching implications for the entire family and particularly the marital relationship itself. As the marital relationship is weakened by the overly close mother-child relationship, trust and intimate communication between husband and wife is threatened or destroyed [23]. Many fathers are pushed out of participation in the care of their ill children, and the mother's life becomes focused entirely on "her" sick child.

If this type of maladaptive situation develops, the father is most often left alone without his wife, his sick child, and frequently without his other children as well if they have been farmed out to relatives or friends. Adding to the separation already formed is the fact that many children with cancer are treated at medical centers that are long distances from their homes, leaving fathers at home to try to keep the rest of the family together and functioning.

Most fathers find themselves overwhelmed by this situation and unable to cope with the impenetrable, abnormal bond that has developed between the mother and the sick child. If the father goes to the hospital to be with his ill child, he is often made the dumping ground for all of the frustrations and anxieties of his wife, his child, and sometimes even the staff. When the child is cared for at home, the father again is usually bombarded with anxieties and frustrations about clinic visits, progress reports, laboratory data, discipline problems, and so on. If this father tries to treat his child as normally as possible during remission, his wife—and the sick child—may accuse him of being cruel, insensitive, and unaware of just how sick his child is.

Thus, many fathers in this intolerable and abnormal situation simply withdraw, drawing both relief and further criticism from their children and wives. Many fathers begin to work more hours or take a second job, supposedly to cope with the great financial demands. However, longer working hours and increased immersion in the job gives the father a seemingly legitimate excuse to withdraw. Sometimes subtly and sometimes openly, he may be told that he fails as a father. In this way, at least he can avoid failure as a breadwinner.

As the father becomes more and more immersed in his work and the mother becomes more and more immersed in "her" sick child, a vicious cycle begins with far-reaching catastrophic effects on the entire family. The ill child becomes overly dependent, increasingly regressed, and cannot bear to be away from the mother, even to go to school. The siblings withdraw into depression or begin to exhibit hostile behavior in order to get the attention that they need. Approximately 80 percent of siblings of children with cancer develop achievement or behavioral problems at school as well as discipline problems at home. Subsequently, home discipline fails. Interpersonal and sexual problems often develop between husband and wife as both parents feel increasingly impotent to control their family. The father may feel a great deal of anger toward his wife and the hospital staff for "preventing" his participation in care of the sick child. Since most fathers remain silent and withdrawn, the mother often feels an equally great resentment toward her husband, perceiving that she must grieve alone [7, 12, 13, 22, 28, 33, 42].

The key nursing intervention into this maladaptive parent-child dyad is early prevention. No one person, not even the mother, should be expected or mandated to shoulder the entire burden of care. All health professionals and educators must be willing to accept some responsibility for support of the family and for care of the child. By strongly encouraging both fathers and mothers to view themselves as part of the treatment team and to also attend to the needs of each other as well as the other children, this maladaptive dyad will be less likely to develop. Most parents want to know as much as possible about their child's diagnosis and treatment, so involvement of the parents (as well as the child, when appropriate) in nurse-physician-family conferences is vital. Although parents can be expected to retain little information from the first meeting after diagnosis, honest teaching must be provided and repeated as necessary regarding the disease process, treatment plans and side effects, treatment alternatives, and prognosis.

Discipline of the Sick Child

Maintaining regular discipline and setting behavioral limits for the child with cancer is crucial to the maintenance of optimal normalcy for that child. *Parental support* refers to those parental behaviors that set limits for the child, define structure in the child's psychosocial environment, and/or direct the child's actions. *Parental punishment*, or punitive behaviors, refers to the use of physical or non-physical punishment with little concern for the needs or feelings of the child. *Parental encouragement of autonomy* refers to those parental behaviors that enhance the child's capacity for independent thinking and action [43].

Ill children, like healthy children, look to their parents to see who is in control and to see if the parents care enough to expect reasonable behavior. Failure to maintain discipline can provoke extreme anxiety. The sick child may interpret a lack of normal discipline to mean that he or she has been "written off" and that discipline is of no significance because death is expected soon. Abnormal permissiveness and pampering will only frighten the child and leave him or her with the idea that parents have lost control of the child's situation. In addition, unnatural permissiveness leaves the child with cancer vulnerable to sibling jealousy and hostility as they see the sick child "getting away" with behavior for which they would be punished.

On the other hand, abnormal restrictiveness, punitive behavior, and overprotection may be the result of the parent's tendency to set too many limits owing to fear or worry about the ill child's health or safety. Abnormal restrictiveness and punitive actions tend to have negative effects on the child's self-concept, resulting in dependent children who have much anxiety and internal stress [43].

Children with cancer who have a high level of self-confidence and independence seem to have one of two types of parental support: (1) parents who are more supportive, less punitive, and who focus on constructively building the child's self-concept or (2) parents who encourage autonomy in their children. These children have an increased sense of control over their environment, reducing helplessness, abnormal dependency, and other maladaptive behaviors [43].

Approximately two-thirds of parents who have a child with cancer have discipline problems with that child. More than half of parents reporting discipline problems said that the difficulties resulted from parental lack of knowledge either about reasonable expectations of the child or about how to help the child effectively adapt to the demands of the cancer experience [6]. Since most discipline problems are basically problems with socialization of the child, an effective intervention is to normalize the ill child's social environment as much as possible. This social normalcy includes, among other things, the return of the ill child to school, avoidance of home tutors, attending to the needs of siblings and spouse, and similar interventions. Normal discipline and a normal social environment carry messages of both hope and expectation for the child with cancer: hope that he or she will get better and the expectation that the ill child will, as much as possible, maintain his or her normal position in the family as a valued member of a dynamic, social unit.

Effect of the Childhood Cancer Experience on the Parents' Marital Relationship

When their child's malignancy is first diagnosed, parents usually openly share their feelings but, for a variety of reasons, few couples continue to do this consistently. Communication between the spouses tends to revolve solely around the daily progress of their sick child. Rarely does the couple any longer talk about themselves as a couple, their hopes, plans, relationship, and often not even about their other children. Both husband and wife often feel misunderstood and neglected by the other, and even the closest couples will begin to drift apart owing to physical separation, very real fatigue, the fear that they will both fall apart at the same time, denial, anger, or depression.

Mothers are frequently expected by health professionals, the ill child, and the larger society to take on the major responsibility for provision of care. Fathers are usually directed back to home and work, often by nurses and physicians, in order to attend to both financial needs as well as the needs of the healthy children at home. Even if the abnormal parent-child dyad that was discussed earlier does not develop, this all-too-frequent pattern of expectation and behavior results in one parent being overwhelmed by the sick child's needs yet advanced in grief work, and the other parent able to avoid the painful daily experience of childhood cancer but far less able to adapt to the child, the disease, and the implications of the disease. If the parents continue to live in their separate worlds, the rift between them will widen and marital alienation may occur.

Conflicts between parents impede their communication and mutual support, resulting in reduced support for their ill child. Fathers frequently resent the physician-mother-child relationship, viewing it as threatening his own decision-making power within the couple relationship and the family; mothers often resent the father's ability to escape from the intense and painful world of childhood cancer. Minor stressors can cause major conflict and mutual withdrawal, and marital stability is often threatened. Parents of children with cancer have more marital discord than do the parents of children with other chronic diseases. However, even though the parents' stress is high and prolonged, preliminary studies indicate that these parents resort to divorce no more frequently than the general population [23]. A primary nursing intervention is to assist parents to resolve their major disagreements and to promote communication between them.

Negative Effects on Family Financial Status

Financial reserves of parents who have a child with cancer are rapidly depleted. In 1979, it was estimated that parents suffered a median loss of 26.6 percent of their weekly income owing to medical expenses not covered by third-party payors [23]. For example, in 1978, the average cost of a bone marrow transplant was $60,000 [8], and one should remember that bone marrow transplantation is usually reserved as one of the *final* treatments to attempt to prevent death from acute childhood leukemia.

External Support Systems for Parents

Unfortunately, most parents discover that external support systems are limited and that many of the people from whom parents might expect support actually turn *to* the parents for assistance in their own grieving for the sick child. Grandparents, for example, are often nearly immobilized by their threefold grief: grief for themselves, for their son or daughter, and for their ill grandchild. The grandparents themselves may not be in good physical health and thus are limited in ways that they can help with the physical care of the sick child or the siblings. Their limitations often extend to the ways in which they can assist the family with the emotional strain of the illness. The grandparents frequently believe erroneously that they should have all the answers, should be able to cope better than the parents of the child with cancer, and should be an example to the rest of the extended family. The grandparents inevitably fail at their unrealistically high self-expectations and often actually become afraid to care for their ill grandchild. Thus, grandparents are likely to feel left out and helpless, and view themselves as intense failures as both parents and grandparents.

Friends of the parents of a child with cancer may either abandon the parents or cause even more distress for the family by their own reactions to the diagnosis of cancer. Distant relatives, friends, and business contacts of the parents often respond to the child's diagnosis with great fear, leaving a profound impact upon the family. If the cancer experience is ignored by well-meaning friends or relatives, the child's reality is distorted and the child is not accepted for exactly who she or he is: a child who has cancer. On the other hand, if the friends focus primarily on the malignancy, the normal aspects of the child that need to be recognized are ignored. Either way, the child is made more vulnerable to despair and the parents may feel forced to "play games" with their friends and relatives, adding to an already heavy burden. When the child is diagnosed with cancer, friends of the parents are suddenly and acutely aware of both their own and their children's mortality and vulnerability to death and disease. Playmates may no longer want or be permitted to play with the sick child. In school, the child may be excluded from class activities without an adequate reason or may be subjected to teasing and other biological-personal-social insults secondary to the adults' fear of contagion. As a result, families with a child who has cancer quickly become very lonely families and often are eventually isolated from their former support systems. Since this most frequently occurs before the family has established other adequate support systems, the effect on the family of a child with cancer is devastating.

Community health nurses are a potential source of parental support, but they will be effective only if they receive specialized, quality education in all aspects of the childhood cancer experience. A mere referral to community health nurses will assure neither quality care of the child nor effective support to the family. The goal of the community health nurse in caring for a family struggling with the burden of childhood cancer is to promote the family's normal life style. In order to achieve this goal, the community health nurse must assess the family's emotional and physical needs, assess the family's readiness to learn about home care, provide teaching about the child's home care, and involve community resources when appropriate [3, 19].

SIBLINGS

Siblings are often called "the forgotten grievers." The brothers and sisters of the child with cancer learn very soon that their needs and desires are usually subordinate to those of the ill child. Their parents spend much time at the hospital; and when the parents are home, they are frequently irritable, tired, and distracted. Thus, the entire familiar family structure is disrupted, and the sibling's needs for nurturing are not adequately met. Often, their questions are not answered, and so they may fantasize that the sick child is having a great deal of fun in the hospital. They may perceive their parents as overindulging the ill brother or sister; and when family or friends come to visit, no one asks about how *they* are. Most siblings fear that they will also develop cancer [13]. Because of the occasional normal wish to be an only child and thus the center of their parents' attention, the siblings may believe that they "caused" the malignancy to occur. At school or family activities, siblings are often angry and embarrassed by the strange and frightening physical changes in their ill brother or sister. All of these stressors will often lead to maladaptive responses from the siblings, yet these well children are rarely willing or able to verbalize their negative feelings.

In at least 50 percent of the families in which a child had died of cancer, siblings with apparently normal previous behavior later developed maladaptive behavioral patterns [2]. Common maladaptive problems exhibited by siblings of children with cancer are outlined in Figure 10.2.

Interventions to minimize maladaptive responses and to promote adaptive coping by the siblings of a child with cancer must begin with honest information. If the child is old enough to ask the question, he or she is old enough to receive an honest answer. The siblings must receive candid information about the malignancy, treatment, side effects, and expected outcomes or prognosis. Additionally, the nurses must help the parents to emphasize that the disease is not contagious, that the cause of the disease is unknown, and that the siblings did not cause their brother or sister to develop cancer. Siblings should be encouraged to visit the sick child in the hospital. In these ways, fears and fantasies will be dispelled, and the siblings will be more likely to maintain a near-normal relationship with the ill child.

Siblings need an environment conducive to the expression of feelings. They need to cry, be happy, ask questions, and view and touch again. The well children in

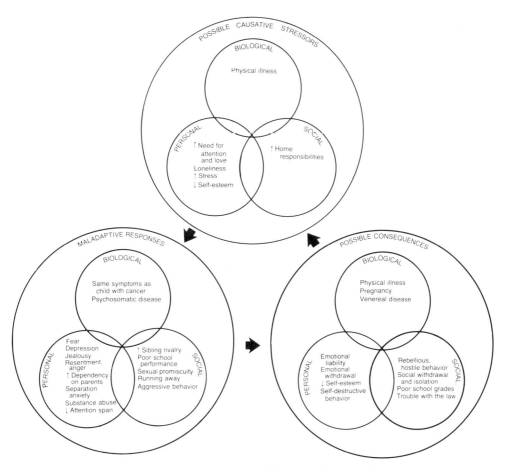

Figure 10.2. Maladaptive Responses of Siblings of Children with Cancer

this family in crisis need the comfort of knowing that they are still loved, accepted, and valued despite the painful experience of childhood cancer. Many parents need nursing help in order to achieve this.

PEERS OF THE CHILD WITH CANCER

Peers of the child with cancer are subdivided into two distinct groups: (1) healthy peers with whom the child had developed a relationship before diagnosis of the disease and (2) peers who also have cancer with whom the child developed a relationship after the diagnosis of cancer. Discussion of the peers who also have cancer may be found in Concept X.

Healthy peers of the child with cancer with whom the child had developed a relationship before the diagnosis of the disease include schoolmates, neighborhood children, children of the parents' friends, and children within the extended family group. Few of these children receive any kind of explanation for the mysterious and frightening changes that they see in their friend. These healthy children eavesdrop and wheedle in order to obtain information from adults; then they fill in the gaps with their own fantasies. Their questions may seem cruel, gruesome, or trivial to adults but are actually born of their natural curiosity and usually genuine concern for their friend.

School-age children who are able to maintain a near-normal relationship with their healthy peers feel increased security and an enhanced sense of self-worth. In adolescents, peer belonging is crucial, and feelings of inadequacy and loss of self-esteem often occur during the experience of cancer. Major body changes, such as weight gain or loss, alopecia, scars, radiation markings, or amputation of a limb, add to the stress of personal, social, and sexual maturation. Embarrassment resulting from these changes may result in social withdrawal and isolation, depression, and despair.

School or community health nurses are the health professionals who have the most contact with the healthy peers of children with cancer. General information about the disease, treatment, side effects of treatment, and prognosis may satisfy the questions of the healthy peers as well as protect the privacy of the child with cancer.

THE FATALLY ILL CHILD WITH CANCER

CONCEPT VII:
Although many of the aspects of nursing care for the fatally ill child are similar to those for the dying adult, children are not just "little adults" and thus there are therapeutic measures unique to the treatment of the dying child.

If long-term remission or cure is not achieved, childhood cancer becomes a progressive disease marked by hopeful intervals, medical treatment that is effective only on an intermittent basis, an uncertain outcome for a long period of time, and finally a bitter ending to the struggle against cancer. Ironically, increased survival times have been a double-edged sword, increasing the life-span of the sick child but also prolonging and intensifying the suffering of the child and family. Management of the care of the child with advanced and probably terminal malignancy involves many important yet nebulous questions dealing with human values, ethics, and quality of life. As with fatally ill adults, "we can" is *not* synonymous with "we ought," and for the child with advanced cancer, there comes a time when a decision must be made about what more ought to be done for the sick child.

Alternatives for medical treatment of fatally ill children are comprised of three basic treatment plans [10]. The first is no medical treatment at all other than those to provide comfort. Nursing treatment is also geared solely toward enhancing the physical, personal, and social comfort of the dying child. This first alternative implies that the best course of action is to send the child home to die without pain in its broadest sense and within the security of the familiar home environment, family members, friends, and pets. If the child's family opts for this first alternative yet keeps the sick child in the hospital, it implies that visiting privileges are extended beyond normal hospital policy; diagnostic and treatment measures, such as intravenous feedings, laboratory tests, X-rays and scans, and antineoplastic medical measures, are all completely discontinued. Both nursing and medical treatments are focused solely on enhancing relief from physical, personal, and social pain. To completely discontinue daily blood work or chemotherapy, for example, is a very difficult option for the treatment team to accept, for it implies that the caregivers as well as their treatments have failed. Their best skills and their best knowledge have not been successful in warding off death, and the discontinuation of any further treatment attempts blatantly shouts "Failure!" at the treatment team. Whether or not the child is cared for at home or in the hospital, the child and the family must be assured that they will not be abandoned to fare as best they can on their own. Comfort measures, such as a manageable diet, pain control and prevention or treatment of skin breakdown, must be focused upon; and these comfort measures are the *only* form of medical or nursing treatment provided. If the child is cared for at home, the parents must feel free to bring the child back to the hospital or to call the nurse or physician at any time should disquieting situations arise.

The second treatment option is that of palliative care, which also places the highest priority on control of pain in its broadest sense. Certain medications, chemotherapy protocols, irradiation, and even surgery may eventually result in a higher quality of remaining life for the child even though extension of life is not the goal of palliative care. Chemotherapy, radiotherapy, and surgery can all decrease the child's long-term physical pain experience by reducing tumor pressure on nerves or vital structures. However, this pain control is paid for by the child in terms of short-term physical pain associated with diagnostic and treatment procedures and the personal-social pain associated with longer hospitalization, stress, and isolation from family and friends. Sequelae of the palliative procedures, such as the inability to talk because of a tracheostomy, must be evaluated in terms of its worth to the child. The decision to implement this second treatment option can be very difficult to make. The enhanced quality of life after the palliative procedure must be real and valid when measured against the procedure's inherent discomfort, and recovery time must not use up long portions of the child's remaining life.

The final treatment alternative is that of administering investigational treatments, and is by far the most controversial of all choices. This option involves using new drugs, combinations of drugs, or new treatment procedures that offer a slight chance for cure and very frequently cause a significant increase in the child's suffering, pain, and morbidity. The child is vulnerable to severe and oftentimes unknown toxicities of the experimental treatment. These toxicities, along with hospitalization and the isolation of the child, often result in the untimely and premature death of the child. This treatment alternative may cause severe physical, personal, and social hardships on the child, the family, and the staff. However, this option is the only one that offers any chance at all of cure. Even if the treatment is not successful, many parents console themselves with the knowledge that everything possible was done for their dying child, that they helped to add to the body of knowledge about cancer treatment, and that other children may benefit from this knowledge.

Primary goals for nurses and physicians who work with fatally ill children and their families are multiple. Goals include maximizing normal function in the lives of the child and family; facilitating communication within the family; providing overall comfort for the child (especially pain control); effectively involving community agencies, community health nurses, schools, and counseling services as appropriate; and providing family follow-up care after the child's death. For further discussion of general aspects of care for the fatally ill child, refer to Chapter 12.

CONCEPT VIII:
Biological aspects of care for the dying child are similar to those relevant to the dying adult.

Biological aspects of care for the child dying of cancer are similar in most ways to those particular aspects of care for the dying adult. Refer to Chapter 12 for general information on biological care of the fatally ill child.

Pain control is of primary importance to both the child and parents. For general information regarding pain assessment and pain control during the terminal phase of illness, refer to Chapters 11 and 12. The nursing and medical goals for pain control in the dying child include achievement of a state wherein the child is awake, alert, and interested in the external environment *because* of freedom from pain. Thus, a PRN scheduling of dosing is no more appropriate for these children than for dying adults.

CONCEPT IX:
Personal aspects of care for the dying child are significantly different from those relevant to the dying adult.

One out of every twenty children will face the death of a parent during their childhood [5]. Virtually every child will experience the death of a grandparent, pet, or friend; and thus the child with cancer has probably had some experience with grieving and loss. Mourning is not just feeling sad, but is the specific psychological process by which human beings, including children, are able to release some of the feelings they have invested in a person whose death is impending (e.g., themselves) or in a person who has died (e.g., a peer with cancer). Mourning also implies that the child or adult is able to extend their love to the living after the mourning process has been completed. Mourning includes the child's struggle with feelings of guilt that they were somehow to blame for development of the disease and with feelings of anger that their life is coming to an end before they grow old. Dying children who are mourning for the loss of their parents, siblings, friends, and even themselves need love, caring, and depth of response from parents and caregivers rather than the loss of the presence of these significant others. The mourning, dying child may exhibit emotional lability, increased sensitivity to minor remarks from others, and/or acting-out behavior. So this child will experience approach-avoidance conflicts, needing and wanting the nurturing offered by parents and staff yet simultaneously not permitting others to know of this need since this would only increase their dependency.

THE CHILD'S CONCEPTS OF DEATH

The concept of death is acquired through the sequential development of cognitive abilities. The adult concept of death as being irrevocable, universal, and irreversible is not usually attained until preadolescence. Unless nurses understand how children in various age groups and developmental stages perceive death, they cannot effectively intervene into the presence of maladaptive responses. There are three distinct concepts of death in children, depending on the age and developmental stage of the child [17].

Infants, Toddlers, and Preschoolers

Death has the least significance for infants, toddlers, and preschoolers. In infants less than six months of age, death seems to have little, if any, meaning to the child. However, once the parent-child relationship has been firmly established, even the actual or threatened temporary loss of that parent elicits great resistance from the child. Prolonged separation between parent and child during the first few years produces more deleterious effects on the child's physical, personal, and social growth and development than at any subsequent age. For the toddler, the very nature of wakefulness and sleep establishes a cycle of being and nonbeing, and the toddler and preschool years are periods of excessive nightmares and fear of the dark. The majority of children aged five years or younger react to their probable death by the expression of separation anxiety. The impending death of a toddler or preschooler (less than five or six years old) is perceived as an event that is reversible, temporary, and/or as a punishment for real or imagined misdeeds. For example, the very young child may "bury" seeds in the ground and then witness the flowers' rebirth and regrowth in the spring. Most of these children really believe that they too will be buried in the ground and then will be reborn in the spring just like the flower. Preschoolers, in particular, are noted for precausal, or magical, thinking, in which they believe that there is a definite cause-and-effect relationship between their thoughts and behavior and the external event that happens. This belief in their own perceived self-power and magical thinking is particularly significant if the child develops cancer, for she or he may view the disease, impending death, and the sorrow they see in their parents as being the result of their own "wrong" or "bad" thoughts and their actual or imagined misdeeds in the past. This situation engenders an enormous sense of self-guilt in the child.

The School-Age Child

The school-age child (ages six to ten) has a deeper sense of death in a very concrete way. Death is frequently personified as God, the devil, the bogeyman, and so on, and there is a definite destructive connotation to death. School-age children particularly fear the mutilation and punishment they frequently associate with their own impending death. Younger school-age children still associate misdeeds and "bad" thoughts with causing their own death from relentless cancer and with causing their parent's grief, and they feel intense guilt and personal responsibility. However, because of their increased cognitive skills, they respond well to logical explanation. By the age of eight, awareness of their own mortality is apparent. By the age of nine or ten, most children have formulated the adult concept of death: that it is universal, irreversible, and inevitable. At this age, the child will often develop a ghoulish sense of humor in order to master their fear of death. Their response to this adult concept of death is greatly influenced by a number of significant adult others, especially the parents. In school-age children who are dying, there is a tendency to fear the unknown much more than the known. For this reason, cognitive preparation is necessary and very effective in all phases of treatment in order to achieve reasonable adaptation by the child. These older school-age children respond well to thorough explanations of the disease process in terminology they can understand, treatment plans and expected side effects, and names of drugs. Since the developmental task of this age is industry, these children with cancer can achieve independence, self-worth, and self-esteem if the nurse and parents will help the child to maintain as much control over their internal as over their external environments. By facilitating an understanding of what is going on inside the child's body and by participating in what is done to him or her, the child can achieve some measure of self-control.

Adolescence

In the adolescent stage, between prepuberty and early adulthood, the individual exhibits little evidence of the bland acceptance of death that is characterized by a virtual void of feelings as described by Kubler-Ross [21]. This acceptance, which may indeed be seen in adults, occurs when the person has worked through the grief necessary to accept the loss of self and has largely dissolved emotional ties with others [35]. This type of quiescence, if it appears, may be difficult to differentiate from the organic effects of progressive critical disease. It is also possible that peaceful acceptance of one's impending death may be more difficult for the younger adolescent than for older adolescents. Of all people, adolescents have by far the most difficulty in coping with their own death. Although they fully understand the adult concept of death, they are the least likely among both the pediatric and adult groups of cancer clients to accept the end of their own life. The adolescent's developmental task is to establish an adult identity, so any small aspect of being different from their peers is a tremendous threat. A kind of adaptation may occur, but it is not the peaceful acceptance of one's inevitable death. This type of adaptation in adolescents instead occurs when it is simply easier to die than to live.

SUMMARY: CONCEPTS OF DEATH AMONG DYING CHILDREN

There is some awareness and comprehension of their impending death in fatally ill children regardless of their age and even in those situations when "truth" is withheld from the child. The majority of children five years of age and younger usually demonstrate separation anxiety, whereas most children older than age ten exhibit death anxiety. The drawings of fatally ill children contain many symbols of death, especially the use of dark colors such as black or brown. Younger children tend to express their separation anxiety symbolically and physiologically. Most older boys tend to express their death anxiety by acting-out behavior, and the majority of older girls seem to become depressed and withdrawn in response to death anxiety.

CONCEPT X:
The fatally ill child's stages of awareness are on a continuum and are significantly different from adult stages of awareness of possible death [4, 5].

The lack of direct expression of the awareness of his or her progress and prognosis does not mean that the dying child has a lack of awareness. The dying child's stages of awareness are on a continuum, and certain tasks at one stage must be accomplished before progression to the next stage will occur (see Figure 10.3).

PASSAGE FROM NORMAL HEALTH TO STAGE 1

During this transitional passage, the child quickly learns the difference between "them" and "us." The "us" are the ill children and their parents who take orders and speak only when spoken to. The "them" are the nurses and physicians who give the orders, come and go as they please, inflict pain, and bring bad news. Before diagnosis is confirmed, the child still considers himself or herself to be a normal, healthy child. After the diagnosis is confirmed, the child concludes that she or he is very ill. Questions from the child at this stage tend to be concrete inquiries about what is happening and whether a particular procedure will hurt. The more probing questions dealing with "why" occur only after the child reaches Stage 1 and continue until Stage 5. During Stage 5, the child usually stops asking questions altogether.

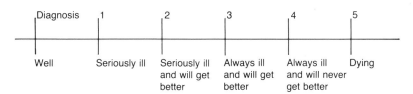

Figure 10.3. The Fatally Ill Child's Stages of Awareness (From Myra Bluebond-Langner, *The Private Worlds of Dying Children.* Copyright © 1978 by Princeton University Press. Fig., p. 169, reprinted by permission of Princeton University Press.)

STAGE 1

The message offered by the child is "I'm pretty sick, you know!" Exhibition of sickness to nearly everyone is characteristic of this stage. The child's conclusion that he or she is "pretty sick, you know" is drawn from carefully selected evidence such as changes in peoples' behavior toward the child, physical changes (e.g., alopecia, weight loss, and so on), and the exhibited wounds as mentioned before.

PASSAGE TO STAGE 2

The transitional passage to Stage 2 is usually very rapid. During this transitional time, the child experiences great separation anxiety regarding parents. Conversely, parents also fear the ultimate separation from their child (death) and so do not force any separation between themselves and their child, even when the parents wish to be alone. Thus, the sick child can manipulate their parents fairly easily at this time. The ill child greatly fears the strange, threatening, unknown environment of the hospital or clinic, but as the environment becomes more familiar, the sick child begins to socialize with new peers who also have cancer. At this point, separation from parents becomes easier. Play groups with the new peers gives the child the opportunity to observe and question other children who are in similar situations, learning about antineoplastic treatments and their side effects and what diagnostic procedures to expect. The child does not pass into Stage 2 until he or she experiences the first remission and is able to relate the antineoplastic treatment to getting better. Passage between Stage 1 and Stage 2 is relatively longer than the transition between normal health and Stage 1.

STAGE 2

Stage 2 is the time of the first remission. During this stage, the sick child continues to accumulate knowledge about antineoplastic treatments and expected side effects. Their information is cumulative, and most children with cancer know a great deal about the drugs, side effects, blood counts, and so on. The ill child begins to seek support that the drugs will make him or her better. The child and parents exhibit a strong sense of hope with less focus on the illness, and a near-normal life pattern resumes. The child remains at Stage 2 until the first relapse—the incident that makes him think that he may always be ill.

PASSAGE TO STAGE 3

Passage to Stage 3 is also comparatively longer than the passage to Stage 1. The ill child becomes aware of the existence of a cycle of relapse-remission, and the child is frustrated and depressed to see that, once again, the same symptoms, the same procedures, the same treatments, and the same gloomy parental reactions occur as in Stage 1. Hospital staff exhibit a maladaptive phenomena during this transition time. They speak less openly with the child and tend to give only brief and concrete explanations for treatments. The staff usually avoid extended inter-action with either the child or the parents, keeping staff contact at a level that will prevent close, intimate involvement.

During this time, the child becomes desirous of building relationships with peo-ple other than mother. These children want people around to talk with and to question. The ill child will invite others to watch television or play with toys in order to coerce them into staying, and then will begin to ask the questions. Since she or he realizes that adults are reluctant to answer questions, the child relies heavily on overheard conversations among adults. When adults talk outside of the child's room, the child often becomes very quiet in order to hear, even directing others in the room to be quiet so that he or she can listen.

STAGE 3

During this stage, the child with cancer believes that although he or she will get sick many times, recovery will always occur. This is the time of the second remission, and the child clings to this belief until another relapse occurs.

PASSAGE TO STAGE 4

During this transitional time, the child's sense of well-being begins to fade. There seems to be no freedom from pain, and parents stop planning things because plans are so often cancelled at the last minute because of one more of a long series of physical complications experienced by the sick child.

The child with cancer becomes increasingly aware of being different from nor-mal, healthy children. School attendance often becomes sporadic, resulting in both physical and social deleterious effects on the child. The child's universe becomes more and more focused on the hospital and less and less home-centered. Each new disease experience feeds the doubt that he or she will ever get better.

STAGE 4

While in Stage 4, the ill child still attempts to make contacts with the outside well world. The child does not want to be in isolation, for example, because he or she fears that other well people will not visit any longer.

Regarding the child's peers with cancer, as long as there is a valid reason as to why the friend stopped visiting (e.g., he really did go home), the sick child remains in Stage 4. Passage to Stage 5 begins upon hearing of the death of a friend with cancer. Only then does the ill child realize that the relapse-remission cycle does not continue for an indefinite period of time. The cycle has a definite end: death.

PASSAGE TO STAGE 5

The death of another child affirms to the sick child that he or she will also die. Before this point, the death of another child has no connection to the ill child's life, since she or he had always believed that recovery from the current relapse would occur.

STAGE 5

A characteristic of Stage 5 is that direct reference to a dead peer is taboo after the death has been discussed once. There is now minimal play with toys; and when the child does play, there is strong emphasis on disease and death. Death imagery in play is heavy at this time—a little girl may "bury" her dolls, for example.

Some children refuse to converse openly about death. Instead they simply make a statement indicating their awareness of impending death and then abruptly terminate the conversation. For example, a school-age child may announce, "I'm not going to school anymore," and then turn away and refuse to converse further at all. Another child might blurt out, "I won't be here for my birthday," and then run out of the room or crawl under the sheets.

Many statements from children with cancer in Stage 5 have a dramatic and startling quality. For example, a six-year-old boy who woke up from his nap to see two physicians standing by his bed smiled and said, "I fooled you. I didn't die." Another little boy was lying on his back and was asked if he would like to be turned. He responded with the statement, "No. I'm practicing for my coffin." [5].

Conversation and information-gathering about drugs and side effects virtually stop, since the dying child realizes that drugs are not the answer. Additionally, the child is very concerned about the time left to him. He becomes impatient if other people take too long to do things, since time is a precious commodity and is no longer endless. Withdrawal from family and friends may also occur. Finally, in this stage just before death, parents and staff should not be surprised if the child stops asking questions altogether. After all, the child knows the answers.

CONCEPT XI:
Personal responses from the child with cancer and from the family are diverse, but the most common ones are anxiety and anticipatory grieving.

ANXIETY

Anxiety—the vague, nebulous sense of fear and feeling of impending doom—is a nearly universal experience for both families and their children with cancer. Familial anxiety has been discussed in some detail, but the ill child's anxiety must be further addressed.

Children with cancer have significantly more anxiety, death anxiety in particular, than healthy children or children with nonmalignant chronic disease. To tell or not to tell: that is the question faced by every parent of a child with cancer. Yet, despite attempts to shield children from the grim truth of probable impending death, these children are perceptively aware of conspiracies. They realize that something is very wrong merely by the reactions of the adults. The most difficult aspect of cancer with which the child must cope is impending death, and the child must cope with this information which represents forces and events beyond his control. The child's range of coping behaviors, as in adults, is wide, ranging from crying and depression to hostility or overintellectualization. The child may attempt to cope with death anxiety by hostile, externally directed behavior, such as biting or noncompliance with treatment, or by self-protective and internally directed behavior, such as guarding the door of the room, crying, and cringing at the approach of a staff member or running out of the room before a treatment procedure. If the parents play the "don't tell" game, the child's anxiety is doubled, for he or she will have the tremendous anxiety of feeling the necessity for protecting their parents and other adults from the fact that the child knows that she or he is dying. This fact of impending death is often a burden that is nearly impossible to be borne alone, yet the child is forced into this highly anxious position if the "don't tell" game is being played.

ANTICIPATORY GRIEF

The anticipatory grief experienced by the child with cancer is similar to that experienced by adults, but a child's anticipatory grief is tempered by developmental stage and cognitive abilities. The difference between the anticipatory grief experiences of the child and of the adult is that often the child's anticipatory grief is hidden and must be experienced alone. This is because the child is often put into the position of protecting the adults from the reality of his or her knowledge of impending death. Every relapse intensifies the child's anticipatory grief. The lack of direct expression, the comparative silence, and the infrequency of the communication of anticipatory grieving does *not* mean that the child is unaware of the prognosis and the implications of what is happening to his or her body.

The dying child goes through what can often be a long and painful process to discover what the childhood experience means. During this process, the child assimilates, integrates, and synthesizes a great deal of information to discover what it all means, and, as mentioned before, the information is gathered from a variety of sources. With the arrival at each new stage comes a greater understanding of the disease, its implications, and its probable prognosis. This leaves the child with a great burden of coping—often alone—and it is indeed a part of the anticipatory grief process.

CONCEPT XII:
Communication problems with the dying child are multiple and diverse, especially if the prognosis is hidden from the child.

Dying is difficult to do alone, and yet in so many ways, the experiences of the dying process must be done alone and cannot be shared with anyone else. If anyone is aware of this, it is the child who is dying. He or she is aware of the perceived restrictions against sharing feelings about impending death. If the child breaks this taboo, it is rarely done directly and is done instead by highly symbolic methods. They realize from the reactions of others that something is very wrong. Yet they also know that parents do not want to talk about the situation, so the children silently agree to the "don't tell" conspiracy and protect others by not asking questions. However, this destructive game between parents/staff and child denies dying children the opportunity to discuss their fears, questions, and thoughts. They are not given the truth and often their fantasies are more frightening and bizarre than even the grimmest truth.

To tell a child that he or she is suffering from a hopeless, incurable disease does indeed dispel hope and often even life itself. But to tell the child about his disease and the reason for treatment instills hope and allows for support from others. Exactly how, when, and what to tell the child about impending death is a delicate and very individual matter, depending, among other things, upon the child's developmental stage and cognitive abilities as well as the actual prognosis. There is as much danger in telling the child too much as in telling too little.

The way in which children ask questions will give clues to the nurse about the kinds of questions the child is asking. Few children ask questions such as, "Am I going to die?" So, the child instead asks indirect questions, such as "what if the bad cells won't go away?" or what happens if there are not more medicines. In this manner, they always leave room for hope [5].

Children with cancer are not always overtly talking about dying even when the prognosis is openly known. Much of the time is spent becoming aware and getting things together. When the child probes for more information, that information is seldom given in ways that are easy enough for the child to understand. With children, it is far easier for the nurses and physicians to evade questions or to give only partially true answers. Children may thus feel more directly open with some staff members than with others. Health professionals must remember that even the dying child has the right and frequently wants the responsibility of being informed of the progression of his or her disease. These children have two basic types of questions: (1) Am I going to die," and if the answer is affirmative, (2) When, where, how, and why am I going to die?"

Nursing measures appropriate to the personal and social problems include those appropriate to the unique needs of the individual child and the dynamics of the family to which the child belongs. With the child, nurses can expect conversation to be heavily laced with death imagery, such as questions about what dying will be like, when to expect the death event to occur, and the nursing and medical care of the child will continue to receive, especially in the area of pain control [4]. It is especially important for the nurse to remember that, in this situation, children often speak in symbolic or nonverbal language/communication. Even when asked direct questions and given the opportunity to verbally respond in a direct manner, children may respond in a symbolic way that must be interpreted with consideration of their developmental stage, age, and cognitive abilities. It is important for the nurse to point out the things that *can* be done: comfort measures, pain control, no more diagnostic or treatment procedures (if clinical course A is selected), and the opportunity for the child to be surrounded by the people and things that he or she loves (e.g., parents, siblings, friends, and even pets).

PARENTAL COMMUNICATION WITH THEIR DYING CHILD

In long-term and potentially fatal illness, such as childhood cancer, parental grief for the anticipated loss begins long before the actual death of the child (see further discussion of parental anticipatory grief later in this chapter). The parents' reactions during the terminal stage of their child's illness are influenced by their previous acceptance or denial of the child's disease process. This is a period of intense anticipatory grieving; and as the child's condition worsens, many fears are intensified [5]:

1. *Fear of death.* What will my child die from? What will happen when my child dies? How will we know when the death event is imminent?
2. *Fear that their child is in pain.* Often the parents will report that the child is in pain even though nursing assessments conclude that the child appears to be comfortable and free from pain. The nurse and paranursing professionals must remember that watching one's child die is a pain for the parent that is immeasurable, and that these feelings subjectively color the parent's perception of their child's pain experience.
3. *Fear of loss of emotional control.* Often the parents may attempt to hide their loss of emotional control by requesting that the child be heavily sedated, which is usually not therapeutic for the child. Supporting the family by being physically present at the time of impending death, by making the child as comfortable as possible, and by continuing to talk to the child, especially if he or she is still awake, will help the parent and family feel in control without sedating the child.
4. *Fear of isolation and loneliness.* The parent often fears that their child will die alone and when the parent is not there. The nurse should strongly emphasize to the parents that, if death approaches sooner than expected, the nurse will notify the parents immediately.

Nurses should encourage parents to verbally communicate with their dying child, as closure is enhanced by open communication and a life review. Verbal communication from the parents to the child should continue even if the child is comatose or during the actual death event, for as far as we know, the sense of hearing is the last of the senses to fade.

For further reference to general concepts of the personal aspects of care for the child who is fatally ill, refer to Chapter 12.

CONCEPT XIII:
Social aspects of the childhood cancer experience have a deleterious effect on all of the fatally ill child's life experiences.

SCHOOL

As has already been described, continuation of school is appropriate even for the dying child as much as is feasible. School is a child's work, and continuation of that work helps the child to overcome feelings of helplessness and hopelessness. Children are most comforted by the physical presence of those who they know and love in a familiar environment and routine, and this includes school attendance and activities until the child is totally incapacitated and unable to attend the regular school. The child looks forward to the social contacts and stimulation provided by school, even when they are very weak. The school's expectation must not be for the dying child to maintain predisease levels of academic achievement, for to do so would be devastating to the child's self-esteem and would initiate a sense of failure. Instead, the school's goal for this child is to provide distraction from the disease by focusing the child's attention on academic and social activities at any level at which the child is capable [24]. Teachers need detailed information about the dying child's disease, therapy, prognosis, and daily activities.

School administrators and teachers may be reluctant to allow the dying child back to school owing to reasons previously discussed in this chapter. The health team must correct misinformation and help school professionals deal with their concerns. Classmates may also be resistant to the dying child returning to their schoolroom because of (1) the fears that the sick child will get acutely ill or even die during class, (2) the many fantasies and questions regarding the ill child's experiences in the hospital, (3) the strange, mysterious physical changes they see occurring in their friend, and (4) the fear of contagion. If classmates are denied this information, they may respond by ignoring or ridiculing the sick child. An effective nursing intervention is for the school nurse to have a special classtime teaching experience—with teachers and administrators in attendance—to clear up misunderstandings and dispel unwarranted fear.

In summary, school attendance even by children fatally ill with cancer serves multiple positive purposes. School attendance by the ill child increases social contact, development, and stimulation; distracts the child's focus of attention on illness, symptoms, and pain; increases the child's sense of dignity; and normalizes the child's life style as much as possible. Although home tutors are never appropriate for the child in remission, home tutors can help continue the school experience and the child's cognitive development for those fatally ill children who are too debilitated to return to regular school.

PARENTAL RESPONSE TO THEIR DYING CHILD: ANTICIPATORY GRIEF

Unlike parents who suffer a sudden loss of a child owing to illness or injury, parents of a fatally ill child with cancer are unable to resolve their grieving until the child is dead or pronounced cured. However, the prolonged anticipatory grieving process allows the family to complete unfinished business and to help their sick child and siblings to understand and cope with a fatal prognosis. Anticipatory grieving begins almost immediately after the diagnosis of their child. For these parents, the child dies twice—once at the time of actual diagnosis and one at the actual demise. Much of the parents' anticipatory grieving remains until the child begins to physically improve and moves toward the first remission. During this initial anticipatory grieving and accompanying emotional shock, parents have great difficulty making decisions and yet are forced to make a great many of them. When remission ends and the child enters relapse, there is a return of the anticipatory grieving: once again the parents must face the loss of their child. Depression and loss of hope are common, and nurses can help parents to formulate realistic short-term goals and to establish reasonable priorities of care.

The family in which a child is dying is under enormous stress. If not acknowledged and intervened into, this stress (of which anticipatory grief is a major part) can result in significant biological, personal, and social disorders in the survivors. The family and the child define the needs that must be addressed so that an effective nursing plan of care can be made. Anxiety, fear, depression, and grief are all normal in these families and are all part of the process of anticipatory grief. Anticipatory grief allows the parents, as well as the siblings and other family members, to better tolerate bereavement after the actual death of the child.

The two major factors that determine whether or not parental anticipatory grief will help or hinder the child's progress are (1) the premorbid family personality and (2) the time of onset of parental anticipatory grief [26].

Definition of the premorbid family personality includes the aspects of the preillness family structure, individual interactions and personality of family members prior to the onset of the child's symptoms and diagnosis of disease, and previous experience with anticipatory grieving. If the premorbid family personality exhibited a marginally adjusted, unstable, and hostile family, the diagnosis of cancer in one of the children may result in the family disintegrating into hate, guilt, self-incrimination, and despair. As was previously stated, the childhood cancer experience does not always bring the family closer together. If the premorbid family personality is unstable, the anticipatory grief response may mushroom into further maladaptive responses such as pain, depression, and inability to function. Superficial overindulgence may alternate with bursts of outright hostility which plunge both healthy and sick children into despair since they may perceive that it is their fault that the one familiar and secure entity in their lives is falling apart *because* of the children. In this situation, anticipatory grief becomes a destructive force rather than a healthy process, separating parents and all of their children rather than pulling them closer together.

In the families exhibiting maladaptive anticipatory grief, hope is a thing of a fragile nature, and escape from the grim reality of the situation is possible only by extensive denial and/or rationalization. To these families, the child with cancer is perceived as already doomed or treated as though he or she is already dead, and these families often believe that treatment is of no avail. These reactions only intensify and prolong the ill child's suffering. The child is generally significantly depressed. These children often exhibit inability to function, and are slow, disorganized, tired, and uninterested in any external event. Any aspect of the disease and its treatment easily overwhelm these children. Parents feel unable to stop the disease process, fail to carry out treatment regimens, and experience an overwhelming sense of helplessness. These families can be helped by assisting them to realize that, although life activities may be more limited or different than before, family life need not be empty or meaningless. Although treatment may not effect cure, it can extend the child's periods of useful life and normal function. These families, above all, must be helped to maintain a meaningful, active, and loving relationship with all their children, including the child with cancer.

Steps in the Anticipatory Grief Process

The first step in anticipatory grief by parents is the initiation of the process of grief and mourning. The loss, or threatened loss, of their child is very real, with nothing imaginary about it.

Step two is that of anticipatory grief work. This process involves the increasing realization of the significance of what is to be lost. For the child, especially the older child and adolescent, "life" is not merely a biological abstraction but his own personal life as he or she has lived it. So the child and the family together turn their eyes away from the present and toward the past, reviewing the life of the child, the people in it, the child's accomplishments, and the child's experiences. In order for this grief work to be successful, two requirements must be fulfilled. First, the outcome of the life review must be good, the child being able to say, "All in all, my life has been good." Second, having arrived at the first conclusion, the dying child and the family must concede that the same is true of life in general. Such a state of being signifies the end of grief work for both the dying child and the family. The acceptance of the child's death means, first of all, acceptance of the child's life in particular and of life itself in general.

Anticipatory Grieving in the Father

The father, in the role of protector of his wife and children, often experiences tremendous stress when faced with the reality that his child has fatal cancer. The responsibility of holding everyone else up and together, of being the pillar of strength, is a heavy burden—for who is there to hold him up? He may totally deny grief, sadness, and depression, for in our culture these attributes are accepted more readily in women than in men. The most accepted stage of grief work for fathers to exhibit openly are those of anger and acceptance, for these imply strength.

Anticipatory Grieving: Mothers and Fathers Together

Even though parents rarely give up hope altogether, they usually begin to prepare themselves for the inevitable death of their child. Rarely, if ever, are mothers, and fathers in the same stage of anticipatory grief at the same time. The mother usually arrives at the acceptance stage long before the father does, primarily because she has faced many daily crises and may welcome death as a relief and an end to the suffering for their child [13]. Although there will be a heightened, stressful grieving reaction with each major crisis experienced by the child, many parents will have the bulk of their grief work completed by the time the child actually dies [7, 11, 31].

As mothers and fathers progress through the anticipatory grief process, the ideal is to achieve some level of acceptance of the impending death of their child. There are, however, obstacles that impede achievement of this ideal [38]:

1. Protracted, maladaptive denial of the disease and its fatal prognosis.
2. "Shopping around" for medical opinions. Although second opinions are certainly valid and physicians and nurses should not be threatened by this parental choice, prolonged "shopping around" may delay treatment until it is too late.
3. Parental manipulation of the treatment team to cause overt disagreement among the professionals, thus justifying parental unrealistic hope.
4. Willingness by the parents to spend unreasonable amounts of money in the attempt to cure a child who is certainly going to die.
5. Overprotection and/or overindulgence of the ill child.
6. Failure to permit the child to be as independent as is age-appropriate.
7. An inappropriate focus on the dying child to the exclusion of everyone else.
8. Complete realignment of the normal family structure so as to revolve exclusively around the dying child, usually to the detriment of the marital relationship and siblings.
9. Refusal to tell the dying child or the siblings of the expected outcome of the disease.
10. Attempts by the parents to assign guilt to themselves or to others.
11. Exaggerated parental concern over biological, personal, or social minutiae.
12. Focus on one facet of the clinical picture (for example, the platelet count) and letting parental hope rise or fall with the fluctuations of that one clinical facet.
13. Premortem death of the child, or treating the child as if he or she were already dead.

THERAPEUTIC INTERVENTIONS INTO MALADAPTIVE ANTICIPATORY GRIEF

Parents are usually stunned by palpable evidence that their child is almost certainly going to die, and this in itself may break through the pathological denial. The overall nursing goal is to keep the family involved in caring for their moribund child. Nurses must provide the support and teaching necessary to help the family cope with the stress involved in caring for their dying child and in coping with life without the child. Moderate parental anxiety when dealing with a dying child is not necessary maladaptive but seems to serve the purpose of mobilizing resources and ultimately integrating the dying experience into the total family life situation. Overwhelming anxiety, on the other hand, results in family disorganization and prevents effective coping mechanisms from being utilized. The most effective nursing treatment in this situation consists of what is known as emotional hyperalimentation, or 200 percent support. Nursing intervention into maladaptive anticipatory grief focuses primarily on preventive measures aimed to minimize postdeath family distress.

CONCEPT XIV:
Bereavement after the death of the child affects the whole famiy and often results in a long period characterized by biological, personal, and social maladaptation.

PARENTAL BEREAVEMENT

The death of a child causes the role and status of parenthood to be lost to the bereaved parents. Regardless of whether there are other children in the family, the parental nurturing role toward the dead child is gone forever. The death often produces feelings of guilt and a sense of failure for not protecting the child from the death situation, with a resulting loss of parental self-esteem. Additionally, there is an inability to fulfill the expectations of society (i.e., raising the child to adulthood) combined with the failure to meet one's own expectations as a parent. These personal and societal stressors on the parent produce a highly anxious state. Since both parents are experiencing the loss of their child, as well as the anxiety and enormous sense of failure, they often are not able to respond adequately to each other's needs for comforting and loving reassurance.

At the time of the child's actual death event, some fathers in particular cannot force themselves to stay in the room. They feel useless and helpless, unable to bear to watch their child die, and the fathers may fear that they may break down or lose emotional control. If he is able to verbalize his feelings, he frequently expresses tremendous guilt, frustration, anger, and self-hatred. The nurse should never force, shame, or coerce him to stay in his dying child's room but instead should encourage him to be present and give him special support to do so. If he still refuses to stay in the room, the nurse must accept his decision nonjudgmentally and keep him informed on the child's condition.

When the child dies, there is a reaction of shock by the entire family that the death event has finally occurred. Most family members, especially the parents, will review their relationship with the child at this time, providing a prime time for the nurse to validate that the parents and the rest of the family loved their child well and did their best to support the now-dead child and to fight the disease. Death of the child will bring its own new grief reaction. However, if anticipatory grieving has been adaptive and healthy, then the postdeath grieving is usually shorter and less intense than it would be otherwise [16, 21]. Nurses must remember that surviving family members, especially the parents, need a great deal of support after death of the child, and that providing this support is a preventive measure to minimize postdeath familial dysfunction. A follow-up conference including the family, nurses, and physicians will allow the parents to discuss their feelings about what should or should not have been done during the treatment of the child's disease. *Grief and its pain must be experienced in order to be healed.* If the grieving process is arrested, illness or death will occur. In other words, one cannot choose whether or not to experience grief; one merely chooses how to do so. Persons *will* grieve, either psychically or somatically.

Although the extended family and friends of the bereaved parents are most supportive and sympathetic during the first few months after the child's death, this external support begins to wane after a relatively brief period of time. The time when external support is strongest (i.e., during the first few months) is also the time when parents are experiencing relief from the strain of their dead child's long illness. The most difficult phase of bereavement often begins several months after the child's death and resolves only gradually over a period of as long as two years. Both acute and chronic symptoms of grief occur and there may be sporadic recurrences of the grieving symptomatology. Parents need to be reassured that this pattern is normal and will eventually dim with time.

CONCEPT XV:
Siblings of the child with terminal cancer have significant coping problems yet receive little attention from either parents or health professionals.

Siblings are often the forgotten mourners. Unless parents give a reasonable explanation for their continued absences from home, the siblings will regard the dying child as responsible for disruption of the family. Being honest with the siblings and including them in family discussions will allow them to be a contributing, rather than neglected, part of the family. Siblings commonly feel anger toward the dying child and the parents for their temporary loss of parental attention. Although they are forced to cope with a disrupted family life, they are usually given no rewards and, often, no or inadequate explanations. Their perception is that of a brother or sister who has the complete attention of the parents and grandparents, who enjoys many new gifts, and who is the focus of concern for parents, extended family, and family friends. Helping siblings to understand the reasons behind the change in family routine and facilitating as much contact as possible between the sibling and the dying child will help the healthy brothers and sisters to cope with the crisis situation.

Parents are nearly always the ones who must tell the siblings of the impending or actual death of their sick brother or sister. Because of the still strong death taboo in our society, parents usually have much difficulty with this task. Even after they know that death is impending for their brother or sister, many siblings never tell their parents about their problems or about physical and/or emotional distresses that they might have [13]. Sometimes the well children hide their distress in order to protect their parents from further worry; yet often if they do tell their parents, the parents resent the physical complaints and may even overtly communicate that the well child is malingering just to get attention while the parent's primary focus is on the child who is dying. These parents do not seem to realize that their well children only need to be allowed to talk, cry, and be loved. Many, if not most, parents have the attitude that, by virture of the siblings' healthy status, they must just "make do" during this time of crisis. This parental behavior often leads to acting-out behavior, withdrawal, and labile emotions in the siblings. Because of the siblings' lack of understanding and because of the physical and emotional absence of the parents from home, siblings often feel a great deal of rejection. Even when the ill child dies, the siblings at least temporarily lose their parents because of the parents' immersion in grief. This feeling of rejection and isolation on the part of the sibling often leads to panic and self-hatred.

When the ill child does die, siblings are often not allowed to go to the funeral. The sibling loved his sick brother or sister. Yet now, there are no thank you's for the sibling's sacrifices, no chance to say goodbye to the loved child, but only criticism for "being bad" or for misbehaving or asking too many of the "wrong" questions. The funeral for the deceased child is as important a ritual to the siblings as for the adults. The funeral gives recognition to the deceased child's life, enables the survivors to share their grief, and facilitates closure between the dead child and the survivors. A funeral is rarely grim—it is only sad. The refusal of the siblings' requests to attend the funeral of their brother or sister only impedes the ability to effect closure in the relationship. Siblings *should* be allowed to attend the dead child's funeral, for in this way, fantasies will be dispelled. Additionally, if the siblings attend the funeral, they are able to share their grief with others instead of being alone with it, and will be able to obtain emotional support from extended family members and friends at a time when parental grief is so intense that they may be unable to attend to the needs of their other children.

CONCEPT XVI:
Although a large percentage of fatally ill children die in the hospital, home care for these children is an option being chosen by an increasing number of families.

DEATH IN THE HOSPITAL

An acute care hospital is a difficult place for a child to die in. Visiting hours, restrictions on who may and who may not visit, the propensity (especially in teaching hospitals) for unnecessary laboratory work or X-rays, and the very experience of not being in the child's own bed in the child's own home are all disadvantages that make it very difficult for the fatally ill child to achieve a healthy death in the hospital.

If, however, the parents choose the acute care hospital as the site for their child's death, nurses must act as strong client advocates to ensure that the impersonal busyness of the hospital intrudes as little as possible upon the child and the family during this time. As a general rule, visitors (regardless of their age), telephone calls, and length of visitations should not be restricted. The nurse should encourage the parents to bring in familiar toys, blankets, pillows, photographs, and so on in order to surround the dying child with as many familiar and beloved objects from home as possible. In their role as advocates for the child, nurses must strongly encourage physicians to provide adequate pain control as well as to limit painful diagnostic tests to only those that are absolutely necessary. It is of no benefit to the dying child to draw painful laboratory specimens, for example, if no corrective measures are planned for the aberrations that may be found.

There are, however, some advantages to the hospital as the site for the child's death. A large amount of the burden of physical and personal care is lifted from the parents owing to the availability of nurses, occupational therapists, and other professionals. The progressive deterioration and accompanying "small" physical crises that so commonly occur with impending death do not have to be dealt with by the parents alone, for nursing and medical help is readily available. The sick child may also feel more secure in the hospital and even may be frightened to leave the security of the hospital's health equipment and professional assistance.

DEATH AT HOME

It is certainly feasible and may even be desirable for fatally ill children to die at home rather than in the acute care hospital setting. In one study of parents who kept their dying children home to die, only one of the fifty-eight families studied would have chosen to have readmitted their child to the hospital for the death event. In this study, response from the nurses and physicians involved was strongly positive; and a primary benefit of the child's death experience occurring at home was that the child was able to live in the familiar and secure home setting in a full and meaningful way right up to the moment of death [29].

If the dying child and parents choose to go home for the dying experience, the parents, instead of nurses and physicians, become the primary caregivers. Since the parents are in control of giving care to their dying child and because the parents are able to do everything they can to make their child comfortable, happy, and pain-free, parental guilt may be minimized after the child dies.

There are many advantages to keeping the child home for the dying experience [29, 30]. Besides the tremendous reduction in the financial cost of care, the personal benefits to the entire family are varied, in depth, and broad in scope. The dying child who is at home and receiving primary care from his or her parents receives much more individualized and loving care than if he or she were in the hospital. The sick child is in a warm, secure, familiar environment; and since the entire family is able to spend more time with and around the child, separation anxiety is reduced. Both the dying child and the well siblings feel less loneliness because of the fact that their family is all together under one roof again. At home, the dying child can relax and participate to a maximal degree in normal family activities. The child, as well as the parents, enjoy increased privacy. In addition, dying children can also have the pleasurable distractions of visits from neighborhood friends and school classmates, a pleasure that would require special one-time arrangements in most hospital settings. All of the above pleasurable activities tend to lift the child's spirits and provide distraction from the unpleasantries associated with the childhood cancer experience, thus decreasing the sick child's depression and pain.

Parents, too, reap many benefits from having their dying child at home. Because physical separation is no longer a stressor, intimacy, trust, and open communication within the marital relationship is enhanced. Both parents are able to share in the care of their dying child, relieving a virtually intolerable burden on one parent (usually the mother) and enhancing intimate participation in the child's care by the other parent (usually the father). Additionally, there is more privacy for the family as a whole and for the spouses in particular.

Although the siblings may be both glad and afraid to have their dying sister or brother at home, they soon become aware that this situation can be very positive for them, too. The well children in the family can also enjoy the security of staying in their own home instead of being farmed out to friends or relatives during the dying child's final hospitalization. Since the whole family is together again, siblings receive more care and attention from both their parents, and home activities begin to become more and more normal as all family members adjust to the situation of having their dying child in their midst. In addition, the siblings can learn to help take care of the sick child, increasing their own sense of importance and of belonging and banishing the frightening fantasies that so often appear in their minds if the dying child is hospitalized and thus separated from them. Although the death of the child with cancer certainly has a psychological impact on the well children in the family, there seems to be no increase in sibling distress or behavioral problems when compared with siblings of children who die in the hospital. Indeed, most siblings report that after the death of their brother or sister at home, neither death itself nor the predeath experience is as frightening as it was before [29].

Just as with any other situation, there are significant disadvantages to home care for the dying child that must be resolved if the home care situation is to be effective. First, there is the unpredictability of the child's actual life-span. This plus the usual inflexibility of the parents' work schedules can negatively affect planning of home care. The older child with cancer may recognize the increased responsibilities of the parents, and this recognition may precipitate guilt in the child. Balancing this, however, is the normal expectation from children that their parents will take care of them, especially when the child is ill. Although most children prefer to be home rather than in the hospital, the dying child may feel some insecurities about being away from the hospital and its professional staff and might wonder whether the family will know what to do in a crisis situation.

There may also be negative social responses to the situation of the child being brought home to die. Friends of the family may feel uncomfortable about changes in the child's appearance or by the fact that the dying child knows of his or her prognosis. Other family contacts may precipitate guilt in the parents by implying that the parents are not "doing enough" for the child and that the child should be in the hospital. Friends, relatives, and grandparents may let it be clearly known that they do not support the parents' decision to bring the child home to die. In addition, nurses and physicians may give the parents only partial support and may demonstrate lack of flexibility, both of which make it much more difficult for the parents to effectively manage their child's home care.

In order for home care of the dying child to be successful, a subtle yet significant reversal of roles must take place: parents must become the primary caregivers and decision makers, and nurses and physicians must act in the roles of consultants and facilitators. First and foremost, the parents must truly realize that their child is dying and that a sudden change in the child's condition does not necessarily warrant a rushed trip to the hospital. Physicians must be flexible in prescribing medications, and nurses must teach parents what to expect as the child's condition deteriorates and what to do about changes in the child's clinical condition. Community health nurses and other community resources can be used to provide nursing assistance, medical equipment, and supplies. The parents also need to clearly understand that hospitalization is always an acceptable option if the burden of the physical and emotional care of their dying child becomes too heavy. Finally, as with home care before the disease was diagnosed as terminal, parents must feel free to call the hospital nursing unit or the physician's office for advice.

CONCEPT XVII:
Health professionals must assist families to adapt to life without one of their children.

Although nurses and physicians may assume that families will adjust to the tragedy of their child's death in a rational and sensible manner, this is not often the case. Watching one's child die, whether at home or in the hospital, is a stressor that renders parents irrational, illogical, and not at all objective. The tasks of physicians and nurses before, during, and after the child's death generally consist of supportive interventions. Health professionals must view their primary task as continuing to provide appropriate physical, personal, and social care to the dying child while simultaneously attending to the family's needs. It is important that both nurses and physicians are flexible in responding to the needs of the child and family for reassurance and self-respect despite the wide emotional fluctuations common at this time.

DIRECTIONS OF CARE FOR NURSES AND PHYSICIANS

1. Always be truthful when sharing information about child's prognosis with the parents and extended family. Very few parents wish to be deceived, and dishonesty destroys trust.
2. Give information and emotional support in a manner that will minimize disruption of the normal schedule of the child and parents. Routine, familiar daily patterns of living provide comfort and security.
3. Be truthful in answering the parents' questions. An honest "I don't know" is more acceptable than an evasive response.
4. Nurses must offer information so that both the child and parents will be familiar with the hospital environment and will know what to expect regarding hospital routines and diagnostic or treatment procedures.
5. Attempt to minimize the time that the child and family must spend waiting for test results.
6. Assist the parents to prepare for questions that the child might ask.
7. Facilitate closeness and communication within the marital relationship.
8. Help parents to be aware that their healthy children at home need

truthful answers, nurturing, and—above all—parental attention and love.

9. Reassure parents that a decrease in sexual desire during this difficult time is normal and temporary. Fatigue, the grieving response, and psychic pain secondary to their child's dying experience all contribute to the spouses' needs for physical closeness, touching, hugging, and holding rather than sexual intercourse *per se.*

10. Encourage parents to become involved in a mutually supportive, self-help group of parents who also have children with cancer. At the very least, parents will discover that they are not traveling this dreadful road alone.

11. Help parents to understand that other relatives and family friends are often at a loss for comforting words. Silence does not imply not caring.

12. Become involved with the dying child and his or her family. Dispense once and for all with the nonsense of objective professional distancing, and do not be afraid to express feelings and concerns.

13. Relinquish the idea that "M.D." means "Member of the Deity." The attitude of "Dr. God" only intimidates the recipients of care who, after all, are a dying child and two grieving, frightened parents.

14. Be sensitive to the supportive relationship between the parent and child. For example, the child may cooperate during a treatment or diagnostic procedure if the parent stays with the child, whereas panic in the child may be the result if health professionals insist that the parent "step out of the room for a few minutes." Trust between the parent and child can be seriously damaged by an insensitive nurse or physician.

15. Be honest and specific regarding treatment goals, side effects, and expected outcomes. Prevent nasty and distressing surprises.

16. Realize that some parents panic easily. Help these parents to maintain control by expressing their feelings in a constructive, healthy manner, and help them to control and contribute to their child's care. *Tell* the parents if their fear and anxiety is truly justified.

17. Listen to parents. Most parents have an intuitive sense of small changes—positive or negative—in their child's condition even though they may not be able to identify the specific physical, personal, or social change.

18. Let the child know that his or her nurses and physicians feel love and concern for him or her. Dying children need to know that the treatment team is really trying to help them as much as possible for as long as possible. If the child understands and believes this, painful procedures are much easier for the child to tolerate.

CONCEPT XVIII:
Since parents are part of the treatment team, guidelines for the parents are also appropriate.

GUIDELINES FOR PARENTS

1. Answer the child's questions truthfully. If the child is old enough to ask the question, the child is old enough to receive an honest and candid answer. Parents must realize that their dying children know when they are being lied to or given evasive answers.

2. Realize that if parents do not panic, neither will the child. Parental panic will only initiate, exacerbate, and perpetuate the child's panic.

3. Express a sense of humor. Besides lifting the spirits of both child and family, laughter is thought to actually decrease the child's perception of physical pain through the release of endorphins, the body's "natural morphine."

4. Parents should treat the sick child as normally as possible, maintaining routine discipline and behavioral limits. Even the dying child hates to be "different" and a change in the parents' normal behavior only increases the sick child's fears. It is not a loving thing to do to spoil the ill child for two primary reasons: (a) being overly permissive will make healthy siblings deeply resent the sick child, and (b) the ill child will feel less "different" if he or she is expected to behave in a socially acceptable and responsible manner.

5. Although parents will focus priority attention on the care of their sick child, a sensitive balance must be maintained between that focus of attention and the awareness of other crucial aspects of the parents' lives. Parental responsibilities must be fulfilled toward the other children, marital responsibilities must be fulfilled toward one another, and job responsibilities must be fulfilled at the place of employment. If the parental focus is solely on the dying child, these other relationships will die. Parents must remember the old adage that quality of time spent with the sick child is far more important than quantity of time. *All* relationships must be in optimal harmony in order to facilitate a healthy death for the child.

6. Remember to give love, nurturing, attention, and time to the healthy siblings. Ensure that the brothers and sisters at home receive the parental love and attention that they need in order to better cope with the family disruption with which they are faced.

7. Parents must realize that well siblings may worry that they too will develop cancer. Reassuring them that, as far as we know, cancer is not contagious will do much to dispel these fears.

8. Parents must understand that bitterness and anger are normal and appropriate feelings at this time. However, the manner in which any one of the family members *expresses* this bitterness and anger can be maladaptive and destructive. A healthy way to deal with these feelings is for the individual to release and communicate the feelings toward a member of the helping professions or treatment team rather than toward each other, members of the extended family, the other well children, friends, or the dying child. After adequate ventilation of feel-

ings, the family member can more effectively go about the business of supporting the dying child, the spouse, and the well children.

9. Parents must reevaluate their priorities. For example, before the childhood cancer experience, career work and job advancement may have been a very high priority for the parent. Now, however, the new situation of having a child who is dying from cancer demands a new assessment of what is really important. Priorities usually must be changed, at least temporarily.

10. Be aware of the dying child's withdrawal, if it should occur. Encourage the child to express feelings through verbal or nonverbal means, and accept the child's feelings nonjudgmentally and with compassion. After all, parents will be losing a child; grandparents, a grandchild; and siblings, a brother or sister; but the dying child is losing everything—including the future for which he or she may have planned.

11. Fathers must be encouraged to express feelings. Failure for him to do so may result in the maladaptive responses discussed previously.

12. Become involved in a mutually supportive, self-help parents group. New insights, ventilation of feelings, and the awareness that one is not walking this terrible road alone are some of the benefits to be garnered from a parents support group.

13. Make funeral arrangements and a decision about an autopsy prior to the actual death event. If the process of making funeral arrangements is simply too painful for the parents to do, a relative or trusted friend may take care of these matters. These arrangements will eliminate an enormous amount of emotional trauma at the time of the child's death.

SUMMARY

CONCEPT XIX:
Nurses and physicians must help families to cope with childhood cancer: a chronic, life-threatening illness usually requiring long periods of treatment.

Common aspects of the childhood cancer experience include (1) long months or years of antineoplastic treatment, (2) frequent, severe, and distressing side effects of treatment, (3) complications of the disease process or progression of the disease, (4) years of ''being married'' to a doctor's office, outpatient clinic, or hospital, (5) accompanying personal and social stressors, and (6) often the bitter ending of the child's death despite years of treatment. Although more and more hope can be offered as time goes on, there are no guarantees of cure. Thus, the family finds itself in the position of desperately wanting to hope and believe in a cure for their child, yet still needing to face the reality of possible relapse and death.

After years of living with the childhood cancer experience, parents will either turn it into a positive experience of growth and love or will find that the family's basic foundation is destroyed. Sadly, a large proportion of families have serious and

Table 10.1. Familial Dysfunction After Death of the Child [18]

Familial Dysfunction	Percentage of Families
Biological Dysfunction	
Health problems, including ulcers and hypertension	95%
Personal Dysfunction	
Morbid grief reactions, including daily cemetery visits, enshrining the effects of the dead child, and the inability to make referral to the dead child within family conversation	88%
Difficulty with management of home responsibilities	43%
Serious drinking by at least one parent	40%
At least one member of the family receiving psychiatric treatment for the first time	35%
Social Dysfunction	
Parent-child relationship problems and school problems among the well children	75%
Increased marital discord	70%
Adult family members with major job-related problems	60%
Other	
Multiple familial biological, personal, and social problems	88%
More serious problems needing professional intervention occurring simultaneously	75%

significant problems after the death of the child, and a large majority of families exhibit multiple and simultaneous problems [18]. These postdeath problems are serious enough to warrant professional intervention (see Table 10.1), yet few families receive any, much less adequate, professional intervention. What is especially significant is that 80 percent of the familial dysfunction present in these families did not exist before the dead child was diagnosed with cancer. This aspect of family care makes it all the more important to include postdeath bereavement care for the family that has lost a child to malignant disease.

In summary, the child with cancer and his or her family may or may not cope well with the stress of the disease experience. The child-parent unit that copes well does much more than merely survive. The entire family unit grows, develops, and enjoys the life that is left—and they do it all together. Adaptation to childhood cancer does not mean that regression, anger, and other so-named maladaptive responses will not occur. These reactions may be the only ways that the child can exert some kind of control over a life situation that is largely controlling him. If the caregivers make it a priority to give back as much life control as possible to the child-family unit, the continuation of maladaptive responses is unlikely.

REFERENCES

1. Bartholome, W. G. The Shadow of Childhood Cancer and Society's Responsibilities. In American Cancer Society. *Proceedings of the National Conference on the Care of the Child with Cancer.* New York: American Cancer Society, 1979. Pp. 168–171.

2. Binger, C. M., Ablin, A. R., Feuerstein, R. C., Kushner, J. H., Zoger, S., and Mikkelson, C. Childhood Leukemia: Emotional Impact on Patient and Family. *N Engl J Med* 280:414, 1969.

3. Bloomquist, L. M. and Lewis-Hunstiger, M. J. To Care for the Child at Home: Discharge Planning for the Child with Leukemia. *Cancer Nurs* 1:303, 1978.

4. Bluebond-Langner, M. I Know—Do You? A Study of Awareness, Communication, and Coping in Terminally Ill Children. In B. Schoenberg, A. C. Carr, A. H. Kutscher, D. Peretz, and I. Goldberg (Eds.). *Anticipatory Grief.* New York: Columbia University Press, 1974. Chapter 20.

5. Bluebond-Langner, M. *The Private Worlds of Dying Children.* Princeton, NJ: Princeton University Press, 1978.

6. Blumberg, B., Flaherty, M., and Lewin, J. *Coping with Cancer: A Resource for the Health Professional,* N.I.H. Publication No. 80–2080. Bethesda, MD: National Institutes of Health, 1980. P. 145.

7. Bozeman, J. F., Orbach, C. F., and Sutherland, A. M. Psychological Impact of Cancer and its Treatment. The Adaptation of Mothers to the Threatened Loss of Children Through Leukemia: Part I. *Cancer* 8:1, 1955.

8. Cahan, M. P. and Lyddane, N. P. Bone Marrow Transplantation at U.C.L.A. *Cancer Nurs* 1:47, 1978.

9. DeChristopher, J. Children with Cancer: Their Perceptions of the Health Care Experience. *Topics Clin Nurs* 2(4):9, 1981.

10. Exelby, P. R. Part II: The Child with Advanced Cancer. In American Cancer Society. *Proceedings of the American Cancer Society Second National Conference on Human Values and Cancer.* New York: American Cancer Society, 1978. Pp. 51–56.

11. Friedman, S. B., Chodoff, P., Mason, J. W., and Hamburg, D. A. Behavioral Observations on Parents Anticipating the Death of a Child. *Pediatrics* 32:610, 1963.

12. Futterman, E. H. and Hoffman, I. Transient School Phobia in a Leukemic Child. *J Am Acad Child Psychol* 9:477, 1970.

13. Gyulay, J. The Forgotten Grievers. *Am J Nurs* 75:1476, 1975.

14. Hartmann, J. R., Rudolph, L. A., Trull, P., Johnson, F. L., and Hutchison, F. The Child and the Adolescent: Part I. Introduction. In American Cancer Society. *Proceedings of the American Cancer Society Second National Conference on Human Values and Cancer.* New York: American Cancer Society, 1978. Pp. 15–19.

15. Hersh, S. P. Meeting the Psychosocial Needs of the Cancer Patient. In American Cancer Society. *Proceedings of the American Cancer Society Second National Conference on Human Values and Cancer.* New York: American Cancer Society, 1978. Pp. 20–28.

16. Hodge, J. R. They That Mourn. *J Religion Health* 11:229, 1972.

17. Hostler, S. How the Child Perceives Illness and Death. In U. S. Department of Health and Human Services. *Proceedings of the First National Conference for Parents of Children with Cancer,* N.I.H. Publication No. 80–2176. Bethesda, MD: U. S. Department of Health and Human Services, 1980. Pp. 19–27.

18. Kaplan, D. M. The Family When the Child Dies. In American Cancer Society. *Proceedings of the American Cancer Society Second National Conference on Human Values and Cancer.* New York: American Cancer Society, 1978. Pp. 78–82.

19. Klopovich, P., Suenram, D., and Cairns, N. A Common Sense Approach to Caring for Children with Cancer: The Community Health Nurse. *Cancer Nurs* 3:201, 1980.

20. Komp, D. M. and Crockett, J. Educational Needs of the Child with Cancer. In American Cancer Society. *Proceedings of the American Cancer Society National Conference on Human Values and Cancer.* New York: American Cancer Society, 1978. Pp. 57–58.

21. Kubler-Ross, E. *On Death and Dying.* New York: Macmillan Co., 1969.

22. Lansky, S. B. Childhood Leukemia: The Child Psychiatrist as a Member of the Oncology Team. *J Am Acad Clin Psychol* 13:499, 1974.

23. Lansky, S. B. and Cairns, N. U. The Family of the Child with Cancer. In American Cancer Society. *Proceedings of the National Conference on the Care of the Child with Cancer.* New York: American Cancer Society, 1979. Pp. 156–162.

24. Lansky, S. B., Pearson, J., and Cairns, N. U. Alternatives for the Care of the Dying Child. In American Cancer Society. *Proceedings of the American Cancer Society Third National Conference on Human Values and Cancer.* New York: American Cancer Society, 1981. Pp. 195–201.

25. Levine, A. S. and Hersh, S. P. The Psychosocial Concomitants of Cancer in Young Patients. In A. S. Levine (Ed.). *Cancer in the Young.* New York: Masson Publishing, 1982. Chapter 15.

26. Lorin, M. I. Implications for Therapy in the Pediatric Patient. In B. Schoenberg, A. C. Carr, A. H. Kutscher, D. Peretz, and I. Goldberg (Eds.). *Anticipatory Grief.* New York: Columbia University Press, 1974. Chapter 21.

27. Mandle, C. The Need for Self-Control, Self-Determination, and Responsibility. In H. Yura and M. B. Walsh (Eds.). *Human Needs and the Nursing Process: 2.* Norwalk, CT: Appleton-Century-Crofts, 1982. Chapter 2.

28. Marten, G. W., Goff, J. R., Powazek, M., and Payne, J. S. Psychosocial Evaluation of Children with Cancer. In American Cancer Society. *Proceedings of the National Conference on the Care of the Child with Cancer.* New York: American Cancer Society, 1979. Pp. 45–49.

29. Martinson, I. M. An Approach for Studying the Feasibility and Desirability of Home Care for the Child Dying of Cancer. In M. C. Cahoon (Ed.). *Cancer Nursing.* New York: Churchill Livingston, 1982. Chapter 2.

30. Martinson, I. M., Armstrong, G. D., Geis, D. P., et al. Facilitating Home Care for Children Dying of Cancer. *Cancer Nurs* 1:41, 1978.

31. McCollum, A. T. and Schwartz, A. H. Social Work and the Mourning Parent. *Soc Work* 17:25, 1972.

32. Neill, K. Behavioral Aspects of Chronic Physical Disease. *Nurs Clin North Am* 14:443, 1979.

33. Pearse, M. The Child with Cancer: Impact on the Family. *J Sch Health* 47(3):174, 1977.

34. Pinkel, P. Cure of the Child with Cancer: Definition and Prospective. In American Cancer Society. *Proceedings of the National Conference on the Care of the Child with Cancer.* New York: American Cancer Society, 1979. Pp. 191–200.

35. Plumb, M. M. and Holland, J. Cancer in Adolescents: The Symptom is the Thing. In B. Schoenberg, A. C. Carr, A. H. Kutschner, D. Peretz, and I. Goldberg (Eds.). *Anticipatory Grief.* New York: Columbia University Press, 1974. Chapter 23.

36. Taylor, M. C. The Need for Self-Esteem. In H. Yura and M. B. Walsh (Eds.). *Human Needs 2 and the Nursing Process.* Norwalk, CT: Appleton-Century-Crofts, 1982. Chapter 4.

37. Taylor, M. M. and Williams, H. A. Use of Therapeutic Play in the Ambulatory Hematology Clinic. *Cancer Nurs* 3:433, 1980.

38. Toch, R. Management of Parental Anticipatory Grief. In B. Schoenberg, A. C. Carr, A. H. Kutschner, D. Peretz, and I. Goldberg (Eds.). *Anticipatory Grief.* New York: Columbia University Press, 1974. Chapter 18.

39. Van Eys, J. The Outlook for the Child with Cancer. *J Sch Health* 47:165, 1977.

40. Waechter, E. H. Developmental Correlates of Physical Disability. *Nurs Forum* 9:90, 1970.

41. Waechter, E. Children's Awareness of Fatal Illness. *Am J Nurs* 71:1168, 1971.

42. Wright, L. An Emotional Support Program for Parents of Dying Children. *J Clin Child Psychol* 3:37, 1974.

43. Yanni, M. I. Y. Perception of Parent's Behavior and Children's General Fearfulness. *Nurs Res* 31:79, 1974.

PART IV

SPECIAL TOPICS IN ONCOLOGY NURSING

Chapter 11

The Person in Pain

CONCEPT I:
Pain is a phenomenon that consists of (1) a private, subjective sensation of hurt; (2) a stimulus that signals current or impending tissue damage; and (3) a pattern of responses intended to protect the person from harm [43].

Pain is a complex process that has biological, personal, and social dimensions. All pain is real, regardless of its cause, and most pain is a combination of psychogenic and physiological factors. It is a phenomenon deeply intertwined with human existence and often precipitates questioning of the meaning of life itself [4]. The concern of caregivers is not to deal with painful malignant lesions per se but to deal with people who are experiencing pain. The negative result that is most often feared and most often verbalized by persons with cancer is pain [31]. Caregivers must never underestimate the influence that mental and emotional status has upon the pain experience, including occurrence, severity, tolerance, and expression of pain.

Analgesia is defined as relief from the sensation of pain, in the broadest meaning of the word, without loss of consciousness [13]. Analgesia, or relief from pain, results in the ability of the ill person to expend energy in coping, living, and perhaps facing death, rather than expending energy in battling pain. Failure of pain relief can reduce the client to a life of dependency and despair, and force the individual to adapt to a repetitious and progressively less effective life style. Health professionals, especially nurses and physicians, are in a unique position that enables them to effectively interrupt this destructive cycle [39].

No overall approach to the management of cancer pain is sufficient [2]. Thus, overall analgesic therapy must include attention to the frequency, severity and duration of pain, the nature of the disease, probable life expectancy of the client, psychological status, and the social aspect of occupational, domestic, and economic factors. Management of the chronic, progressive pain of cancer may be aimed toward one of two goals: eliminating the cause of pain (tumor) or controlling the pain without eliminating the cause.

CONCEPT II:
Although cancer is not always accompanied by pain, a high percentage of clients eventually experience significant pain, necessitating nursing and medical intervention.

Pain does not always accompany cancer, and it is rarely a symptom of early cancer. However, the nature of cancer is highly unpredictable and life-threatening with continual physical and mental threats and insults. For many clients, cancer eventually gives rise to pain that becomes progressively more severe and finally develops into a relentless suffering that greatly potentiates the person's physical and personal deterioration. Severe pain is experienced by 60 percent to 80 percent of hospitalized clients with advanced malignancy [7]. The client's physical and personal deterioration produced by relentless pain results in increased family stress which, in turn, further contributes to the client's suffering.

PAIN AND LEVELS OF NEED

The continuous, destructive nature of the severe, chronic pain often associated with cancer interferes with gratification of needs on all five levels. The client becomes dominated by the pain experience and the striving to avoid or reduce it. The very experience of chronic, severe pain reduces motivation to a narrow, singular focus: relief of pain; the client's universe narrows until it includes only the client and the pain.

At the *physiological level,* chronic severe pain precludes rest, sleep, and physical comfort. Food and fluid intake is often decreased secondary to the nausea and anorexia accompanying chronic pain and concurrent parasympathetic stimulation. Activity and exercise are also commonly decreased.

Safety needs are continuously threatened by severe chronic pain. Although acute pain serves to warn the person of current or impending damage to bodily integrity, the client suffering from the chronic pain of cancer is helpless to eliminate the source of pain. Thus, security is diminished by the ceaseless, hostile presence of pain.

Needs for love and belonging are inadequately gratified when chronic pain becomes the client's primary focus. In order to cope with the pain, the individual directs all energies and consciousness toward the pain and away from significant others. Clients become isolated in a closed world composed solely of themselves and pain. Chronic pain of this nature frustrates the family, friends, and caregivers, leaving them feeling helpless and angry, and thus perpetuating the vicious cycle of pain, withdrawal, and loneliness.

Needs for self-esteem and *self-actualization* are thwarted by the client's growing dependence on others. Dependency on others becomes increasingly necessary as the pain consumes ever-escalating amounts of energy. The client cannot control the external or internal environments but is instead controlled and dominated by pain, perpetuating the phenomena of helplessness, hopelessness, low self-esteem, and the inability for self-actualization.

In a word, the chronic severe pain often associated with advanced cancer interferes with living. One study revealed that 24 percent of the clients with cancer pain experienced slight interference with living, 64 percent a moderate interference, and 12 percent reported a severe interference with living. Thus, over three-quarters of the clients studied experienced a significant disruption in their lives because of the chronic pain associated with cancer [34] (see Table 11.1).

Table 11.1.   Pain's Interference with Living in Persons with Cancer [34]

Disruption in Living	Percent of Subjects
Depression	88%
Difficulty with physical movement	84%
Anxiety	83%
Irritability	80%
Difficulty sleeping	76%
Difficulty concentrating	60%

THE MANAGEMENT AND MISMANAGEMENT OF CHRONIC CANCER PAIN

The pain of cancer deserves a systematic plan for *control,* rather than mere relief. The plan for pain control must aim to conserve the client's physical, mental, and moral resources and social usefulness for as long as possible. Yet the management of chronic cancer pain is an area within cancer care that has been woefully neglected. When compared with the money allocated for research on other aspects of the cancer problem, expenditures have been minimal [35]. In fact, the National Cancer Institute, the major federal agency supporting cancer research, spent only 0.022 percent of its national budget in a recent year on cancer pain research [7]. Overall, there has been a paucity of research on cancer pain. The amount of this research has only recently begun to increase [1].

Effective management of cancer pain must consider several factors, including the severity and duration of pain, the nature of the disease process, the client's probable life expectancy, psychological status, and social background. Stressors in all three spheres of personhood—biological, personal, and social—can and do significantly affect the client's pain experience. Thus, the limitation of pain management to the singular intervention of administering a drug will always fall far short of effective control.

The chronic, progressive pain associated with advanced cancer is often mismanaged for a variety of reasons. For the client and family, pain is one of the primary and most feared aspects of the disease process. Unfortunately, most persons with cancer have had at least a few negative and distressing experiences related to their pain experience prior to the diagnosis of cancer. Most of these persons have experienced the disbelief of health professionals regarding the legitimacy of their reports of pain [23]. This unfortunate yet common experience increases clients' fears and anxieties concerning pain, thus actually increasing the pain experience.

Another factor in the mismanagement of pain associated with malignancy is the inadequate application of available knowledge about cancer pain. This results from a variety of causes, including the lack of organized teaching to health professionals on the topic of effective management of cancer pain, a lack of time in busy clinical practices which precludes health professionals from giving optimal pain relief, and relatively meager published data on the subject. Specialization by caregivers magnifies the problem since, with many physicians and nurses involved in the client's care, accountability for pain control becomes clouded and the buck seems to stop nowhere. Even when there is a good nursing/medical plan for controlling the client's cancer pain, it is often subject to mismanagement merely because of inadequate communication of the plan to all caregivers. In the study previously cited [34], only 30 percent of the subjects participating in the research reported complete pain relief although all subjects received analgesic drugs. The remaining 70 percent reported that the medication reduced pain severity but did not ameliorate the pain. Seventy-eight percent of the subjects experienced pain reduction for less than four hours, yet the most frequently prescribed dosing interval was every four hours.

In addition, 22.5 percent of the subjects in this study—nearly one-quarter—reported that they did not receive their analgesic medication soon after it was requested. Of these individuals, 42.5 percent stated that they had to wait five to twenty minutes before the medication was administered, 27.5 percent waited twenty to forty-five minutes, and an astounding 10 percent reported a delay of one to two hours [34]! What caregivers don't seem to realize is that even a delay of ten minutes can subjectively seem like an eternity to the client experiencing severe pain.

"Snowing" of the client denotes lack of understanding of the problem of chronic pain and often exacerbates the disease process, respiratory depression, stupor, anorexia, nausea, and vomiting [7]. With some clients, potent narcotics are used initially for mild chronic pain that could be easily and effectively controlled by nonnarcotics combined with sedatives. "Snowing" of the person with chronic cancer pain seems to reflect a nursing/medical attitude toward pain control of "peace at any price," the quiet and sedated client being the type considered as a "good patient."

However, "snowing" of the client is not nearly so common as the trend toward undertreatment of chronic cancer pain. There seems to be a trend in the United States and Canada toward the undertreatment of chronic cancer pain, especially when the pharmaceutical treatment includes narcotics. This trend seems to have been in progress since at least 1970, resulting in much needless suffering. One major form of undertreatment is the underprescription of analgesic drugs by physicians [23]. With many clients, analgesics may be adequately prescribed but are then improperly withheld because of the caregivers' fear of creating "addiction." Another factor in undertreatment is inattention to the differences between clients: because awareness and allowances for individual body weight and drug tolerance are seldom made, clients are frequently undermedicated [14]. In one study, 73 percent of the subjects participating in the research remained in moderate to severe distress from physical pain as a result of less than optimal doses of prescribed medication [21]. The causative factors of this phenomenon appear to be the fear of causing respiratory depression [23], the fear of producing addiction in the client, and the failure of both nurses and physicians to apply basic pharmacological knowledge to the problem of chronic pain [21, 23].

Physicians and nurses—the persons who prescribe and decide when to administer the analgesics—tend to undermedicate clients because of a lack of knowledge about narcotic analgesics and the fear of producing addiction. Yet, studies have shown that drug addiction of any medical consequence is very low among persons with chronic cancer pain. With the proper treatment (the right drug, the right dosage, and the right dosing interval), it is possible to alleviate the client's *fear* of pain, protect the client from drug-seeking behavior, and consequently minimize the incidence of tolerance and dependence [5, 53].

TOLERANCE, DEPENDENCE, AND ADDICTION

It has been established that morphine and other narcotics invariably result in tolerance when given in routine, regular doses. *Tolerance* must *not* be confused with *addiction*. Tolerance refers to a decreased responsiveness to *any* pharmacological effect of *any* drug as a consequence of prior administration of that drug, necessitating larger doses of that drug to produce an equivalent effect to that of the initial dose. In general, tolerance occurs to the depressive and analgesic properties of the narcotics but not to the stimulating effects of the drug. For example, in the case of morphine, tolerance develops primarily to analgesia, euphoria, drowsiness, and respiratory depression but not to the effects of the gastrointestinal tract depression or miosis. In the clinical setting, the first sign of developing tolerance to the analgesic effects of the drug will be a decreased duration of action or decreased efficacy of the analgesic effect. However, it must be remembered that tolerance is not an absolute, and that an eventual lethal dose exists regardless of the extent of the individual's tolerance to the narcotic, although the lethal dose is apparently very high [13].

Again, it has been established that routine, regular administration of morphine and the other narcotics will eventually result in physical dependence. And again, *physical dependence* must *not* be equated with *addiction*. Physical dependence is defined as an abnormal physiological state resulting from repeated administration of a drug which then makes necessary the continued use of that drug to prevent the appearance of a withdrawal syndrome [13]. Health professionals would not recommend or condone the abrupt discontinuance of a corticosteroid because of the adverse withdrawal syndrome, yet health professionals do not refer to this situation as "addiction" to corticosteroids. Still, there is a great fear that physical dependence on narcotics is synonymous with "addiction."

Addiction is a frequently used but vague term, representing the extreme of a combination of physical/psychological dependence on a drug, especially a narcotic, manifested as a behavioral pattern of compulsive drug use *without* a pain experience. So, iatrogenically induced physical dependence in a client is not correctly identified as "addiction"; the client is not an "addict." Of primary concern is the comfort and well-being of the client. Of secondary importance is the issue of the development or presence of tolerance and/or physical dependence. After the cause or source of the pain has been eradicated, the secondary problems of tolerance and physical dependence can be appropriately treated as independent medical/nursing problems. Regardless of the potential degree to which tolerance and/or physical dependence may have or has actually developed, narcotic administration should not be discontinued abruptly nor other nonnarcotic, nonanalgesic drugs such as tranquilizers or sedatives be administered in their place out of fear of "addicting" the client in chronic pain. Even worse would be discontinuance of the narcotics and/or substitution of tranquilizers or sedatives in the narcotic-dependent client [13]. Physical dependence is not of concern in the relatively short-term situation;

nor is it of concern in clients with chronic pain [26, 46]. Need for increased dosage probably indicates a change in disease status rather than a problem with physical dependence.

CONCEPT III:
Acute pain has been described as a temporary, self-limiting event.

Acute pain is inherently a protective mechanism, warning the body to protect itself from actual or potential harm. It is generally quite adequately controlled by relatively short-term narcotic or nonnarcotic drug therapy, and it is more easily tolerated if the client has realistic hopes for a quick resolution to the pain. Acute pain almost always initiates a sympathetic nervous system response, with a subsequent increase in oxygen and glucose demand and consumption, hypertension, tachycardia, and tachypnea. Thus, it is of crucial importance to adequately control acute pain in those clients whose oxygenation and metabolic systems are compromised.

CONCEPT IV:
Chronic pain has been described as a situation, rather than an event, in which the pain is continuous or regularly recurs for an indefinite period of time.

Pain is unpleasant and has an urgency that makes it difficult to ignore. In chronic pain, the client is continually alerted that something is causing harm to the integrity of the body, yet is unable to eliminate the source of pain. The resulting anxiety and fear significantly increase pain perception and make pain control much more difficult to achieve.

Chronic pain can be viewed as a circular experience without a known duration of time. The pain seems to be meaningless as well as endless, and the fearful anticipation of continued pain results in anxiety, depression, and insomnia which further increase the pain experience. Chronic, constant pain is also associated with loss of ego strength, loss of libido, and feelings of guilt, futility, helplessness, hopelessness, and worthlessness [32].

Only by preventing the recurrence of chronic pain can anxiety and fear of its return be reduced or eliminated. Once pain returns, it is far more difficult to control than if analgesic measures had been employed before pain recurrence.

Although acute pain is associated with a sympathetic nervous system response, chronic pain usually results in none of the behavioral responses and changes in vital signs seen in acute pain because of the adaptation of the person to the persistent presence of pain [33]. Since most health professionals receive pain education on the acute-pain model, this lack of "traditional pain symptoms" in the person with chronic pain often lead caregivers to doubt the actual existence of pain and thus to provide inadequate treatment. Suffice it to say that a diagnosis of malingering is an accusation that will only serve to destroy a therapeutic relationship between caregiver and client.

CONCEPT V:
The attitudes of health professionals profoundly influence the success or failure of pain control measures for the person with cancer.

It has been shown that the person who is "stoic" and who "can take it (pain)" is preferred by health professionals even if severe pain is obvious and evident. Hospital nursing units with these attitudes seem to have a "raw guts" approach to pain, with the attitude that suffering is "good for the person." Other hospital nursing units exhibit the "peace at any price" approach, administering inappropriately large amounts of analgesics and sedatives and thus ensuring that the complaining client will be quieted and "peace" will be restored [12].

It is important to remember that "intractable pain" is not synonymous with "untreatable pain." Intractable merely refers to pain that is not easily treated by modalities used for acute pain or for mild to moderate chronic pain. For clients with chronic pain resulting from cancer, when all nonnarcotic modalities and strategies have failed to control the pain, the narcotic analgesics may be the one method left to relieve suffering [36]. There is a great deal of misinformation apparent among health professionals regarding the mode of action, relative potencies, onset of action, duration of effect, and realistic side effects of analgesic drugs. The fear of "addicting" a client is quite real in the minds of many nurses, physicians, and pharmacists, despite the significant amount of professional literature indicating that the addiction potential of most narcotic analgesics is very often overestimated.

Another result of professional misinformation is the indiscriminate switching from one narcotic to another when pain control is not achieved. Misinformation about pharmacological facts regarding the available analgesic drugs may result in switching to a less effective drug, causing an increase in the client's pain experience.

CONCEPT VI:
Various theories have been proposed in an attempt to explain the phenomenon of pain but none of the theories completely accounts for the myriad dimensions, contributing factors, and manifestations of the pain process.

SPECIFICITY THEORY [27, 51]

The specificity theory of pain proposes that pain receptors in the skin transmit sensory messages to a pain center in the brain, possibly the thalamus and hypothalamus, thus resulting in pain perception. This theory attempts to provide the rationale for certain surgical procedures aimed at the relief of severe intractable pain (e.g., cordotomy). It fails, however, to account for such phenomena as phantom limb pain. The specificity theory is not a holistic theory since it fails to take into account the nonphysiological factors affecting pain perception.

PATTERN THEORY [27, 51]

The pattern theory proposes that intense peripheral stimulation causes a pattern of nerve impulses that are then interpreted by the brain as pain. This theory explains phantom limb pain as a phenomenon resulting from intense peripheral nerve stimulation, with amputation stimulating abnormal firing patterns. These volleys of nerve impulses are then interpreted by the brain as pain. The pattern theory is not a holistic theory since it fails to take into account the nonphysiological factors affecting pain perception.

AFFECT THEORY [51]

The affect theory takes into consideration the psychogenic and emotional dimensions of pain and regards them as the primary component of the pain experience. This theory postulates that the amount and quality of the person's pain are determined by many psychological variables, such as anxiety, suggestion, and the meaning of pain to the client in the specific situation. According to this theory, responses to pain are learned and patterned according to cultural norms of behavior, and the pain sensation itself is simply a part of the pain experience and may not even be the primary feature. The affect theory is not a holistic theory since it minimizes physiological dimensions of the pain experience.

GATE-CONTROL THEORY [27]

The gate-control theory of pain is one of the most important of the pain theories and is widely accepted by health professionals. The theory proposes that the perception of painful stimuli can be reduced by a gating effect at the spinal segmental level.

The gate-control theory refutes the proposition that the human nervous system contains specialized pain fibers that always produce pain, and nothing but pain, when stimulated. Although a small number of nerve fibers may exist that respond only to intense stimulation, it is more likely that they represent the extreme of a continuous distribution of receptor-fibers rather than a specialized category of "pain fibers."

In addition, this theory postulates that there is not a distinct anatomical area in the brain for pain perception. According to the gate-control theory, the whole brain, rather than just one spot, is the "pain center." The thalamus, hypothalamus, limbic system, brainstem, reticular formation, parietal cortex, and frontal cortex have all been implicated in pain perception; and perception of pain seems to occur as an interaction among all of these brain parts.

Transmission of Pain Information

Pain information is transmitted from the skin to three spinal cord systems: (1) cells of the substantia gelatinosa in the dorsal horn, (2) the dorsal column fibers that project upward toward the brain, and (3) the first central transmission (T) cells in the dorsal horn. The substantia gelatinosa functions as a gate-control system that modulates the afferent pattern of stimulation before the pattern of nerve stimulation reaches and influences the T-cells. The T-cells activate neural mechanisms that make up the action system responsible for the brain's perception of and response to pain. Pain phenomena are a result of interactions among the three spinal cord systems.

The substantia gelatinosa consists of small, densely packed cells that form a functional unit extending the entire length of the spinal cord, and it acts as a gate-control mechanism that modulates the synaptic transmission of nerve impulses from the periphery to the central cells.

In the peripheral nervous system as well as the spinal cord, both small-diameter and large-diameter nerve fibers may be found. Small-diameter fibers tend to be tonically active, adapt slowly, and hold the spinal cord gates open, thus enhancing transmission of painful messages to the brain. Volleys of impulses from small-diameter fibers activate a positive feedback mechanism, exaggerating the effect of subsequently arriving impulses from small-diameter fibers, keeping the spinal cord gate open, and thus increasing pain perception. Large-diameter nerve fibers adapt even more slowly than do small-diameter fibers, elicit a negative feedback mechanism, and tend to close the spinal cord gate, thus stopping the flow of painful messages to the brain. Both positive and negative feedback mechanisms are mediated by the substantia gelatinosa. So, pain perception is significantly affected by the relative balance between large and small fiber activity.

The T-cells are the first central transmission cells in the dorsal horn, and they activate neural mechanisms that comprise the action system responsible for the brain's perception of and response to painful stimuli. Predominance of small-diameter nerve fiber activity increases T-cell output, keeps the gate open, and thus allows the brain to perceive pain. If, on the other hand, the large-diameter nerve fiber steady background activity is artificially raised (for example, by vibration), T-cell output is diminished and pain perception decreased owing to closing of the gate.

Once the integrated firing of T-cells surpasses a preset, critical threshold, the T-cell firing activates a sequence of responses by the action system, which is responsible for the brain's perception of and response to pain. Triggering of the action system by the T-cell denotes the start of the sequence of sensory, cognitive, and behavioral activities that occur when the body sustains damage. Interactions between the gate-control mechanism and the action system may occur at various synaptic levels located at any level of the central nervous system in the course of filtering sensory input.

Central Control Trigger

It is thought that the nervous system contains a mechanism, termed the central control trigger, which activates the particular selective brain processes that exert control over the sensory input transmitted by the spinal cord. Of the two known systems, one or both may be involved: (1) the dorsal column-medial lemniscus system and (2) the dorso-lateral path.

The dorsal column-medial lemniscus system provides a direct route from the spinal cord to the thalamus and somato-sensory cortex. Sensory information ("pain messages") is transmitted rapidly from the skin to the cortex by this route. The separation of signals evoked by different stimuli and precise localization are maintained throughout the system, and conduction of information is relatively unaffected by analgesic drugs.

The dorso-lateral path originates in the dorsal horn and proceeds through the lateral cervical nucleus to the brainstem. This pathway has a small, well-defined receptive field, and sensory conduction along the pathway is extremely rapid, even faster than in the dorsal column-medial lemniscus system.

Both pathways carry precise information about the nature and location of stimuli, and both conduct so rapidly that they may not only affect the receptivity of cortical neurons for further afferent impulses but may also act on the gate-control system itself by way of central-control efferent fibers. Both pathways activate selective brain processes that then influence the modulating properties of the gate-control system

Stimulation of the brain activates descending efferent fibers that can influence afferent impulse conduction at early synaptic levels. Thus, central nervous system activities, such as attention, emotion, and memories of past pain experiences, may exert control over sensory input. It is thought that these central influences are mediated through the gate-control mechanism. Some central activities, such as anxiety or fear, open the gate for all sensory input from every site on the body. Other central activities, such as relaxation and distraction, apparently close the gate and thus reduce pain perception. So, the gate-control mechanism may be profoundly influenced by central activities as patterns of sensory input are analyzed and acted upon by the brain. Therefore, the gate-control theory is a holistic theory because it fully attends to both physiological and psychogenic factors involved in the development of pain.

The concept of interacting gate-control and action systems can account for all types of pain. For example, the phenomenon of hyperalgesia requires two concurrent conditions to be present: (1) enough conducting peripheral nerves to generate input sufficient to activate the action system, and (2) a marked loss of the large-diameter peripheral nerve fibers, which may occur after traumatic peripheral nerve lesions or in some neuropathies. Thus, the normal presynaptic inhibition of pain messages does not occur, and sensory input is transmitted unchecked through the open gate by small fibers, and then interpreted by the brain as pain.

The above factors also explain the phenomenon of increased pain during emotional distress. Increased sensory firing of the large-diameter nerve fibers occurs secondary to increased sympathetic output, and sensory input is again transmitted unchecked through the open gate by small-diameter nerve fibers, resulting in central nervous system interpretation of the input as pain.

Implications for Pain Control

Stimulation of all nerve fibers at a less than acutely painful level by vibration or massage, for example, will stimulate both small-diameter and large-diameter nerve fibers. Small-diameter nerve fibers, however, adapt more quickly to the stimulation than do large-diameter nerve fibers; and large-diameter fibers continue to fire, thus closing the gate. Thus, pain control may be achieved by closing the gate through selective stimulation of large-diameter nerve fibers. This concept of pain and pain control quite adequately explains the analgesic success of acupuncture, acupressure, backrubs and massage, therapeutic touch, distraction, the La-Maze technique, and transcutaneous electrical nerve stimulation (TENS).

Summary

The gate-control theory of pain proposes that the presence or absence of pain is determined by the relative balance between the sensory input from small-diameter and large-diameter nerve fibers and the central inhibitory or excitatory influence on the gate-control system. Analgesia can be effected by stimulation of large-diameter nerve fibers at a less than acutely painful level, thus closing the gate at the level of the spinal cord and blocking pain perception.

ENDOGENOUS PAIN CONTROL THEORY

According to the endogenous pain control theory, suppression of pain can occur at three levels: midbrain, medulla, and spinal cord. The theory postulates that analgesia may be induced by naturally occurring endogenous hormones that decrease perception of pain by decreasing the output of pain-transmission neurons. The endogenous analgesic hormones are identified as: (1) enkephalins (morphine-like hormones), (2) serotonin (a hormone that inhibits the activity of pain-transmitting neurons, and (3) endorphins ("natural morphine" from the pituitary) [51].

These endogenous hormones have been identified in the central nervous system, gastrointestinal system, and plasma of human beings, and they mimic the action of morphine sulfate and are nullified by the presence of a narcotic antagonist such as naloxone (Narcan). These endogenous hormones are more highly concentrated in the areas of the central nervous system that are believed to mediate neural transmission of pain.

Although "endorphin" may be used in a generic sense to include all of the endogenous opiate-like peptides, there are certain distinctions between endorphins and enkephalins that may prove to be clinically significant. Endorphins are related to long-chain peptides [6] and are apparently composed of two components: fractions I and II. Lower concentrations of endorphin fraction I is found in persons with chronic pain as compared to persons not experiencing pain. This phenomenon might be secondary either to hypoactivity in endorphin production or release or to high endorphin consumption [42]. Enkephalins, on the other hand, are related to short-chain peptides and have been found in the peripheral nervous system as well as in the same areas where endorphins are located [6].

The endogenous opiate-like hormones are located in the synapses between nerve fibers, and they likely transmit, modify, and inhibit noxious stimuli. Their inhibitory role is probably secondary to their ability to inhibit the release of another peptide (substance P) that transmits noxious stimuli. The brain contains many specific sites to which opiates, both endogenous and exogenous, form chemical attachments. These opiate binding sites are located in both cognitive areas of the brain and in areas associated with emotion, as well as the substantia gelatinosa in the spinal cord's dorsal horns [50]. This finding supports the long-held assumption that opiates relieve pain by altering pain perception rather than by actually eliminating the pain event itself.

Implications for Pain Control

The endogenous opiate-like hormones may relieve pain even without administration of exogenous analgesic drugs. Persons experiencing less pain than might be clinically expected probably have high levels of endorphins. Endorphin release may potentiate other analgesic methods, since increased endorphin levels have been demonstrated after transcutaneous electrical nerve stimulation and acupuncture [50].

Increased release of endorphins may be responsible for the placebo effect. Evidence supporting this hypothesis includes the fact that naloxone (Narcan), a narcotic antagonist, reverses the placebo effect, the effects of endorphins, and the effects of exogenous narcotic agents [19, 50]. It is also thought that endorphins have an antianxiety effect, perhaps partially because of their effect on psychological aspects of pain. Endorphins have been called the "happiness peptides" because of their ability to induce euphoria. Endorphins have also been implicated in the analgesic effect of distraction since distraction probably precipitates release of endorphins stimulated by a descending impulse from the brain [50].

It is thought that continuous pain depletes endorphin levels, worsening the client's pain experience, anxiety, and depression. It has been demonstrated that persons with chronic pain and/or depression have lower levels of endorphins than do persons not experiencing those situations [20].

Summary

The endogenous pain control theory postulates that the suppression of pain can be achieved through the body's natural opiate-like hormones: endorphin, serotonin, and enkephalin. These hormones mimic the action of morphine and have been demonstrated to potentiate other analgesic methods, reduce anxiety, and induce euphoria. The endogenous opiate-like hormones have been implicated in the analgesic effects of distraction and the placebo effect. The reduced tolerance for and increased perception of pain so commonly observed in persons with chronic pain may be partially due to depletion of endorphins.

PLACEBO EFFECT [19]

The placebo effect is a real, demonstrated method of pain control and is not merely a case of "tricking the person with a sugar pill." In a variety of painful conditions, a constant of approximately one-third of persons experiencing the pain will obtain significant pain relief from a placebo. Placebo analgesia and narcotic analgesia seem to have similar mechanisms of action. With repeated use of the placebo, tolerance occurs with diminution of the analgesic effect, and there is a tendency to increase the "dose" of the placebo over time. Withdrawal symptoms occur when the placebo is suddenly withdrawn from a client who has received the placebo for a period of time, and naloxone (Narcan) reverses the analgesia induced by the placebo. Interestingly, prior administration of naloxone will decrease the probability of a positive placebo response. As was previously discussed, an increased release of endorphins apparently mediates placebo analgesia.

CONCEPT VII:
Care provided by health professionals for the person experiencing cancer pain must be holistic in nature, attending to the biological, personal, and social causes and manifestations of that pain.

As has been previously discussed, the concern of caregivers is not to deal solely with painful malignant lesions but instead to provide effective care for persons who are experiencing pain. The long-term goal for these clients is maintenance of maximal comfort and freedom from pain so that the client may live as normally as possible for as long as possible. Short-term objectives for cancer clients experiencing pain include the removal or reduction of the perception of painful stimuli. In order to achieve these objectives and the long-term goal, caregivers should:

1. Assess the client's pain on a regular basis.
2. Minimize fear, anxiety, and dependency on others.
3. Minimize the pain associated with treatment and diagnostic procedures.
4. Provide general comfort measures to reduce the pain burden.
5. Preserve the client's energy for enjoyable activities.
6. Alleviate and prevent progressive, continuous pain.

ASSESSMENT

Assessment of the cancer client's pain experience is absolutely essential to effective planning and intervention. Both quantitative (objective) and qualitative (subjective) data is necessary. The general assessment must include location, type, and intensity of pain; physical examination and X-ray findings, which may be negative; and emotional or social components affecting the client's pain experience.

Pain assessment is a difficult task since pain is a highly subjective experience, and it must be remembered that not all persons manifest pain in the same way. Thus, guidelines regarding assessment of the signs and symptoms associated with pain cannot be generalized to include all persons experiencing pain. In mild to moderate superficial pain, a sympathetic nervous system response is usually elicited, with hypertension, tachycardia, and tachypnea. In severe or visceral pain, a parasympathetic nervous system response is more characteristic, with hypotension, bradycardia, vomiting, weakness, and/or fainting. If the client's pain has persisted longer than one month, late-stage chronic pain has developed and no change will be noted in vital signs because of bodily adaptation to the pain [33].

When assessing physical appearance of the person experiencing pain, the nurse must keep in mind that different persons exhibit their pain in different ways and that there is not a singular, characteristic "pain behavior" that can be observed in every person who is experiencing pain. The individual may appear to be anxious, distressed, and tense with a constant frown, clenched teeth, a dull pained look in the eyes, and profuse perspiration. On the other hand, the client may lie very still and quiet, responding in this manner to the pain. The person may have attempted to cope with previous pain by using relaxation techniques, distraction, etc., and so will perhaps appear to be quiet, calm, and relaxed. This behavior must *not* be interpreted as necessarily indicating the absence of pain.

Qualitative, subjective data may be obtained by eliciting client reports of the type, location, and intensity of the pain, as well as information about the amount of distress or suffering being experienced by the client as a result of the pain. Information about the type of pain being experienced may be obtained simply by asking the client to describe the pain—what it feels like—through informal, spontaneous questioning or by use of a specific tool such as a Pain Questionnaire (see Figure 11.1). Location of the pain may be determined by asking the client to put an "X" or to shade in the area(s) where pain is perceived on an outline drawing of a human figure. Pain intensity may be assessed by asking the client to "place" the pain on a Pain Intensity Scale (see Figure 11.2), and subjective distress may be evaluated by a similar use of a Pain Distress Scale (see Figure 11.3).

In addition to these data, the nurse must assess whether the pain is continuous or intermittent, what seems to precipitate or exacerbate the pain, the frequency and duration of intermittent pain, what seems to improve or worsen the pain experience, what associated symptoms are present, what strategies have proven effective in controlling previous pain, and what personal or social adverse effects stem from the pain. Each one of these items is an important piece of data that will aid the caregiver in structuring an overall picture of the client's pain and its meaning.

Finally, nurses must realize that the usual pain trajectory, or pain pattern, fluctuates for many clients. They experience significant and severe pain at some times and no pain at all at other times, resulting in uneven pain control. This pain trajectory can even be induced, most often by the "PRN" system of analgesia and pain relief: clients must experience pain and request medication before they can achieve a pain-free state.

DETERMINING CAUSATIVE FACTORS

Clarification of the cause of pain is essential for optimal pain control; however, the causative stressor(s) is not always clearly obvious. It is important, though, that caregivers *not* automatically assume that the client's pain results from the disease process when it may be secondary to many other stressors related or unrelated to the malignancy. Many of these secondary stressors can be easily eliminated or minimized, thus reducing the pain experience even for clients with advanced cancer.

PAIN ASSESSMENT

Name _____

Age _____ Diagnosis _____

Factors Influencing Pain _____

LOCATION

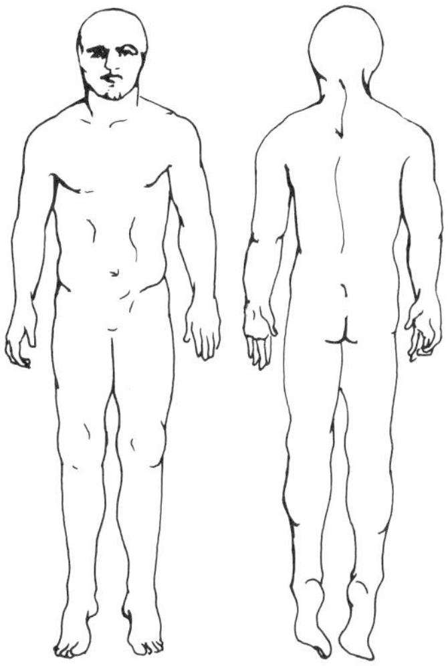

QUALITY (Have patient describe pain in own words)

_____

_____

INTENSITY (Rate pain on a scale of 0-10)

Now _____

1 hour after medication _____

Worst it gets _____

Best it gets _____

FREQUENCY

_____

_____

_____

What makes the pain better? _____

What makes the pain worse? _____

Associated symptoms: _____

PLAN

_____
_____
_____

Figure 11.1. Pain Assessment.

Physiological Mechanisms Contributing to the Pain Experience

Five biological mechanisms have been implicated in the development of chronic cancer pain. The characteristics of the pain will depend on tissue morphology as well as the involved mechanisms.

Bone destruction secondary to infiltration by malignant cells or resulting from metastatic lesions is the most common of the biological mechanisms causing

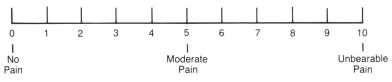

Figure 11.2. Pain Intensity Scale.

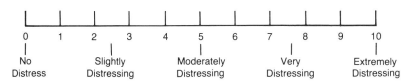

Figure 11.3. Pain Distress Scale.

chronic cancer pain. Bone metastases cause increased release of prostaglandins and subsequent bone breakdown and resorption. The client's pain threshold is reduced through sensitization of free nerve endings [48]. Bone destruction may be assessed by radiological studies, elevation of serum alkaline phosphatase and possibly serum calcium, and the appearance of localized, continuous pain. Maladaptive outcomes of bone destruction may include sharp continuous pain that increases upon movement or ambulation and pathological fractures. Bony metastases are usually quite effectively treated with external beam radiotherapy, and pain intensity generally is significantly decreased by day 4 of treatment in over 90 percent of affected clients [33, 48].

Obstruction of a viscus is another physiological factor in the development of chronic cancer pain. Viscus obstruction is most often due to the obstruction of an organ lumen by tumor growth. In the gastrointestinal or genitourinary tracts, obstruction will result in either a severe, colicky, crampy pain or true visceral pain, which is dull, diffuse, boring, and poorly localized. If a vein, artery or lymphatic channel is obstructed, venous engorgement, arterial ischemia, or edema will result, respectively. In these cases, pain is described as dull, diffuse, burning, and aching [33].

Yet another physiological factor producing chronic cancer pain is the infiltration or compression of peripheral nerves. This phenomenon results in continuous, sharp, stabbing pain generally following the pattern of nerve distribution. Hyperesthesia or paresthesia may also result [33].

Infiltration or distension of integument and/or tissue is a physiological phenomenon resulting in chronic severe cancer pain. This produces severe, dull, aching, and localized pain, with pain severity increasing concurrently with increase of tumor size. This type of pain is secondary to the skin or tissue being painfully stretched because of underlying tumor growth. Distention of tissue or integument may also produce painful ascites [33].

Finally, chronic cancer pain may be precipitated by the inflammation, infection, and necrosis of tissue. Inflammation with its accompanying symptoms of redness, edema, pain, heat, and loss of function may progress to infection, necrosis, and sloughing of tissue. If the inflammatory process alone is present, the pain is characterized by a sensitive tenderness. If, however, necrosis and tissue sloughing have occurred, pain may be excruciating, especially during dressing changes and other manipulative procedures [33].

Personal Mechanisms Contributing to the Pain Experience

Cancer may also produce very real pain or enhancement of physiological pain through personal etiological factors. The influence of personal factors depends upon the client's reaction to the pain. In other words, how people react to pain is highly dependent upon how they perceive it as threatening their lives [17]. It must also be remembered that client responses to pain will vary from time to time, depending on the presence of other stressors and the current situation. It is the *interpretation* of the *threat* of pain that produces the affective aspect of pain, which is synonymous with the phenomena of distress, suffering, and mental anguish. Three categories of personal, or psychological, stressors have been identified: (1) injury or threat of injury, (2) loss or threat of loss, and (3) frustration of drives [10].

FOUNDATION OF GENERAL NURSING INTERVENTIONS

General nursing interventions directed toward all persons experiencing the pain of cancer and cancer treatment are an appropriate foundation for the control of pain. This foundation will relieve much of the pain burden experienced by the person with cancer and allow for further individualized, creative treatment plans to be developed for each person's unique pain experience.

Minimize Pain Related to Antineoplastic Treatment

Prepare clients for any pain expected during diagnostic or treatment procedures. By honestly preparing the client for expected pain and by setting realistic parameters for the duration of expected pain, the nurse will remove the element of surprise and allow the client to mobilize coping resources. Describing the expected pain will reduce distress, not increase it.

Administer analgesics before performing painful treatments or diagnostic procedures. Dressing changes, wound debridement, moving the client to a cart, long periods of time spent lying on a table for cobalt treatments or radiological examinations, and bone marrow aspirations are all frequent and significant sources of pain. In order for this intervention to be successful, the nurse must know when the peak action of the drug occurs so that it will coincide with the painful treatment.

General Comfort Measures

The goal of providing general comfort measures is twofold: (1) to prevent painful complications secondary to the disease process and its treatment, such as immobility, infection, bleeding, and cachexia, and (2) to prevent further trauma, such as pathological fractures and trauma resulting from treatment procedures. General comfort measures include maintenance of good body alignment, supporting painful body parts with pillows, and maintenance of the patency of tubes (e.g., indwelling urinary catheter, nasogastric tubes, chest tubes, surgical drains, etc.). Keeping things within the client's easy reach if movement exacerbates pain is helpful, as is massage and backrubs to increase circulation and relaxation. Other effective general comfort measures include gentle active, passive, or assisted range of motion exercises; reduction of fatigue by administering an analgesic and/or a sleeping pill before bed; and relaxation exercises with or without guided imagery. Since pain results in decreased energy and increased fatigue—both of which, in turn, further worsen perceived pain—relaxation exercises with or without guided imagery may interrupt this vicious cycle by increasing the client's energy and sense of control over the pain experience, as well by decreasing muscle tension and fatigue. Thus, pain perception is reduced.

MANAGEMENT OF SEVERE, CHRONIC PAIN

For constant severe pain, nursing and medical goals must be focused on *prevention* rather than on *relief* of pain. "Pain relief" implies that the client must experience the pain before pain relief mechanisms (e.g., administration of an analgesic) are initiated. Prevention of constant pain, however, demands that analgesics, especially the narcotics, be administered routinely in order to maintain constant analgesic blood levels [38, 47]. The idiom "PRN" brings into play the attitudes held by the involved health professionals that someone other than the client is to determine whether or not pain relief is necessary [12]. The traditional "PRN" pain management routine demands a great deal of attention and time from clients, nurses, and physicians without producing a steady state of comfort for the clients. Thus, for clients with chronic and constant pain, the nurse must manipulate the "PRN" in order to keep the client comfortable and pain-free without loss of consciousness. With a "PRN" prescription from the physician, the nurse may give the medication if, in his or her independent judgment, the client will optimally benefit from the analgesic at that time. If, for example, the medication is prescribed to be given every four hours "PRN" and the person has continuous pain, nurses must *not* wait for the client to ask for the analgesic but should instead give it routinely every four hours along with an ongoing pain assessment and evaluation of analgesic effectiveness. Prompt pain relief plus the reliability and security of the non-PRN dosing schedule results in decreased fear, decreased anxiety, and, thus, decreased pain.

Worldwide experts in the control of chronic, unremitting pain advocate the *prevention* of pain by the administration of oral narcotics at regularly scheduled intervals to maintain constant analgesic blood levels. If clients receive prompt relief from the start and know that they can rely on the next dose appearing on time, they do not increase their own pain by fear and tension [26, 30, 38, 46, 47]. In a two-year study, clients suffering from the chronic pain of malignant disease were treated with a regimen of regular analgesia. Over the two-year period, there was a marked change in the physicians' prescribing habits, with a shift toward using the oral narcotics—the drugs of choice—for the management of chronic pain and away from the use of parenteral administration of narcotics and the use of less effective nonnarcotics. Clients enjoyed an improved quality of life and were relatively free from pain most of the time. This increased level of comfort meant that the clients were able to turn their attention away from their pain and toward more positive personal matters. As an added benefit, the program proved to be cost effective even though the use of medications increased [9].

In the aforementioned study, nurses provided an unanticipated source of resistance to change. They were reluctant to give narcotics to clients who did not ask for them or who denied pain at that moment. However, as the nurses increased their skills in pain assessment, evaluation of analgesia, and dosage adjustments, these concerns appeared to diminish [9].

Despite the many carefully controlled studies indicating that adequate control of chronic severe pain is most often achieved by regular administration of adequate doses of narcotics, a recent study of the medical and nursing management of chronic, severe cancer pain revealed that only 5 percent of drug orders were routine rather than "PRN." In addition, the two drugs most frequently ordered were acetaminophen with codeine or propoxyphene (Darvon). The stronger, more effective narcotics—the drugs of choice for this very common situation—were ordered only infrequently [34].

Negative attitudes toward the use of narcotics need to be replaced with sound knowledge of the actions and effects of these drugs. Although dangerous side effects of the narcotic analgesics do sometimes occur, their frequency and significance are many times overestimated and consequently the narcotics are inappropriately withheld. Staff expectations regarding the usual pain trajectories of clients with chronic cancer pain need to change so that the comfortable, pain-free, yet alert client becomes the norm. When caregivers find themselves saying to clients, "You'll have to expect a little pain," they might ask themselves a question: *"Why?* Why must that client expect some pain?" Careful assessment, a wise and judicious plan encompassing both pharmaceutical and nonpharmaceutical interventions, perceptive evaluation of the plan, and, above all, the expectation that the client's pain *can* be controlled and relieved will aid in establishing the comfortable client as the norm.

CONCEPT VIII:
Pharmaceutical interventions have been successful in reducing the pain experience for cancer clients.

For the management of *chronic pain* often associated with cancer, drugs with longer durations of action are preferred primarily because of convenience for the client. Oral or rectal drugs are preferred for clients remaining at home, again because of convenience and because of the lack of necessary in-depth client/family teaching regarding administration of parenteral drugs. Intramuscular and subcutaneous administration of routine drugs is to be avoided because of the inevitable tissue damage and subsequent decreased absorption of the drug.

Analgesics for control of cancer pain are divided into two basic categories: narcotics and nonnarcotics. Narcotics have greater efficacy and are the drugs of choice for the relief of pain of a more severe nature [18, 20, 30, 41]. In fact, the efficacy of narcotic analgesics is such that, in sufficient dosage, they are able to relieve virtually every level of pain. On the other hand, nonnarcotics, although capable of significant pain relief, are limited to the relief of mild to moderate pain (for example, headache, muscle and joint pain) regardless of the dose administered. Neither tolerance nor physical dependence is associated with nonnarcotic analgesics. Narcotics seem to produce analgesia through the central nervous system; nonnarcotics relieve pain by interfering with peripheral nervous system mechanisms, probably by interference with biosynthesis of prostaglandins.

NARCOTIC ANALGESICS

The narcotic analgesics, also referred to as opiates or opioids, are structurally homogenous agents that are associated with two distinguishing characteristics: (1) the development of tolerance to analgesia and certain other effects of the drug and (2) the development of physical dependence, not to be confused with "addiction." Development of tolerance results in the need for escalating dosages to relieve pain, whereas development of physical dependence is reflected by a withdrawal syndrome if the narcotic is abruptly discontinued or if a narcotic antagonist (e.g., naloxone, or Narcan) is administered. This latter situation is called induced or precipitated withdrawal.

Morphine Sulfate

All information regarding morphine sulfate applies in general to all narcotics. The incidence of adverse side effects and intensity of action of the narcotics as a group vary but little when compared at equianalgesic doses.

Composition.   Morphine sulfate is a natural alkaloid of the opium plant and was first isolated in 1803. Since then, many semisynthetic derivatives of the morphine molecule (e.g, heroin, hydromorphone, oxymorphone, hydrocodone, and oxycodone) and entirely synthetic derivatives (meperidine, fentanyl, methadone, and propoxyphene) have been manufactured. These structurally diverse compounds all share with morphine the ability to induce analgesic effects by central nervous sytem alteration, along with the side effects of respiratory depression, gastrointestinal spasm, and physical dependence. None are significantly different from or superior to morphine, and morphine is the "yardstick" by which other narcotics are evaluated.

Action.   Morphine's mechanism of action is as yet poorly understood, although the site of action is probably within the central nervous system. Central nervous system action is reflected by the exhibition of central nervous system effects. It is speculated that morphine changes the person's *response* to pain rather than actually eliminating the painful stimuli themselves.

Effects.   Therapeutic effects of morphine sulfate include analgesia, depression of gastrointestinal activity, certain therapeutic uses of respiratory depression, antitussive effects, and the inducement of euphoria and an increased sense of well-being. It must be remembered that morphine's side effects are dose-related, being increased with increased dosages, and that adverse or life-threatening effects are merely extensions of adaptive responses to the drug.

In the production of analgesia, morphine apparently increases the central nervous system's threshold for pain rather than actually eliminating the pain source in the body. In other words, the pain source itself does not disappear, but the brain does not interpret the "pain messages" as pain. Although this mechanism of action is generally accepted, actual research data have been inconsistent in "proving" this to be true. Analgesia induced by morphine seems to be selective in that other sensory modalities (for example, vision and hearing) are unaffected at therapeutic doses. Morphine is generally considered to be more effective against continuous dull pain rather than sharp, intermittent pain. The standard dosage of 10 mg. per 70 kilograms of body weight given parenterally will relieve moderate to severe pain of any type in the majority of clients [13].

Morphine is not nearly as effective by the oral route as the parenteral route of administration. Approximately six times the parenteral dosage is considered to be equianalgesic for oral administration. In other words, 60 mg. of oral morphine is equianalgesic to 10 mg. of parenteral morphine. Pain sensitivity also decreases with the client's advancing age, so an elderly person would obtain pain relief with a smaller dosage of morphine than would be necessary for a younger person.

Other central nervous system effects of morphine are a combination of overt stimulation and depression of various central nervous system areas. Either dysphoria or euphoria may occur, as may drowsiness, respiratory depression, suppression of the cough reflex, miosis, inhibition of ACTH and gonadotrophin release, increased antidiuretic hormone release, and initial stimulation of the medullary chemoreceptor trigger zone that controls vomiting followed by depression of the vomiting center [13]. Loss of consciousness secondary to profound sedation does not occur with therapeutic doses of morphine. It must always be remembered that chronic pain is an extremely fatiguing experience and that adequate pain relief will allow the person to sleep. The client may be easily aroused from this sleep, which is both necessary and very much needed, thus demonstrating that the client is sleeping rather than sedated. Euphoria after the administration of morphine is more likely to be seen in the client experiencing acute pain. It is important to note, however, that these statements regarding the effects of morphine are generalizations and not applicable to all clients because every person has unique physiological and psychological manifestations of their pain experience and because some people have idiosyncratic responses to morphine despite the degree and severity of their pain.

The effects of morphine sulfate on the smooth muscle of the gastrointestinal system is one of the more important of the drug's effects. For many years, opium, which contains 10 percent morphine sulfate, has been used therapeutically for the treatment of diarrhea and dysentery. Indeed, this use of morphine antedates by centuries its use as an analgesic. The overall action of morphine on the smooth musculature of the gastrointestinal tract is one of decreased peristalsis and thus produces a constipating effect. Discussion of the maladaptive effects of morphine on the gastrointestinal tract may be found later in this chapter and in Chapter 12.

Respiratory depression is an often overestimated effect of morphine sulfate and may even be used as a therapeutic side effect. As with the other side effects of morphine, the degree of respiratory depression is dose-related and is secondary to two physiological phenomena: (1) initial reduction of the responsiveness of the brainstem respiratory center to circulating blood levels of carbon dioxide and (2) direct depression of pontine and medullary centers regulating respiratory rhythm [13]. Therapeutically, this side effect of morphine sulfate may be utilized for those clients who are extremely short of breath because of anxiety and/or pain. It is very frightening to have to fight for breath, and this vicious cycle of anxiety-pain-shortness of breath may be interrupted by the slight respiratory depression induced by therapeutic dosages of morphine and actually improve gas exchange. Discussion of the maladaptive effects of morphine-induced respiratory dysfunction may be found later in this chapter and in Chapter 12.

The cardiovascular system is not appreciably affected by morphine sulfate, with blood pressure, pulse, and cardiac workload virtually unchanged. Blood pressure remains normal even after toxic doses of morphine, until hypoxia secondary to respiratory depression induces a fall. Additionally, there is no direct effect on cerebral vasculature and circulation [13]. Maladaptive cardiovascular responses to morphine are discussed later in the chapter.

Morphine sulfate is an effective antitussive and cough suppressant, although codeine is generally considered to be better in this regard. For antitussive action, a subanalgesic dose is effective [13].

Adverse side effects of morphine sulfate on the gastrointestinal system may be unpleasant and even life-threatening. Nausea and vomiting are a direct effect of morphine's stimulation of the central nervous system's medullary chemoreceptor trigger zone. After repeated doses of morphine, however, the vomiting center is eventually depressed, and the nausea and vomiting disappear. Nausea and vomiting occur more frequently in ambulatory clients than in those who are recumbent, demonstrating a probable vestibular component to this side effect. Nausea and vomiting may be prevented or treated by concurrent administration of antiemetics or agents used to treat motion sickness. The constipating effects of morphine sulfate are a direct result of the slowing of peristalsis in the intestines. Morphine sulfate may also cause severe painful spasms of the smooth muscle of the biliary tract, occurring even at therapeutic doses and resulting in sharp rises in intraductal pressure. Clients receiving morphine sulfate, especially those who are receiving the drug on a routine basis, *must* also receive concurrent doses of stool softeners in order to assure that the side effect of constipation will be countered. Further discussion of these adverse gastrointestinal side effects may be found in Chapter 11.

Cerebral vasodilation may result from even mild respiratory depression and the subsequent retention of carbon dioxide in the circulating blood. Carbon dioxide is a powerful vasodilator; and because of this cerebral vasodilation, increased intracranial pressure results. Thus, morphine and the other narcotics are contraindicated in cranial trauma and/or head injury, conditions in which the client is vulnerable to the life-threatening sequelae of increased intracranial pressure.

Morphine and most other opiates also release histamine, producing vasodilation in the cutaneous vasculature, often resulting in an overall feeling of warmth or itching of the face and/or nose. Additionally, the histamine and resultant vasodilation may result in orthostatic hypotension in recumbent clients.

Codeine [13]

Like morphine, codeine is a naturally occurring alkaloid of opium. Unlike morphine, it is very effective when taken orally and is relatively nonaddicting [32]. However, the widespread concept that codeine is a mild analgesic incapable of providing analgesia equivalent to morphine is a generally accepted but erroneous idea. Codeine is prescribed for oral administration and often prescribed for ambulatory outpatients, generally being classified along with aspirin as a mild analgesic with few side effects. Morphine is twelve to thirteen times as potent as codeine when given intramuscularly, which simply means that approximately 120 mg. of parenteral codeine are necessary to produce an analgesic equivalent to 10 mg. of morphine. However, oral doses of codeine larger than 65 mg. are rarely used.

As an antitussive, 15 to 20 mg. of oral codeine is generally accepted to be an effective dose. For inducing analgesia, 30 to 65 mg. of oral codeine is a therapeutic dose. With the use of therapeutic doses, side effects are few and usually transient. Nausea, constipation, dizziness, and/or slight sedation or drowsiness are common transient adverse effects of codeine.

Codeine is unique among the narcotics in that *it can be routinely taken for long periods of time with little risk of significant physical dependence.* The use of 65 mg. of codeine every four hours daily for several months is not associated with a significant risk of narcotic physical dependence. Tolerance to codeine, however, will gradually develop over time, sometimes necessitating an increase in the dosage [13].

Meperidine (Demerol)

Meperidine is a wholly synthetic agent structurally dissimilar to morphine but not significantly different from morphine in its pharmacological actions. In therapeutic parenteral dosages, which are 80 to 100 mg., meperidine produces analgesia, sedation, and mild respiratory depression as well as the other central nervous system effects of narcotics.

Morphine is approximately eight to ten times as potent as meperidine; but when given in equianalgesic doses, meperidine produces the same analgesia, sedation, and respiratory depression. Differences between meperidine and morphine include the following: (1) meperidine's duration of action is shorter, averaging only about three hours, thus necessitating shorter intervals between administration and more frequent administration for adequate pain relief, (2) meperidine usually produces less severe gastrointestinal side effects than does morphine and is not useful in the treatment of diarrhea, and (3) toxic doses of meperidine may cause different effects than does morphine. Toxic doses of meperidine are characterized by central nervous system excitation, widely dilated pupils, tremors, and convulsions. These are in contrast to the profound narcosis and coma associated with morphine and the other opiates [13].

Oral administration of meperidine is extremely ineffective. In order to achieve analgesia with oral meperidine equal to that obtained with 75 mg. of parenteral meperidine or with 10 mg. of parenteral morphine, *300 mg.* of oral meperidine are necessary. This is inconvenient and costly, making oral meperidine of little clinical use in pain control. These data about oral meperidine are unfortunately not widely known, and a significant number of physicians prescribe oral meperidine to ambulatory cancer clients suffering from significant pain. The usual prescribed dosage of 50 mg. of oral meperidine is equianalgesic to 10 grains (or two tablets) of aspirin and therefore is completely inadequate for control of significant cancer pain [12].

Methadone (Dolophine) [13]

Methadone is a synthetic narcotic analgesic qualitatively similar to morphine sulfate, producing analgesia, sedation, respiratory depression, miosis, and antitussive activity as well as subjective effects similar to those seen with morphine.

Methadone is equianalgesic by the oral and parenteral routes, making it significantly more effective than morphine by the oral route. Methadone also has the advantage of causing minimal euphoria and thus is minimally addicting.

Methadone's duration of action is similar to morphine after a single administration. However, repeated dosages of methadone results in a cumulative effect within the body, thus effectively increasing methadone's duration of action. This cumulative effect is, however, a double-edged sword since sudden and acute respiratory depression can occur as a result of the accumulation of methadone in the client's body. Thus, if sudden respiratory depression occurs in a client who has been receiving routine doses of methadone, the accumulated methadone should be suspected as the causative stressor. Administration of a test dose of naloxone (Narcan) will confirm or refute the suspicion, with the client suffering from methadone intoxication exhibiting a rapid improvement in respiratory status.

Hydromorphone (Dilaudid)

Hydromorphone hydrochloride is a hydrogenated ketone of morphine and has seven times the analgesic effect of morphine when given by intravenous injection. Hydromorphone also provides significant pain relief after oral administration. The half-life of elimination of hydromorphone is approximately 2.6 hours, and there is rapid but incomplete absorption after oral administration [49].

Propoxyphene (Darvon)

Propoxyphene is a synthetic agent structurally similar to methadone, and cross-dependence and cross-tolerance has been demonstrated between propoxyphene and the other narcotics. The analgesic efficacy of propoxyphene has been debated for many years. Propoxyphene undeniably causes central nervous system effects similar to codeine, but whether significant analgesia is one of those central nervous system actions is not completely agreed upon [13]. Many authorities state that when the standard dosage of 65 mg. of propoxyphene is given, the analgesic effect is equivalent or perhaps even inferior to ten grains (two tablets) of aspirin

[12, 13, 28, 29, 32]. In addition, propoxyphene is much more expensive than aspirin.

Despite this data, propoxyphene is widely prescribed for ambulatory clients, probably primarily because of unjustified overconcern about codeine's dependency potential and the initial claim that propoxyphene was "nonaddicting." Yet, the fact is that there is no difference between codeine and propoxyphene regarding dependency potentials. Common side effects of propoxyphene include nausea, dizziness, and constipation [13].

Pentazocine (Talwin)

Pentazocine is not a narcotic analgesic per se, but it demonstrates enough similar effects that it is included in this discussion. Pentazocine is a partial opioid agonist with weak narcotic antagonistic properties. Although pentazocine can cause a withdrawal syndrome if given in large doses to narcotic-dependent clients, it does not reverse the respiratory depression seen with opiate toxicity. In addition, although there is no cross-dependence with narcotics, pentazocine can cause its own physical dependency.

Fifty milligrams of pentazocine is approximately equianalgesic with 60 mg. of codeine; and if administered parenterally, it is about one-fourth as potent as morphine. Side effects of pentazocine include central nervous system and gastrointestinal effects similar to morphine. Dizziness, nausea, sedation, and hallucinations can occur even at therapeutic doses, and other side effects include hypertension and tachycardia [13]. Pentazocine is primarily used as an analgesic for mild to moderate pain and is frequently prescribed for ambulatory clients.

ACUTE NARCOTIC INTOXICATION

When considering the topic of acute narcotic intoxication, the caregiver must remember that clients with severe chronic pain exhibit higher titers of free endorphins than do clients who are experiencing acute pain or who are pain-free. This phenomenon may explain the different reaction to narcotic administration exhibited by clients experiencing chronic cancer pain as opposed to drug abusers. The former exhibit less euphoria and a tendency to sleep because of pain-induced fatigue, as opposed to the marked euphoria and sedation observed in drug abusers [20].

Death from acute narcotic intoxication in humans results from acute, profound, life-threatening respiratory depression. Signs and symptoms of acute narcotic intoxication include:

1. Deep sleep and stupor proceeding to coma
2. Bradypnea
3. Constricted pinpoint pupils (except with meperidine, which produces widely dilated pupils)
4. Eventual hypotension secondary to respiratory depression
5. Eventual pupillary dilation and shock, both secondary to hypoxia

Unless intervened into promptly, acute narcotic intoxication will culminate in the client's death.

There is some variance among signs and symtoms indicative of life-threatening narcotic toxicity that are associated with specific drugs. Levorphanol (Levo-Dromoran) and methadone (Dolophine) may produce insidious central nervous system and respiratory depression after several days or weeks of routine administration. This phenomenon is secondary to the accumulation of the drug within the body [20] and is more likely to occur in elderly clients [44]. With these two particular drugs, it is better to make necessary dosage adjustments by increasing the dosage amount than by decreasing the dosage intervals. Such intervention will be less apt to result in insidious accumulation of the drug [20]. Toxic doses of propoxyphene (Darvon) often result in confusion, hallucinations, and seizures, as well as central nervous system and respiratory depression [13].

There is a wide range of therapeutic dosage within the narcotic drug group, and so it may be difficult to predict toxicity. Factors of tolerance, physical dependence, and severity of the pain experience must be considered when assessing toxicity potential. Serious life-threatening toxicity from morphine sulfate generally does not occur unless an oral bolus dosage exceeds 120 to 150 mg. or a parenteral bolus dosage exceeds 30 to 40 mg. *and* unless the dosage is given to an opiate-naive person. Individuals with pain and/or with narcotic tolerance can withstand even greater dosages of morphine. Individual variation, however, does exist so it is necessary to continuously monitor clients who are receiving large doses of any narcotic [13].

The primary aim of treatment for acute narcotic intoxication is to restore and maintain adequate ventilation. Naloxone (Narcan), a narcotic antagonist, is the specific drug of choice since it reverses respiratory depression almost instantaneously. However, the duration of action of naloxone is much shorter than morphine and the other opiates. Therefore, the acutely intoxicated client needs continual monitoring and readministration of additional doses of naloxone. In addition, initiation of naloxone administration to the acutely intoxicated, opiate-dependent client must be carried out very carefully. In this situation, inappropriate administration of naloxone can precipitate a withdrawal syndrome so severe that it cannot be adequately treated during naloxone's duration of action [13].

If naloxone is not available, the treatment principle of restoring and maintaining adequate ventilation remains the same, although the treatment methods change. Establishment of a patent airway receives first priorty, and restoration of efficient pulmonary gas exchange follows.

PAIN CONTROL WITH NARCOTICS FOR FATALLY ILL CLIENTS

In terminal illness associated with severe and unremitting pain, the primary aim is to provide pain-free comfort. At no time should an effective dose of a narcotic be withheld from a fatally ill person in pain [16]. The *only* consideration should be that of continued analgesic efficacy should the course of the illness be prolonged. The generally acceptable approach is to provide pain control with a combination of oral nonnarcotic and narcotic agents before utilizing the more potent parenteral opiates. If the disease process is so prolonged as to render the client virtually completely tolerant to narcotic analgesics, or should the pain become so severe that pain control is not possible even with high-dose potent narcotics, then other nonpharmaceutical interventions such as neurosurgery must be instituted. For a more detailed discussion of pain control for the fatally ill, see Chapter 11.

PRINCIPLES OF NURSING INTERVENTIONS REGARDING NARCOTIC ANALGESIA

Optimal doses must be determined by titration. Very large doses of narcotics may eventually be necessary to obtain satisfactory pain control in persons experiencing severe, chronic cancer pain. The nurse must remember that, not only do these clients *tolerate* these high dosages, they also *need* these prescribed amounts of narcotics. These high doses may seem inappropriately large if thought of in terms of the dosages of narcotics usually administered for acute pain, but the person with chronic, severe cancer pain will almost always maintain normal vital signs after administration of the narcotic. These clients will also usually sleep for extended periods of time after receiving adequate doses of narcotics, but this extended sleeping is not indicative of sedation or overdose. Severe pain is exhausting and prevents sleep, and the extended sleep is both appropriate and needed.

It is better to start with a narcotic dose that is a little too high than one that is too low. If a low dose of the narcotic is used initially with the intent to titrate upwards, the client will likely experience increased anxiety because of lack of adequate analgesia, and the anxiety will perpetuate and worsen the pain experience. This necessitates a higher dose of narcotic than would have been the case if a slightly higher dose had been used initially [20].

The most important nursing consideration for helping the person experiencing chronic, severe cancer pain is scheduling of drug administration. By administering the drug on a regularly scheduled basis rather than "PRN," blood levels of the analgesic are maintained so that recurrence of pain does not occur. By preventing recurrence of pain, the client's anxiety regarding return of the pain is lessened and so a lower dose of a regularly scheduled narcotic becomes sufficient. When determining the frequency of drug administration, it is clearly important to know the duration of action of the drug in use and to schedule administration of each dose before the previous dose loses its effect. "PRN" scheduling allows someone other than the client to decide if and when pain relief is necessary and needed. If necessary, the nurse must manipulate the "PRN" prescription in order to keep the client comfortable. "PRN" implies that the nurse may administer the medication if, in his or her independent professional judgment, it would be best for the client to receive the drug at that time. If the narcotic is prescribed to be given every four hours PRN, for example, and the client has continuous pain, the nurse must not wait for the client to request the medication but should administer the narcotic routinely every four hours *while continuing appropriate nursing assessment and evaluation of the client's pain.*

ADJUNCTIVE PHARMACEUTICAL TREATMENT [24]

Two often-prescribed drugs for the "potentiation" of narcotics are hydroxyzine (Vistaril) and promethazine (Phenergan). Yet, data strongly substantiates that neither of the two drugs potentiates the effects of narcotics.

Hydroxyzine (Vistaril) given intramuscularly seems to have a potent analgesic action in itself, with 100 mg. of intramuscular hydroxyzine being equianalgesic to 8 mg. of intramuscular morphine. So, when hydroxyzine is administered together with morphine or another opiate, the increased analgesic effect is merely additive in nature.

Promethazine (Phenergan), on the other hand, has been found to actually *increase* pain intensity and perception. When promethazine is administered concurrently with a narcotic, pain relief is probably reduced. However, promethazine's highly sedating effect results in the situation of the client merely being too sedated to report pain, and health professionals tend to mistake this sedation for pain relief.

The principal adjunctive drugs used in conjunction with narcotics are the phenothiazines, utilized to combat nausea and vomiting. The most commonly prescribed phenothiazines used for this purpose are chlorpromazine (Thorazine) and prochlorperazine (Compazine).

Also, if the client is receiving narcotics on a routine basis, a daily routine dose of a laxative and/or stool softener is mandatory. This intervention will help to prevent the sometimes-fatal complications of constipation, fecal impaction, and intestinal obstruction commonly associated with routine narcotic usage.

Another class of commonly prescribed adjunctive drugs is the psychotropic pharmaceutical agents. Minor tranquilizers are of little value and usually just increase the depression. For reduction of anxiety, recommended drugs include trifluoperazine (Stelazine), thioridazine (Mellaril), or chlorpromazine (Thorazine). For reduction of depression, use of the tricyclic antidepressants is recommended. However, at least fifteen days will elapse before the tricyclic antidepressants will be effective in elevating the client's mood [32].

NONNARCOTIC ANALGESICS

The nonnarcotic analgesics are a large, structurally different group of pharmaceutical agents. In addition to their analgesic properties, many also have antipyretic and/or anti-inflammatory effects as well. Although many of the nonnarcotic analgesics are available without a physician's prescription, their toxicity is frequently underestimated. Tolerance and physical dependence are not associated with the nonnarcotic analgesics.

Acetylsalicylic Acid (Aspirin)

Aspirin is the most effective, most important, and most widely used of all analgesic drugs. It has antipyretic and anti-inflammatory properties in addition to its analgesic effects, is inexpensive, and has a relatively low incidence of adverse side effects when taken in recommended therapeutic dosages. Aspirin has a lower maximal analgesic effect than do the narcotics, with 650 mg. of aspirin being approximately equal to 65 mg. of codeine or propoxyphene (Darvon) in terms of analgesia. Doses of aspirin greater than 650 mg. do not appreciably increase the analgesic effect, although larger doses may prolong its duration of action [13].

Aspirin relieves pain by both peripheral and central mechanisms, both of which are poorly understood. Its peripheral mechanism of action is thought to be by inhibition of prostaglandin biosynthesis. The central mechanism of analgesic action possibly occurs in the anterior hypothalamus, the same site at which aspirin's antipyretic action is effected.

Aspirin lowers body temperature in febrile persons, but not in persons with a normal body temperature. Again, aspirin's inhibition of prostaglandin biosynthesis probably accounts for its antipyretic action. Prostaglandins are postulated to mediate the body's fever response to pyrogens, resulting in an increased synthesis and release of prostaglandins at thermoregulatory centers in the hypothalamus and possibly throughout the entire brain. Aspirin and acetaminophen (Tylenol) both probably reduce fever indirectly by interfering with prostaglandin synthesis and release, thus interrupting the pyrogen-mediated fever response [13].

Aspirin's interference with the biosynthesis and release of prostaglandins also accounts for its anti-inflammatory properties. It has been postulated that, since prostaglandins have been isolated in inflammatory exudates, aspirin's interference with the synthesis and release of prostaglandins results in anti-inflammatory action [13].

Aspirin is indicated for the relief of mild to moderate, low-intensity pain, such as headache, muscle pain, and bone or joint aches. The standard dosage is 325 to 650 mg. by mouth every four hours.

The most common adverse side effect of aspirin is local irritation to the mucosal cells of the gastrointestinal tract, resulting in epigastric distress, nausea, vomiting, and even exacerbation of peptic ulcer. Chronic use of aspirin is ulcerogenic and may cause painless gastrointestinal bleeding. Gastrointestinal irritation can be minimized by taking aspirin with food or milk.

Aspirin also decreases the ability of platelets to aggregate and thus must be used with extreme caution, if at all, in persons predisposed to bleeding. Persons who are thrombocytopenic or who are taking anticoagulant drugs should *not* concurrently take aspirin because of the danger of hemorrhage.

The danger of aspirin toxicity is widely underestimated and acute overdosage may be fatal, especially in children. Acute aspirin toxicity consists of a series of physiological events culminating in deranged acid-base balance, dehydration, hyperthermia, coma, and death [52]. Aspirin toxicity is a continuum ranging from salicylism (mild intoxication) to death. Salicylism, or mild aspirin intoxication, is initially heralded by tinnitus (ringing or buzzing in the ears). Tinnitus is almost always the first sign of salicylism and is generally associated with dosages of at least six grams per day. If the aspirin dosage is not reduced when tinnitus occurs, other signs characteristic of worsening salicylism appear: headache, dizziness, mental confusion, drowsiness, diaphoresis, thirst, nausea, and vomiting. As aspirin toxicity worsens, the signs and symptoms of salicylism are complicated by acid-base imbalance, hyperventilation as a compensatory response to acidosis, delirium, hallucinations, and seizures. Finally, dehydration, coma, and death occur.

In the treatment of cancer pain, aspirin can be a very useful drug as long as the client is not thrombocytopenic. If high doses of aspirin are necessary, crush the tablet (unless it is enteric-coated) and administer the aspirin with large amounts of water or milk. This will lessen gastric irritation by decreasing the particle size of the drug, reducing the gastric acid concentration, and promoting drug dissolution and absorption [13]. When aspirin alone can no longer provide sufficient pain control, the addition of major tranquilizers and/or antidepressants will potentiate aspirin's analgesic effects by changing the client's affective response to pain. These adjunctive drugs have long half-lives, are effective by the oral route, and can be effective at less than the doses necessary for psychotherapeutic purposes [37].

Acetaminophen (Tylenol)

Acetaminophen is an analgesic and antipyretic drug that is approximately equianalgesic with aspirin [32]. It is indicated for relief of mild to moderate pain like that treated by aspirin. Acetaminophen is usually better tolerated by the client, lacking the side effect of gastrointestinal irritation and bleeding commonly associated with aspirin. Unlike aspirin, acetaminophen has only minimal anti-inflammatory action and thus is of limited use in inflammatory conditions. The recommended dose of 325 to 650 mg. by mouth every four hours is well-tolerated by most people. Additionally, acetaminophen does not inhibit platelet aggregation and so is safe to give to thrombocytopenic clients or to persons receiving anticoagulant therapy.

In toxic doses, acetaminophen does not produce the acid-base imbalance commonly associated with aspirin. Instead, acute intoxication with acetaminophen usually produces a potentially fatal hepatic necrosis [13].

Phenylbutazone (Butazolidin)

Phenylbutazone is an analgesic, antipyretic, anti-inflammatory drug in which the anti-inflammatory action predominates and is a result of the inhibition of prostaglandin synthesis. Unfortunately, phenylbutazone is associated with a high incidence of potentially serious side effects, including nausea, vomiting, epigastric pain, nervousness, vertigo, blurred vision, and insomnia. Occasionally, phenylbutazone produces fatal agranulocytosis and aplastic anemia. It is thus necessary to instruct the client to take the drug with food or milk to minimize gastrointestinal side effects and to maintain close client supervision, including periodic hematological evaluation. Because of the high incidence of serious side effects, phenylbutazone is used primarily as a short-term treatment for inflammatory conditions rather than as a primary analgesic [13].

Indomethacin (Indocin)

Like phenylbutazone, indomethacin is an analgesic, antipyretic, and anti-inflammatory drug and is used almost exclusively for its anti-inflammatory properties. Indomethacin also has a significantly high incidence of serious adverse effects similar to phenylbutazone, with approximately 20 percent of clients finding it necessary to discontinue the drug because of the appearance of severe gastrointestinal and/or central nervous system side effects [13].

Ibuprofen (Motrin)

Ibuprofen is a nonnarcotic analgesic that is also used primarily for its anti-inflammatory effects. This drug has no apparent antipyretic action and is fairly well tolerated, causing less gastrointestinal distress or bleeding than phenylbutazone or indomethacin. Nevertheless, the client should be advised to take the drug with food or milk [13].

Fenoprofen (Nalfon)

Fenoprofen is a nonnarcotic analgesic, antipyretic, and anti-inflammatory drug structurally similar to ibuprofen. It is well tolerated, with fewer gastrointestinal side effects than aspirin but still should be taken with food or milk [13].

Methotrimeprazine (Levoprome)

Methotrimeprazine is a phenothiazine derivative that is structurally related to chlorpromazine (Thorazine) and is reportedly an effective analgesic, although it has no anti-inflammatory or antipyretic actions. It has been reported that 20 mg. of methotrimeprazine is analgesically equivalent to 10 mg. of morphine [3].

Table 11.2. Relative Potencies of Analgesics Approximately Equivalent to 10 mg. Parenteral Morphine

Drug	I.M.	P.O.
Morphine	10.0	60.0
Hydromorphone (Dilaudid)	1.5	7.5
Methadone HC1 (Dolophine)	10.0	20.0
Levorphanol tartrate (LevoDromoran)	2.0	4.0
Meperidine HC1 (Demerol)	75.0	300.0
Codeine	130.0	200.0
Oxycodone HC1 (Percocet, Percodan)	—	30.0

Relative Potencies of Analgesics Approximately Equivalent to 650 mg. Oral Aspirin

Oral Drug	P.O.
Pentazocine HC1 (Talwin)	30.0
Codeine	32.0
Meperidine (Demerol)	50.0
Propoxyphene HC1 (Darvon)	65.0
Acetaminophen (Tylenol)	650.0
Aspirin	650.0

The most common adverse effect of methotrimeprazine is orthostatic hypoten-sion, thus limiting its usefulness in ambulatory clients. Like chlorpromazine, it re-sults in significant sedation and antiemesis; but unlike chlorpromazine, it causes no physical dependence. Additionally, since it does not cause respiratory depres-sion, it may be useful in pain management for some cases of cancer [13].

CONCEPT IX:
Nonpharmaceutical and nonsurgical analgesic interventions have been successful in reducing the pain experience for cancer clients.

HYPNOSIS

Introduction and History

Approximately one out of four people will respond well to hypnosis for pain relief [10], yet hypnosis is often dismissed by health professionals as a parlor game without any clinical value. Medical and nursing resistance to hypnosis may be secondary to reluctance by those professionals to become emotionally involved with their clients, especially those who are dying. This close emotional involvement is a prerequisite for effective hypnotherapy because an effective therapist must have conviction in the efficacy of hypnosis as a pain-control treatment, highly intuitive capacities, and the ability to establish a close empathic rapport with the client [15]. Another block to the use of hypnotherapy for pain control may be client attitude. Hypnosis may be difficult in those clients who equate hypnosis and relaxation with "giving up the battle" instead of viewing these therapies as merely another strategy to win their battle against pain and cancer.

Hypnosis can reduce suffering, which is a subjective, emotional, evaluative re-sponse to pain and to the fear of the unknown—which in itself is a debilitating emotion. Suffering is reduced simply because hypnosis deals with imagination, emotions, and value judgments; and suffering involves (1) nonacceptance, (2) fear of the unknown, (3) a pessimistic evaluation about the meaning of the pain, (4) the perception that the pain is endless, and (5) the often-observed emotions of self-destruction, guilt, and resentment [11]. The advantages of hypnosis include reduc-tion or eradication of pain, increased appetite and thus an improved nutritional status, a happier and more relaxed emotional environment, and a sense of in-creased control by the client. Hypnosis prolongs hope and may therefore even pro-long life [15].

In 1821 one of the first attempts to perform surgery while the client was under hypnosis was carried out in France, and in 1829 a mastectomy was performed using hypnosis as the anesthetic agent. Interestingly, no movement or complaints of pain by the client were observed during the 1829 surgery. In 1842, a mid-thigh amputation was successfully performed with hypnosis as the sole anesthetic agent. Since then, many thousands of major and minor surgical procedures have been successfully performed while the client was experiencing deep-trance hypnosis. One factor that may contribute to this success is the phenomenon that a hypnotized client is able to block pain perception emanating from a specific body area; and in responsive subjects, all pain can be removed for a controlled period of time [8].

Clinical Implications

It is possible to teach most clients how to be hypnotized in only a few sessions, and then the client can be taught to hypnotize himself or herself and use hypnotherapy for pain relief without the presence of the therapist. A light hypnotic trance resembles a state of simple deep relaxation, whereas a deep trance resembles a stupor. It is in the "in-between" hypnotic states that the therapist can use the most creative strategies to induce sustained pain relief: the client can displace the pain to another part of the body, the client can alter the painful sensation to a sensation that does not hurt, the client can use images such as turning switches on and off to control pain, the client can disassociate herself or himself from the painful body part, and he or she can create images to replace a reality fraught with physical pain [15].

Although it is thought that hypnosis may close the gate at the spinal level, the mechanism of action is still unknown, and yet the mere induction of hypnosis alone without suggestion for analgesia does not significantly increase pain tolerance [8]. It is important to note that pain relief obtained through hypnosis is demonstrably distinguishable from the placebo response. There seems to be two components involved in hypnotic analgesia: (1) a nonspecific placebo response and (2) a distortion of central nervous system perceptions of pain. This central nervous system distortion of pain perception appears to be specifically induced by hypnosis [25].

Pain, as defined as the neurophysical signal precipitating the perception of physical pain, is not as amenable to hypnotherapy as is the phenomenon of suffering. When suffering is removed by hypnosis, the "pure physical pain" does not hurt so much [11]. Yet, the hypnotized person seems to be able to block pain felt in specified body areas, and *all* pain can be removed with hypnosis for a controlled period of time [8].

In most cases of chronic pain, care must be taken to phrase suggestions in such a manner that not all pain perception is blocked. For example, the therapist may suggest that the pain will become much less and that the majority of tormenting, excruciating, painful sensations will leave, but that there will be a slight degree of discomfort left. In this way, the client will be left with enough pain perception that any change in the course of the disease will be detectable [8].

It must be remembered that hypnotherapy must be initiated *before* severe, continuous pain develops so that the client will have the capacity to devote full attention to learning the hypnosis procedures and techniques without the distraction of severe pain. Additionally, hypnotherapy usually requires periodic reinforcement by the therapist even after the client has gained the skills of self-hypnosis.

Clinical research with hypnotherapy is difficult to carry out, leaving health professionals with a paucity of scientific data from which they may draw more definitive conclusions. The primary reason for this is that researchers cannot test hypnotherapy against some placebo, since hypnotherapy itself may be the most powerful of placebos.

MASSAGE AND BACKRUBS

Massage and backrubs have long been used in nursing practice as a general comfort measure and to induce relaxation in the client. This analgesic therapy is based on the gate-control theory of pain, since large-diameter nerve fibers are stimulated, thus closing the gate and reducing pain perception. Massage and backrubs do indeed increase relaxation, mobility and pain relief. About 85 percent of clients achieve significant reduction in pain [40].

APPLICATION OF COLD

Application of ice packs have generally been of more benefit to clients in pain than has application of heat. Local application of ice may be achieved by the use of ice packs or ice popsicles, made by freezing water in a paper cup after placing a tongue-blade "handle" in the water [40].

RELAXATION WITH GUIDED IMAGERY

Relaxation with guided imagery is a psychophysiological approach that may be a form of hypnosis or self-hypnosis [40]. The therapist guides the client into deeper and deeper levels of physical and mental relaxation, with an emphasis on "letting go" of tensions, fears, anxiety, and muscle tension. It is then suggested to the client that he or she visualize, in a variety of ways, a strengthening of the immune system and the attack of strong immunological cells against weaker malignant cells. Within the concept of relaxation are included the aspects of resolving emotional distress and emphasizing better nutrition. It has already been noted that clients experiencing chronic cancer pain tend to eat poorly with an increase of junk food in their diets. By including nutritional and emotional aspects within relaxation therapy, client nutrition tends to improve and the resolution of emotional distress helps to facilitate emotional relaxation and quietness.

DISTRACTION

Distraction has long been known to be a powerful analgesic since it displaces the client's conscious awareness to nonpainful, pleasurable entities. Distraction may be instituted by physical, mental, or social activities [33].

CONCEPT X:
Neurosurgical procedures have been successful in reducing the pain experience for cancer clients.

Pain pathways can be interrupted at three major levels: the level of peripheral neurons, the level of spinal cord neurons, and the level of thalamic neurons

[45]. Neurosurgery as a measure to control intractable pain in the person with cancer is reserved for those situations in which the pain has been refractory to other analgesic measures.

NEUROSURGERY AT FIRST LEVEL (PERIPHERAL) NEURONS

Nerve Blocks

Nerve blocks may be performed with local anesthetics or neurolytic agents, such as alcohol, phenol, or saline solution. The pharmaceutical agent is injected into a peripheral or sympathetic nerve in order to reduce or eradicate the nerve's capacity for transmission of pain messages. The injected agent may also be introduced paravertebrally into spinal nerves or subdurally into posterior roots of spinal cord nerves. If local anesthetics are used, the resulting analgesia will only last for a few hours. If neurolytic agents are used, analgesia will persist for weeks or months. The side effects of a nerve block—headache, numbness, and paresthesia—are minor and transient, making repeated nerve blocks feasible for maintenance of pain control [37, 45].

Neurectomy

This procedure is a surgical interruption of a peripheral nerve. Unfortunately, the specific nerve fiber responsible for the transmission of the client's pain impulses is difficult to isolate and contains both motor and sensory fibers. Resection of the nerve may thus result in loss of motor function as well as analgesia. Since peripheral nerves regenerate, the neurectomy is a temporary measure. There are enough disadvantages to the neurectomy procedure that it is not considered to be an effective pain control measure [45].

Rhizotomy

A rhizotomy is a surgical interruption of a spinal nerve root at the anatomical location of its entrance into the spinal cord. This procedure eliminates all sensation from the bodily area that is innervated by the nerve root. A rhizotomy is performed by laminectomy and is used for treatment of intractable pain secondary to head and neck cancers [45].

Sympathectomy

This surgical procedure involves interruption of sympathetic ganglia at various points along the sympathetic chain of nerve fibers. Sympathectomy is sometimes used for treatment of peripheral vascular disease and phantom limb pain [45].

NEUROSURGERY AT SECOND LEVEL (SPINAL CORD) NEURONS

Neurosurgery at the second level, or spinal cord, neurons involves interruption of the lateral spinothalamic tract.

Percutaneous Cordotomy

This neurosurgical procedure involves interruption of the spinothalamic tract within the spinal cord. Analgesia usually persists for several months after a percutaneous cordotomy, making the procedure a temporary one. This procedure is used to treat various types of intractable pain. Advantages of the percutaneous cordotomy include the fact that the procedure can be carried out on a conscious, awake client and that it has a low mortality rate. The procedure results in a wide range of analgesia below the surgical site with preservation of the sensory and motor functions. Disadvantages of percutaneous cordotomy include the risks of bladder and/or bowel dysfunction and of sexual impotence, as well as the risk of respiratory failure after cervical cordotomy. Despite the recurrence of pain after a few months, the advantages of the procedure far outweigh the relatively low incidence of adverse effects, making it feasible to repeat percutaneous cordotomy for continued pain control [37, 45].

Tractotomy

Tractotomy is a neurosurgical procedure in which the spinothalamic tract is severed in the mesencephalon. The procedure is usually reserved for intractable pain in the head, neck, and arms. Performed by an occipital craniotomy, the tractotomy is technically intricate with a high mortality rate, making it impractical for widespread use [45].

NEUROSURGERY AT THE THIRD LEVEL (THALAMIC) NEURONS

Neurosurgical intervention at the level of the third order neurons is performed in regions of the thalamus and frontal lobe of the cortex. These procedures are rarely done and are reserved for clients with severe, intractable pain refractory to any other analgesic measures [37, 45].

> **CONCEPT XI:**
> **Nursing management of severe, chronic pain experienced by persons with cancer requires creative, innovative intervention based on a solid knowledge base of medical measures, nursing measures, pharmaceutical data, and the complex interactions between mind, body, and environment.**

Pain is a complex phenomenon and is even more complex in the cancer client because of the added factors of the unique anxiety accompanying cancer, the chronicity of the disease process along with its episodic acute problems, disrupted family and social dynamics, and the tendency to experience feelings of hopelessness, helplessness, and futility. Cancer clients fear intractable, chronic pain even more than they fear death, and the specter of such pain always waiting in the wings makes it even more likely that the individual will indeed experience pain and will perpetuate and intensify the client's pain experience.

Nursing management of cancer pain consists of much more than merely giving a pill or an injection. Instead, the nurse must utilize creativity as well as judicious use of drugs to eradicate cancer pain. The client's perception that the nurse cares for him or her and is concerned about the pain are potent analgesic measures that cannot be overestimated. Successful management of cancer pain is one of the most difficult challenges in oncologic nursing and one that requires a commitment to and employment of holistic care.

REFERENCES

1. Anderson, J. L. Nursing Management of the Cancer Patient in Pain: A Review of the Literature. *Cancer Nurs* 5:33, 1982.
2. Bagley, C. S., Falinski, E., Garnizo, N., and Hooker, L. Pain Management: A Pilot Project. *Cancer Nurs* 5:191, 1982.
3. Beaver, W. T., Wallenstein, S. L., Houde, R. W., and Rogers, A. A Comparison of the Analgesic Effects of Methotrimeprazine and Morphine in Patients with Cancer. *Clin Pharmacol Ther* 7:436, 1966.
4. Benoliel, J. Q. and Crowley, D. M. *The Patient in Pain: New Concepts.* New York: American Cancer Society, 1974.
5. Bibb, P. I. Therapy for Intractable Pain. *Cancer Nurs* 2:247, 1979.
6. Boguslawski, M. Therapeutic Touch: A Facilitator of Pain Relief. *Topics Clin Nurs* 2(1):27, 1980.
7. Bonica, J. J. Cancer Pain: A Major National Health Problem. *Cancer Nurs* 1:313, 1978.
8. Crasilneck, H. B. and Hall, J. A. Clinical Hypnosis in Problems of Pain. In A. K. Jacox (Ed.). *Pain: A Source Book for Nurses and Other Health Professionals.* Boston: Little, Brown and Co., 1977. Chapter 10.
9. Degner, L. F., Fujii, S. H., and Levitt, M. Implementing a Program to Control Chronic Pain of Malignant Disease for Patients in an Extended Care Facility. *Cancer Nurs* 5:263, 1982.
10. Engel, G. *Psychological Development in Health and Disease.* Philadelphia: W. B. Saunders, 1962. P. 289.
11. Ewin, D. M. Relieve Suffering—and Pain—with Hypnosis. *Geriatrics* 33:(6):87, 1978.
12. Frank, R. M. Pain Management and the Appropriate Use of Analgesics. *Cancer Nurs* 3:155, 1980.
13. Gebhart, G. F. Narcotic and Nonnarcotic Analgesics for Relief of Pain. In A. K. Jacox (Ed.). *Pain: A Source Book for Nurses and Other Health Professionals.* Boston: Little, Brown and Co., 1977. Chapter 9.
14. Hackett, T. P. Pain and Prejudice. *Med Times* 99(2):130, 1971.
15. Holden, C. Pain Control with Hypnosis. *Science* 198:808, 1977.
16. Lamerton, R. *Care of the Dying.* New York: Penguin Books, 1980. Chapter 4.
17. Lazarus, R. *Psychological Stress and the Coping Process.* New York: McGraw-Hill, 1966. P. 25.
18. Lee, R. M. (Ed.). International Symposium on Cancer Nursing. *AORNJ* 22:987, 1975.
19. Levine, J. D., Gordon, N. C., and Fields, H. L. The Mechanism of Placebo Analgesia. *Lancet* 1:645, 1978.
20. Lipman, A. G. Drug Therapy in Cancer Pain. *Cancer Nurs* 3:39, 1980.

21. Marks, R. M. and Sacher, M. D. Undertreatment of Medical Inpatients with Narcotic Analgesics. *Ann Intern Med* 78:173, 1973.
22. Mathews, G., Zarro, V., and Osterholm, J. Cancer Pain and Its Treatment. *Semin Drug Treat* 3(1):45, 1973.
23. McCaffery, M. *Nursing Management of the Patient with Pain* (2nd Ed.). Philadelphia: J. B. Lippincott, 1979.
24. McCaffery, M. Patients Shouldn't Have to Suffer: How to Relieve Pain with Injectable Narcotics. *Nurs 80* 10(10):34, 1980.
25. McGlashan, T. H., Evans, F. J., and Orne, M. T. The Nature of Hypnotic Analgesia and Placebo Response to Experimental Pain. *Psychosom Med* 31:227, 1969.
26. Melzack, R., Ofiesh, J., and Mount, B. The Brompton Mixture: Effects on Pain in Cancer Patients. *Can Med Assoc J* 115(2):125, 1976.
27. Melzack, R. and Wall, P. D. Pain Mechanisms: A New Theory. *Science* 150:971, 1965.
28. Miller, R. R., Feingold, A., and Paxinos, J. Propoxyphene Hydrochloride: A Critical Review. *JAMA* 213:996, 1970.
29. Moertel, C. G., Ahmann, D. L., Taylor, W. F., and Schwartau, N. A Comparative Evaluation of Marketed Analgesic Drugs. *N Engl J Med* 286:813, 1972.
30. Mount, B. M., Ajemian, I., and Scott, J. F. Use of the Brompton Mixture in Treating the Chronic Pain of Malignant Disease. *Can Med Assoc J* 115:122, 1976.
31. Mundinger, M. Nursing Diagnosis for Cancer Patients. *Cancer Nurs* 1:221, 1978.
32. Pace, J. B. Psychophysiology of Pain: Diagnostic and Therapeutic Implications. *J Fam Pract* 5:553, 1977.
33. Rankin, M. The Progressive Pain of Cancer. *Topics Clin Nurs* 2(1):57, 1980.
34. Rankin, M. Use of Drugs for Pain with Cancer Patients. *Cancer Nurs* 5:181, 1982.
35. Reed-Ash, C. Pain and the Cancer Patient. *Cancer Nurs* 5:179, 1982.
36. Rogers, A. Drugs for Pain. In American Cancer Society. *Proceedings of the National Conference on Cancer Nursing.* New York: American Cancer Society, 1977. Pp. 39–43.
37. Rowlingson, J. C. Management of Cancer Pain. *Cancer Nurs* 1:317, 1978.
38. Saunders, C. Control of Pain in Terminal Cancer. *Nurs Times* 72:1133, 1976.
39. Shawver, M. M. Pain Associated with Cancer. In A. K. Jacox (Ed.). *Pain: A Source Book for Nurses and Other Health Professionals.* Boston: Little, Brown and Co., 1977. Chapter 17.
40. Shealy, C. N. Holistic Management of Chronic Pain. *Topics Clin Nurs* 2(1):1, 1980.
41. Shimm, D., Logue, G., Maltbie, A., and Dugan, S. Medical Management of Chronic Cancer Pain. *JAMA* 241:2408, 1979.
42. Sjölund, B. H. and Eriksson, M. B. E. Endorphins and Analgesia Produced by Peripheral Conditioning Stimulation. In J. J. Bonica, et al (Eds.). *Advances in Pain Research and Therapy, Volume 3.* New York: Raven Press, 1979. Pp. 587–592.
43. Sternbach, R. *Pain: A Psychophysiological Analysis.* New York: Academic Press, 1968. P. 12.
44. Symonds, P. Methadone in the Elderly. *Br Med J* 1:512, 1977.
45. Terzian, M. P. Neurosurgical Interventions for the Management of Chronic Intractable Pain. *Topics Clin Nurs* 2(1):75, 1980.
46. Twycross, R. Clinical Experience with Diamorphine in Advanced Malignant Disease. *Int J Clin Pharmacol Biopharm* 9(3):184, 1974.
47. Twycross, R. Diseases of the Central Nervous System: Relief of Terminal Pain. *Br Med J* 4:212, 1975.
48. Twycross, R. The Target is a Pain-Free Patient. *Nurs Mirror* 147(24):38, 1978.
49. Vallner, J. J., Stewart, J. T., Kotzan, J. A., Kirsten, E. B., and Honigberg, I. L. Pharmacokinetics and Bioavailability of Hydromorphone Following Intravenous and Oral Administration to Human Subjects. *J Clin Pharmacol* 21:52, 1981.

50. West, B. A. Understanding Endorphins: Our Natural Pain Relief System. *Nurs 81* 11(2):50, 1981.

51. Wolf, Z. R. Pain Theories: An Overview. *Topics Clin Nurs* 2(1):9, 1980.

52. Woodburg, D. M. and Fingl, E. Analgesic-Antipyretics, Anti-Inflammatory Agents, and Drugs Employed in the Therapy of Gout. In L. S. Goodman and A. Gilman (Eds.). *The Pharmacological Basis of Therapeutics* (5th Ed.). New York: Macmillan, 1975.

Chapter 12

Care Of The Dying

CONCEPT I:
For some persons with cancer, the time comes when cure and remission are beyond the capacity of current curative treatment.

Although experiential, personal knowledge of death itself remains unknown, the process of dying is one that must be experienced by each person. In most cases, the very intimate act of dying, like that of giving birth, is a process requiring some assistance. The prevalent attitude toward death in our society is one of denial. This attitude is poor preparation for the personal experience of dying, as the process of dying must be integrated into the remaining life experience of the fatally ill person.

The process of dying should be both human and humane. To be human, it must be consciously assimilated and given a unique quality by the fatally ill person. To be humane, all caretakers who assist the dying person must provide whatever is necessary to relieve pain and to enable the person to have major control over the last act of life [51].

At some point in time, the client may become aware that he or she is dying, although the awareness of impending death is not always conscious. The preconscious premonitions of impending death result from central nervous system interpretation of signals about the rate of physiological decline [61].

HEALTHY/UNHEALTHY DEATH

Achievement of a healthy death implies cohesion within and among the personal and social spheres of being, despite the progressive deterioration of the physical sphere.

Adaptive personal and social responses are possible despite physiological decline, resulting in healthy death (see Figure 12.1). Healthy death is characterized by (1) normal grieving, (2) the ability to look back on one's life with satisfaction, (3) continued hope and orientation to the future, although goals may be short term and simple, (4) absence of unresolved psycho-socio-spiritual conflicts, and (5) an intact family unit demonstrating open communication.

Maladaptive personal and social responses, when coupled with progressive physiological deterioration, will result in the phenomenon of unhealthy death (see Figure 12.2).

Unhealthy death is characterized by (1) abnormal or delayed grieving, (2) an inability to find satisfaction in life review, (3) unrealistic hopes for achievement of temporally distant goals, or abandonment of any hope at all as a result of ''giving

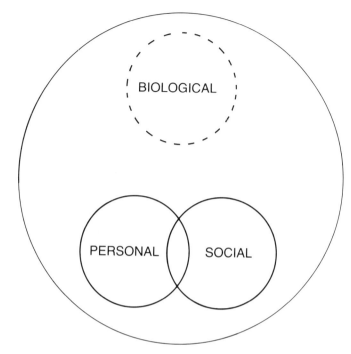

Figure 12.1. Healthy death.

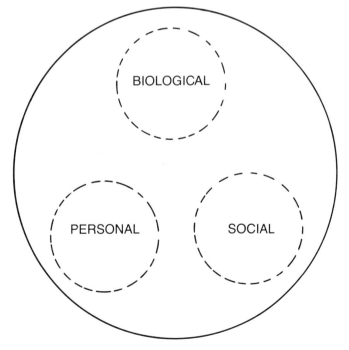

Figure 12.2. Unhealthy death.

up," (4) the presence of unresolved personal or social conflicts, and (5) a disrupted family unit displaying modes of communication that are ineffective in achieving cohesion among family members.

Achievement of a healthy death is thwarted when the fatally ill person is deceived about his or her prognosis. In response to the question, "If you had a fatal illness, would you want to be told about it or not," nine out of ten Americans replied, "Yes, I would want to be told" [8]. Rather than protecting dying persons from the harsh reality of truth, we often simply leave them alone with it instead. Fatally ill persons are unable to complete their unfinished business if they are unaware of their prognosis and are likely to lose trust in the health team if they discover they have been deceived. Most fatally ill persons prefer open and honest communication about their conditions and a desire for maximum information [12]. At any time, the dying person may choose to reject the information offered, yet retains the option to resume the communication at a later time. The nurse and other health professionals must respect the individual client's decision as whether to accept or reject information and must also convey permission to the client for reestablishment of communication when the client desires.

THE SPECIAL RIGHTS AND NEEDS OF THE DYING

The person who is dying holds specific rights (see Figure 12.3), and has special needs, different from those experienced by well persons or by persons ill with nonfatal disease conditions.

Dying persons want to be treated as living human beings, rather than being exhibited as "cases" as if their disease or physical condition were more important than the person. They need relief from distressing symptoms, the security of a compassionate environment, continuation of expert medical and nursing care, and the assurance that neither they nor their families will be abondoned [13]. Fatally ill persons need to know what is happening to their bodies and to talk about this experience with someone who will listen and attempt to understand. They need to participate in decisions affecting their remaining life experiences and the impending death experience. Additionally, an aspect that is often overlooked by health professionals is the need of the dying person to be given permission to "feel bad" instead of having to hide his or her feelings in order to protect the feelings of others [46]. Persons who are dying often experience common fears:

1. the loss of function of senses [47]
2. the loss of an organ, or body mutilation [2, 47]
3. the unknown process of dying [2, 47, 51]
4. pain [2, 47]
5. questioned ability to "stand it" [47]
6. loss of dignity [2, 47]
7. powerlessness [9, 47]
8. abandonment now that they are "dying failures"
9. enforced dependency on others for fulfillment of physical needs [9]
10. isolation from other human beings and resultant loneliness [2]
11. lack of fulfillment or meaning in life [2]

Figure 12.3. The Dying Person's Bill of Rights (From A. J. Barbus, The Dying Person's Bill of Rights, *American Journal of Nursing* 75 (January 1975): 99. Copyright © 1975, American Journal of Nursing Company. Reprinted by permission.)

I have the right to be treated as a living human being until I die.

I have the right to maintain a sense of hopefulness however changing its focus might be.

I have the right to be cared for by those who can maintain a sense of hopefulness, however changing this might be.

I have the right to express my feelings and emotions about my approaching death in my own way.

I have the right to participate in decisions concerning my care.

I have the right to expect continuing medical and nursing attention even though "cure" goals must be changed to "comfort" goals.

I have the right not to die alone.

I have the right to be free from pain.

I have the right to have my questions answered honestly.

I have the right not to be deceived.

I have the right to have help from and for my family in accepting my death.

I have the right to die in peace and dignity.

I have the right to discuss and enlarge my religious and/or spiritual experiences, whatever these may mean to others.

I have the right to retain my individuality and not be judged for my decisions which may be contrary to the beliefs of others.

I have the right to expect that the sanctity of the human body will be respected after death.

I have the right to be cared for by caring, sensitive, knowledgeable people who will attempt to understand my needs and will be able to gain some satisfaction in helping me face my death.

The manner in which most people would choose to die is often very different from their actual dying experience. Most people would prefer to die quickly, painlessly, at home, and with minimal inconvenience to their families [22, 23]. However, most people with terminal cancer have lingering dying trajectories, associated with significant physical distress and family disruption. Less than one-third of fatally ill persons die at home, with an even smaller percentage in major urban areas [51]; the general hospital is the most common location for death [42].

Dying persons often suffer from inappropriate and clumsy terminal care. The dying process is a very fatiguing experience, yet it is at this time that most persons receive less physical and emotional care than at any other point in the treatment process. The terminal period is likely to be managed by strangers in an unfamiliar setting rather than by family members in the home. Hospitals are designed to give efficient care, aggressive therapy, and a commitment to preservation of life, and thus do not offer a good milieu for dying [35, 52].

BLOCKS IMPEDING HIGH-QUALITY TERMINAL CARE

Appropriate and sensitive management of the dying person's care may be precluded by the health professional's sense of failure in the role of healer. As recently as 1968, 88 percent of physicians studied preferred to withhold information about an unfavorable prognosis from persons with advanced cancer [50], and in studies done in 1969, most physicians recommended evasion rather than truth regarding fatal conditions [17, 38]. A 1976 study revealed sharp changes in physicians' attitudes, with 87 percent affirming the value of honesty with persons having advanced cancer [10].

A 1978 study observed that 79.9 percent of nurses believed that nursing places greater emphasis on prolongation of life than on palliative care for the dying person. However, over 90 percent of the nurses studied opposed utilization of extraordinary means of life support for fatally ill persons, as opposed to 63 percent of physicians with the same belief [34].

Fatally ill persons under the care of physicians with high death anxiety were hospitalized an average of five days longer before dying than were those dying clients treated by physicians with medium or low death anxiety. It was postulated that physicians with high death anxiety may be less willing to accept the impending death of their clients, put them in the hospital earlier and/or use extraordinary means to keep them alive [56].

Although attitudes are slowly changing, the reality of terminal care in our current health care delivery system is one of paternalistic treatment in which health professionals "decide" what the dying person needs, and how and when care will be delivered. Institutional health care agencies are still too often insensitive to the client's need for control over important life events, and the traditional physician-client relationship provides the client with little or no sense of control, as the client is expected to rely solely on professional help.

It is not easy to experience the dying process. It is harder still to experience it emotionally and spiritually alone and with a sense of helplessness. The fatally-ill person is the center of the dying experience and somehow must become part of the decision-making process that affects his or her life and eventual death.

THE EMERGING SPECIALTY OF CARE OF THE DYING

Health professionals who, in other types of health care delivery, pride themselves on careful diagnosis followed by rational and scientifically sound treatment often seem to revert to superstition, emotions, and mythology when faced with a dying person [41]. However, the American medical and nursing communities are beginning to be pressured to develop guidelines for determining appropriate care for the dying client, and thus a growing body of scientific knowledge about the dying process has formed the basis for an emerging specialty of care of the dying. The interactions between the client, family, and caregivers form the framework for development of creative and scientifically sound care of the fatally ill person [20].

CONCEPT II:
Medical and nursing interventions must shift to palliative care.

When aggressive curative treatment becomes irrelevant to the client's real needs, then medical and nursing treatment should change to focus on comfort, making the client's life as peaceful, contented, and meaningful as possible until

Figure 12.4.

We need never say:
"There is nothing more
we can do."

death occurs [53]. The distress caused by the symptom can be as important as what causes the symptom. Palliative care requires limited use of technology and apparatus, extensive personal care, and an ordering of the physical and social environments so that they can be therapeutic in themselves. Palliative care implies the attitude of intensive caring rather than intensive care, and is designed to control pain in the broadest sense and to provide personal support for clients and families during the terminal phase of illness.

If a client's consciousness is focused on his or her suffering with such intensity that everything else in life is excluded, then dignity, self-respect, and the capacity for self-control are diminished or lost [13]. Inherent in the concept of palliative care is the concept of "careful neglect." Symptoms are always treated but not always treated with curative intent.

PROMOTION OF A HIGH QUALITY OF LIFE UNTIL DEATH

The nursing care delivered to the fatally ill client can make the dying process one of optimal physical and psychological ease or one of humiliation and pain. Enhancing quality of life implies recognizing and fulfilling the client's physical, psychological, social, and spiritual needs.

The "dying trajectory" is defined as the perceived course of death [26]. A quick trajectory refers to sudden, usually unexpected death. The lingering trajectory refers to an extended, unusually lengthy dying process and is most common for clients with terminal cancer. The client's dying trajectory is perceived to be more immediate than that of the caregiver. The lingering trajectory depletes physical and psychological resources of clients, families, and staff, making all who are involved vulnerable to physical and emotional exhaustion.

Communication between health professionals and fatally ill persons has been identified as existing within four contexts. In the closed-awareness context, the staff is aware of the client's diagnosis but the client is not. In the suspicion context, the fatally ill person suspects the truth yet the staff continues to act as though recovery were expected. In the pretense context, although both the client and the staff are aware of the fatal prognosis and realize that the other is aware, both continue to act as though recovery is expected. Finally, in the open awareness context, both client and staff are aware of the prognosis and openly communicate about it [25].

An open awareness context of communication between staff and client facilitates promotion of a high quality of life until the death event.

The nursing care designed and administered to the fatally ill client may result in the experience either of psychological closeness or of loneliness and fear, so palliation is a legitimate psychological as well as physiological goal. If dying persons are expected to function psychologically and cognitively as adults, feelings of anxiety, of dependency, and of being a burden are decreased, thus improving quality of the remaining life [37].

Perception of time is altered for the dying person [19]. Persons with cancer reported more time pressure even though they also reported more free time. Dying persons tend to be more future-oriented in terms of accomplishments before death yet may report that time passes too quickly and that there seems to be inadequate time for completion of desired tasks. This sense of increased time pressure may be explained by knowledge of impending death, and incorporating this altered perception of time into the nursing care plan will improve quality of nursing care, thus improving quality of the client's remaining life.

The dying person may come to more intensely value activities of daily living and pleasurable sensual experiences, as well as planning for the needs of significant others after death, which may reflect the client's desire to safeguard his own accomplishments [9].

HOSPICE: AN ATTITUDE, NOT A PLACE

The hospice attitude affirms life and provides support and care for fatally ill persons and their families [49]. Within the hospice concept of palliative care, death is neither hastened nor postponed, and health professionals attempt to allow clients and families to attain a personally satisfactory level of mental and spiritual preparation for death.

The hospice attitude promotes independence among dying persons and their families by encouraging self-management of the distresses and disabilities of fatal illness [49]. Family and friends of the dying person are regarded as a central part of the core team; and by giving care to their dying member, assisted and supported by health professionals, families may proceed through preparatory grieving which results in more satisfactory bereavement after the death event.

Management and control of distressing physical symptoms enable the client to function at an optimal level. Attention to psychological, social, and spiritual discomforts are equally important. See Table 12.1.

CONCEPT III:
Palliative care must focus on relieving distressing physical symptoms resulting from relentless progression of an incurable malignancy.

Palliative care requires a willingness to do the distasteful and a commitment to care for persons in unlovely situations. Expert nursing care for the dying must be imaginative, creative, and unhurried. Attention to detail must be continuous, and the client must remain in touch with life as much as possible. Advanced

Table 12.1.   The Standards and Principles of a Hospice Program of Care [49]

No.	Standard	Principle
1.	Appropriate therapy is the goal of hospice care.	Dying is a normal process.
2.	Palliative care is the most appropriate form of care when cure is no longer possible.	When cure is not possible, care is still needed.
3.	The goal of palliative care is the prevention of distress from chronic signs and symptoms.	Pain and the symptoms of incurable disease can be controlled.
4.	Admission to a hospice program of care is dependent on patient and family needs and their expressed request for care.	Not all persons need or desire palliative care.
5.	Hospice care consists of a blending of professional and nonprofessional services.	The amount and type of care provided should be related to patient and family needs.
6.	Hospice care considers all aspects of the lives of patients and their families as valued areas of therapeutic concern.	When a patient and family are faced with terminal disease, stress and concerns may arise in many aspects of their lives.
7.	Hospice care is respectful of all patient and family belief systems, and will employ resources to meet the personal philosophical, moral, and religious needs of patients and their families.	Personal philosophical, moral, or religious belief systems are important to patients and families who are facing death.
8.	Hospice care provides continuity of care.	Continuity of care (services and personnel) reduces the patient's and the family's sense of alienation and fragmentation.
9.	A hospice care program considers the patient and family together as the unit of care.	Families experience significant stress during the terminal illness of one of their members.
10.	The patient's family is considered to be a central part of the hospice care team.	Family participation in caregiving is an important part of palliative care.
11.	Hospice care programs seek to identify, coordinate, and supervise persons who can give care to patients who do not have a family member available to take on the responsibility of giving care.	Not all patients have a family member available to take on the responsibility of giving care.
12.	Hospice care for the family continues into the bereavement period.	Family needs continue after the death of one of their members.
13.	Hospice care is available 24 hours a day, 7 days a week.	Patient and family needs may arise at any time.
14.	Hospice care is provided by an interdisciplinary team.	No one individual or professional can meet all the needs of terminally ill patients and families all the time.
15.	Hospice programs will have structured and informal means of providing support to staff.	Persons giving care to others need to be supported and replenished in order to continue to give care.
16.	Hospice programs will be in compliance with the Standards of National Hospice Organization and the applicable laws and regulations governing the organization and delivery of care to patients and families.	The need for quality assurance in health care requires the establishment of standards for practice and program operation.
17.	The services of the hospice program are coordinated under a central administration.	Optimal utilization of services and resources is an important goal in the administration and coordination of patient care.

(continued)

Table 12.1.   The Standards and Principles of a Hospice Program of Care [49] (Cont.)

No.	Standard	Principle
18.	The optimal control of distressful symptoms is an essential part of a hospice care program requiring medical, nursing and other services of the interdisciplinary team.	Attention to physical comfort is central to palliative care.
19.	The hospice care team will have: a. a medical director b. physicians on staff c. a working relationship with the patient's physician.	Medical care is a necessary element of palliative care.
20.	Based on patient's needs and preferences as determining factors in the setting and location for care, a hospice program provides inpatient care and care in the home setting.	The physical environment and setting can influence a patient's response to care.
21.	Education, training, and evaluaton of hospice services is an ongoing activity of a hospice care program.	There is continual need to improve the techniques of palliative care and to disseminate such information.
22.	Accurate and current records are kept on all patients.	Documentation of services is necessary and desirable in the delivery of quality care.

Source: Reprinted from *Standards of a Hospice Program of Care.* Copyright ©1982, National Hospice Organization. Used with permission.

technical apparatus is rarely warranted in the care of the dying person, and assuring the dying client that all effort will be made toward ensuring a high quality of life is a means of providing hope.

PAIN

Assisting the fatally ill person to achieve a healthy death is impossible unless pain is controlled. The appropriate attitude is one of "pain control" rather than "pain relief." A major nursing and medical goal is to maintain the client in an alert but pain-free state until death, making it necessary to continuously assess the client's pain status in order to maintain an effective pain-control regime.

Health professionals must not assume that the comatose client is not in pain, but instead should institute a routine of analgesics and meticulous physical care to prevent pain. The comatose client's inability to express pain does not mean that he or she is not experiencing pain.

"PRN" analgesics are inappropriate for dying persons experiencing pain, since the "as needed" approach to dispensing pain medication requires that the client experience intermittent pain and that the client rely on nurses to determine validity of complaints of pain. Prescribing and administering analgesics on a routine, preventive approach is more effective and appropriate for dying clients [60]. In persons habituated to narcotics, the side effects of sedation and respiratory depression are uncommon even with relatively large doses of narcotics [41]. Palliative surgery and irradiation are sometimes used to control chronic pain; massages, backrubs, and meticulous physical care will reduce the client's pain experience. Evaluation of the pain-control regime must be an ongoing process, so that nurses and physicians can alter the regime as necessary in response to the changing needs of the client.

CONSTIPATION

Constipation may result from chronic use of narcotic analgesics and/or immobility, causing unnecessary pain and even premature death [41]. An appropriate goal is that the client will have a soft, formed stool every other day. It is important for health professionals to remember that feces continue to form even if the client is not eating, thus even clients who are taking nothing by mouth are vulnerable to the distressing symptom of constipation.

In the constipated client, the abdomen appears distended and gassy, often with an easily palpable descending colon. Bowel sounds are continuous, instead of the intermittent sounds auscultated in normally functioning bowels. There may be a continuous slight overflow of liquid fecal material that leaks past the obstruction caused by constipated feces, often resulting in inappropriate medical and nursing treatment for diarrhea, thus further compounding the problem.

It is preferable to prevent constipation by the routine administration of a stool softener to the client who is immobile or concurrently receiving routine narcotics. Treatment of existing constipation may include administration of oral stool softeners and/or cathartics and enemas, unless contraindicated by leukopenia or thrombocytopenia. Evaluation of the bowel-management regime must be an ongoing process, so that nurses and physicians can alter the regime as necessary in response to changing needs of the client.

NAUSEA AND VOMITING

Nausea and vomiting are distressing symptoms commonly observed in dying persons, and may be due to chemotherapy, irradiation, increased intracranial pressure, intestinal obstruction, and/or medication.

Assessment must include frequency and severity of nausea and vomiting, presence of blood or fecal material in the emesis, presence of resulting anorexia and malnutrition, and disruption of fluid and electrolyte balance. An appropriate goal is that the client will report absence of nausea and vomiting.

Effective medical management is based upon treatment with routine antiemetics. If the causative factor is intestinal obstruction and the client elects to refuse curative treatment, vomiting may continue despite successful control of nausea. If the causative stressor is the use of routine narcotics, concurrent administration of an antiemetic is usually successful.

Appropriate nursing management will decrease the experience of nausea and vomiting:

1. Avoid noxious external stimuli, such as unemptied bedpans or urinals, suction containers within view of the client, etc.

2. Remove lid covers from plates of food prior to entering the client's room.
3. Provide six to eight small feedings per day of foods desired by the client.
4. Avoid gas-forming foods.
5. Provide ice chips as desired by the client.
6. Provide carbonated beverages as desired by the client.
7. Administer antiemetic before administration of chemotherapy, before meals, or as needed.
8. Perform oral care frequently and at least after every meal and after every episode of vomiting.
9. Teach the client to take deep breaths during acute nausea.
10. Observe for signs of potassium deficit.
11. Maintain intake and output records, observing for dehydration.
12. Prevent aspiration of emesis.

Evaluation of nausea and vomiting must be a continuing process, so that nurses and physicians can alter the management regime as necessary in response to changing needs of the client.

PATHOLOGICAL FRACTURES OF BONES WITH OSTEOLYTIC LESIONS

Pathological fractures of bones with osteolytic metastases are often seen in persons with terminal cancer and constitute an unnecessary source of pain. Disrupted bone integrity resulting from bone metastases is evidenced by radiological identification of osteolytic lesions, elevations in serum alkaline phosphatase and/or calcium, and pain in the affected area [15]. Disrupted bone integrity due to bone metastases results in great vulnerability to pathological fractures.

Pathological fractures may be precipitated by minor physical trauma or improper turning and/or ambulation. Occurrence of pathological fractures may be minimized by careful ambulation, by prevention of physical trauma to the client, and by applying pressure near the joints rather than the middle of long bones when turning the client. External beam radiotherapy may also be used to shrink osteolytic lesions, thus reducing bone pain and vulnerability to fracture [15].

Progressive elevations of serum levels of alkaline phosphatase and calcium are indicative of progression of osteolytic lesions, and thus increased vulnerability to pathological fractures. Evaluation of radiological studies, serum alkaline phosphatase and calcium levels, and localized pain must be an ongoing process, so that nurses and physicians can alter the management regime as necessary in response to changing needs of the client.

SHORTNESS OF BREATH AND DYSPNEA

Shortness of breath and dyspnea are common sources of discomfort for dying clients. Causative factors may include bronchial obstruction by metastases, congestive heart failure, pulmonary edema, effusions, and infections. Anxiety generated by the subjective sensation of "fighting for breath" further increases oxygen demand, thus worsening the dyspnea. The goal is to ease shortness of breath and dyspnea, not necessarily to obtain better blood-gas results.

Elevating the head of the bed by 30 to 45 degrees will increase the thoracic capacity and thus reduce shortness of breath. Oxygen may be used with some success but is appropriately administered only by cannula. Use of an oxygen mask increases the client's subjective sense of suffocating, thus increasing anxiety and oxygen demand. Additionally, use of an oxygen mask reduces the client's ability to communicate. Administration of oxygen necessitates lubrication of the mucosa of the nose at least every two hours to prevent drying and possible bleeding.

Control of pain will reduce oxygen demand and thus reduce shortness of breath and dyspnea. Administration of corticosteroids may reduce pulmonary inflammation, again reducing shortness of breath. Bronchodilators also may be helpful. External beam radiotherapy may be prescribed in an attempt to shrink lung metastases, especially if the metastatic tumor is blocking a major bronchus or bronchiole. Thoracentesis may be utilized as a temporary comfort measure to decrease shortness of breath resulting from accumulated fluid, but the fluid usually returns within two to three days so that this particular medical intervention has limited usefulness.

Evaluation of shortness of breath and dyspnea must be a continuing process, so that nurses and physicians can alter the management regime as necessary in response to changing needs of the client.

CHRONIC COUGH

Chronic cough may cause unnecessary discomfort to the fatally ill person. Causative factors may include pulmonary inflammation and/or infection, lung metastases, and effusions.

Maintenance of adequate hydration, if possible, will thin pulmonary secretions, enabling easier expectoration of sputum. Ambulation as possible will assist the client to mobilize and expectorate secretions. A routine of turning, deep breathing, and coughing every four hours will help the immobilized client to expectorate pulmonary secretions. Medications may decrease frequency and severity of cough. Expectorants should be given during the day to increase expulsion of secretions from the lungs, whereas cough suppressants should be given at night to enable the client to sleep.

Evaluation of chronic cough must be an ongoing process so that nurses and physicians can alter the treatment regime to meet the changing needs of the client.

INSOMNIA

Insomnia is often experienced by dying persons, causative factors often being pain, shortness of breath, cough, fear, depression, and loneliness. Treatment of causative factors will usually reduce the frequency and severity of insomnia, so it is important for the nurse to determine the stressor that is causing the insomnia.

An alcoholic drink at bedtime, such as wine or beer, may increase relaxation and the ability to sleep comfortably, and massage and backrubs may relax the client and thus allow for easier sleep. Administration of sedatives as prescribed at bedtime may reduce insomnia.

Evaluation of insomnia must be an ongoing process, so that nurses and physicians can alter the treatment regime to meet the changing needs of the client.

INCONTINENCE

Incontinence of urine and/or feces is a frequent source of discomfort for dying persons and may result in skin breakdown, infection, and embarrassment to the client.

For males, an external catheter is often successful in collecting urine. For females and for males in whom treatment with external catheters has been unsuccessful, an indwelling catheter is successful in most cases. Provide catheter care with soap and water, or with medication as prescribed, at least three times daily to minimize risk of urinary tract infection. Change the catheter as indicated to minimize risk of infection, and monitor for leakage of urine around the catheter which may indicate obstruction of the tube.

Fecal incontinence must be managed by meticulous physical care and the use of absorbent pads or diapers.

Evaluation of incontinence must be an ongoing process, so that nurses and physicians can alter the management regime to meet the changing needs of the client.

SKIN BREAKDOWN AND FORMATION OF DECUBITUS ULCERS

The fatally ill person is vulnerable to significant skin breakdown and decubitus ulcer formation resulting from malnutrition, immobility, skin irritation, possible dehydration, external beam radiotherapy, and decreased tissue oxygenation, although skin breakdown is largely preventable. Anatomical areas that are most vulnerable to skin breakdown and decubitus ulcer formation are the sacrum, coccyx, heels, and hips. Assessment of skin condition must be performed daily, the most convenient time usually being during the bath.

A sheepskin is helpful for the client who is still somewhat mobile and is not incontinent. For those clients who are virtually bedridden and/or incontinent, an alternating pressure mattress is effective in relieving pressure on the skin. The client must be turned at least every two hours, and the skin should be gently massaged to increase circulation of blood in the area. Ensure that sheets are wrinkle-free and that pressure areas are not rubbed against the sheet as the client is moved. Adhere strictly to treatment regimes for existing decubitus ulcers, and assess existing ulcerations daily for signs of improvement or signs of deterioration, e.g., drainage, infection, enlargement of the ulcerated area.

Evaluation of skin condition must be an ongoing process so that nurses and physicians can alter the treatment regime to meet the changing needs of the client.

PRURITUS

Pruritus is a source of discomfort for many dying persons, and causative factors may include jaundice or renal failure.

Nursing management can reduce the discomfort of pruritus by bathing the client with nonperfumed soaps or with no soap at all, using starch-free linens on the bed, and using a bed cradle to lift linens off the client's body. Medical treatment of pruritus may include use of antihistaminics [27].

Evaluation of pruritus must be an ongoing process so that nurses and physicians can alter the treatment regime to meet the changing needs of the client.

RESTLESSNESS

Restlessness is often observed in dying persons who are also experiencing a decreased level of consciousness. Causative factors may include urine retention, constipation, cerebral hypoxia, or the subjective sensation of being too hot. Determination of the causative factor will facilitate resolution of restlessness.

If the restlessness is due to urine retention or constipation, its resolution may be easily achieved merely with catheterization or enemas. If the restlessness seems to be due to the client feeling too hot, simply removing blankets from the bed and cooling the environment may provide relief. Sedation and/or oxygen administration may or may not be effective.

Evaluation of restlessness must be an ongoing process so that nurses and physicians may alter the treatment regime in response to the changing needs of the client.

CONCEPT IV:
Palliative care must include recognition and relief of psychological pain.

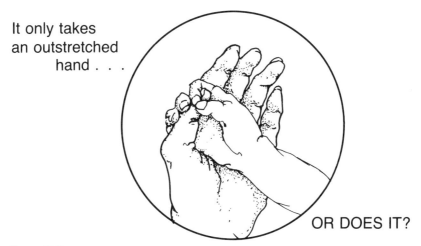

It only takes an outstretched hand . . .

OR DOES IT?

Figure 12.5.

The attitudes and belief systems held by the client largely determine the manner in which he or she copes with the dying process. Modifying factors include course of illness and environmental influences [9], and responses of both family members and health professionals influence the dying person's coping ability [43]. Fatally ill persons who are unable to verbalize fears and concerns may be unable to bring satisfactory closure to parts of their lives.

When the client enters the dying trajectory, he or she may not know the "proper" behavior expected of the dying. Acceptable dying behaviors are learned from past experiences with other dying people, the media, religion, and daily exchanges with health professionals. For example, if the client requests pain medication and the nurse delays bringing it, the client will surmise that his or her request was unacceptable behavior [9].

COPING MECHANISMS

When a person becomes aware of impending death, the result is temporary disintegration of the personality [58]. Each person must rely upon previously used coping mechanisms. Coping mechanisms are not mutually exclusive, but rather are intertwined with one another [9], and those coping mechanisms previously used in other crisis situations are often ineffective in the new situation of dying.

Coping mechanisms may be maladaptive, aggravating rather than relieving the client's psychological pain. At one time or another during the illness, maladaptive coping mechanisms are used by most fatally ill persons [61]. Manipulative or self-pitying behaviors, which are common maladaptive coping mechanisms, may aggravate or impede resolution of psychological pain.

Assessment is necessary before the nurse can determine if coping mechanisms are adaptive or maladaptive. The presence or absence of emotional responses, such as anxiety, fear, depression, hopefulness, helplessness, etc., must be determined. The nurse must determine the client's mode of past and present coping measures, as well as the client's level of comfort with the coping measures currently utilized. Finally, the nurse must determine the extent of anticipated intervention.

Goals for relief of psychological pain and maintenance of psychological comfort are to prevent hopelessness, helplessness, and loneliness, and to preserve dignity. The nurse must support the identified adaptive coping mechanisms and facilitate development of further adaptive coping mechanisms. In order for the nurse to nurture quality of life until death, maladaptive responses must be identified and modified as possible.

Support of adaptive coping mechanisms enhances the client's psychological comfort. The nurse and other health professionals can assist the client to gain perspective on the overall situation. For example, the nurse can give the client permission to express anger or despair, and yet help, not force, the client to attend to the positive aspects of life. The nurse must assure the client that adaptive coping mechanisms are normal and appropriate, since some people are embarrassed or feel guilty about expressing emotions.

When maladaptive coping mechanisms are identified, determine causative factors, if possible, and then institute a carefully planned behavior-modification program. Allow for ventilation of feelings. Support for the effort to reestablish some measure of control over life events may modify maladaptive coping mechanisms [21].

Seeking Self-awareness

Seeking self-awareness is a common adaptive coping strategy [9]. By intensely understanding the feelings precipitated by the dying process, the client may reduce the energy invested in suppression of such insight and may experience an increased sense of worthiness and meaningfulness of life. Self-awareness is enhanced by open and nonjudgmental discussions, active listening, and counseling; yet the development of self-awareness does not necessarily preclude anger, depression, or other maladaptive coping responses from occurring. Clients who have developed self-awareness regarding their dying processes are usually open to others and able to participate in life even while they are dying.

Nurturing Hope

Nurturing hope is a coping strategy often seen in fatally ill persons. Human beings hold an orientation to the future [58]; a person who can perceive no future has no hope. Nurses may thus find it necessary to assist the client to redefine "future" in terms of days or weeks rather than years. The nurse can help the client to change the focus of hope; for example, from hope for cure, to hope for another summer, to hope for control of pain. Hope forms the basis for acceptance of death. Loss of hope implies abandonment of life.

Denial and Suppression

Denial and suppression is a form of seeking self-protection and is the primary coping strategy for most clients with cancer [9]. Seeking self-protection through denial is a strategy for self-defense against internal or external stressors and may be adaptive since the client who uses denial is, in a sense, maintaining hope [9, 61]. If death is denied, a future remains. If a future remains, hope is possible.

Denial is maladaptive if it is overwhelming, results in disorganization, or prevents utilization of more effective coping mechanisms [43]. The client may seem to have complete absence of anxiety or may see no need to complete unfinished business or financially provide for survivors.

Maintenance of denial is more difficult as physiological deterioration progresses, and there are characteristic signs indicating that the client is beginning to move away from denial: (1) effectiveness of treatment is questioned, (2) the word "cancer" is used instead of "tumor" or "growth," and (3) there is an increased ability to socialize with other persons who also have cancer.

Health professionals may be able to intervene into maladaptive denial, although they should never attempt to forcefully break through denial. The nurse can intervene into maladaptive denial by returning as much control over life events and environment as possible to the client, and, as much as possible, by providing continuity of care regarding staff, services, routine care, and environment. Anxiety can be reduced by controlling pain, by anticipation of client needs, and by provision of analgesics before painful procedures. In addition, the nurse can serve as a communication liason between the client, family, and treatment team.

Anxiety

Anxiety in varying degrees is present in all clients with cancer at one time or another. The client who exhibits moderate anxiety seems to fare best [43]. This client recognizes the threat to his body integrity, mobilizes resources, and is able to eventually integrate the cancer situation into the total life experience. As long as the client is uncertain about whether the threat can be controlled, anxiety maintains a search for an effective response [57]. This client usually has strong self-esteem, adequate support systems, and few unresolved conflicts [43]. Usually, only supportive interventions are necessary.

Clients exhibiting overwhelming anxiety, on the other hand, require intervention by health professionals. This client is often immobilized by panic and unable to make decisions regarding treatment or even daily life events. Self-esteem is diminished by diagnosis of cancer and the threat of death, and support systems may be inadequate in assisting this client to reduce anxiety. Interventions are based on "emotional hyperalimentation" [43] and include returning control of life events to the client and providing the opportunity to verbalize feelings.

Regression

Regression is usually seen in fatally ill clients since it is a normal response to any physical illness [61]. Regression is a retreat from responsibilities, and when of mild degree, it is an adaptive response and conducive toward regaining physical strength. Life space is narrowed and perspective of time is contracted. In adaptive regression, the client may partially relinquish adult roles and responsibilities and become more self-centered. Immediate events are more important than events far in the future. The fatally ill client is thus able to be future-oriented in terms of days or weeks instead of years. Adaptive regression reduces anxiety and creates a situation in which hope is possible, and, in addition, permits the client to more easily accept his or her dependency on others for fulfillment of physical needs. Efforts by health professionals or family to expand this client's world may be met with resistance or passivity [9].

Regression becomes maladaptive when used prematurely and exclusively [9]. Participation in and enjoyment of valued personal or social experiences does not occur, and the excessive regression usually alienates family and health professionals, making a therapeutic milieu difficult to achieve. Excessive regression may be interpreted by the fatally ill client as evidence of the complete hopelessness of the situation [61]; thus maladaptive regression requires intervention by the health professional.

Maintaining continuity of care is important since disruption of the daily routine is a serious loss for these clients [9]. Regularly scheduled contacts with health professionals will remove some of the uncertainties in the client's situation and provide a definite event to look forward to. Careful determination of the client's desires is necessary before imposing experiences.

Withdrawal

Withdrawal is related to regression and often observed in fatally ill clients [61]. Withdrawal is a moving away from people; for example, interpersonal relationships, job contacts, and social communication. Withdrawal is adaptive when it gives the fatally ill client time to be introspective without being bothered by external demands. Adaptive withdrawal is a temporary means of ensuring privacy necessary for introspection, allowing the client space and time to sort things out.

The client who exhibits maladaptive withdrawal is unable or unwilling at that time to cope with the reality of dying [9]. Maladaptive withdrawal enables the client to partially escape the reality of the situation and is usually associated with feelings of inadequacy, shame, guilt, and intense depression [61]. The client may be attempting to protect himself or herself from expected ridicule or disgust, as in the case of mutilating surgeries, yet this withdrawal may concurrently result in social isolation at a time when maintenance of interpersonal intimacy is crucial. Family members or caregivers may feel intense rejection from the client, making a therapeutic milieu difficult to maintain. Professional intervention may be preventive by precluding feelings of embarrassment or shame regarding body condition, or it may be curative by maintaining an attitude of intimacy and caring despite the client's inability to reciprocate. Withdrawn clients usually regain the need and desire to experience interpersonal closeness and intimacy after the realities of the situation have been reconciled.

Anger

Anger is a coping mechanism frequently utilized by fatally ill persons, and is a way of attempting to aggressively remove an external threat [61]. Since cancer is an internal threat, the person changes the problem to an external one and thus perceives it to exist outside of himself or herself: for example, in poor medical treatment, inadequate nursing care, and unsatisfactory meals. The fatally ill person's anger often has a realistic basis. The client may be angry at fate or God because of the situation, at the betrayal of his or her own body, at other people who are healthy and not dying, or at the loss of control over life.

Anger must be expressed if it is to be resolved [40]. Not permitting expression of angry feelings—for example, telling the client that she or he shouldn't feel "that way," insisting that the client acknowledge only the positive aspects of life, or dismissing the anger by saying "It's God's will"—will abort the resolution of anger. It is important, also, for the health professional to realize that women in our society have been "taught" that open expression of anger is usually unacceptable behavior, so anger may be expressed by whining or by demanding, manipulative behavior. Allowing the client to express anger and offering nonjudgmental response without defensiveness usually will facilitate resolution of anger.

PERCEIVED HELPLESSNESS

Feelings of helplessness are widespread phenomena among fatally ill persons and may even increase the client's vulnerability to death [57]. Helplessness is the perception that important life events are controlled by powerful others and that internally initiated actions will not be effective in escaping aversive events. The defining characteristic of helplessness is failure to escape from aversive, unwanted events [32].

Independence is a highly valued social attribute. Over two-thirds of males and over one-third of females in one study stated that they wanted to die suddenly and unexpectedly [6]. As control over death in general increases—through intensive care units, organ transplants, and life-sustaining technology—personal control over one's own death decreases, resulting in a feeling of powerlessness. The secure possession of one's own body as a safe entity under one's control overcomes a sense of vulnerability to external forces [4].

When exposed to aversive events that are uncontrollable, the person learns that internally initiated actions are futile, and feelings of helplessness ensue [57]. It has been observed that the negative effects of stress are particularly potent when feelings of helplessness are present [55]. This state of quiescence and helplessness have been commonly observed in fatally ill persons with cancer [31]. The client may perceive institutional demands for passivity as loss of ability to control the environment. Cognitively, the dying client still realizes that independence is valued, but the body cannot comply, and the client may fear dependence on health professionals to determine when and how death occurs. Fear of dependency is often justified, since many clients do depend on the treatment team for physical need fulfillment and manipulation of the environment and events surrounding the death event itself.

Helplessness in the dying person is manifested in varying ways. Coping mechanisms usually become less effective, and the client may exhibit reduced tolerance of external stimuli, such as noise, procedures, or changes in the environment [61]. The client usually exhibits a loss of self-confidence. Anger, resentment, and frustration may be verbally or nonverbally expressed, and the client may attempt to regain control by refusing to adhere to treatment protocols [9]. Self-devaluation, psychomotor retardation, feelings of sadness, and the expectancy that responding is futile have been associated with the phenomenon of perceived helplessness [33]. Perceived helplessness is usually followed by the development of anxiety and depression [57]. Helplessness in the person with cancer frequently results in disengagement from the external environment [54].

Management of maladaptive perceived helplessness is based on returning control over life events to the client as much as possible. For many clients, the prospect of becoming dependent on others for fulfillment of physical needs is unbearable and so they need very matter-of-fact care, as the worst of all responses for them is pity [41]. Health professionals should provide an "ego prosthesis," which refers to maintenance of a constant environmental milieu based on the principle of "same ness" [61]. Belief in environmental control may even prolong life [18, 57].

NORMAL GRIEVING

The fatally ill client experiences a normal grieving process that should not be confused with maladaptive coping mechanisms. For a certain period of time for most clients, anticipatory grief assumes a role of significance in the person's behavior, and the health professional must be aware that time is a crucial variable in the grieving process as the process is normally self-limiting. The client begins the grieving process with the recognition that death represents a loss that is real and inevitable [61], and the person mourns not only for things already lost, but also for losses that are projected to lie ahead. The client mourns for the possible loss of life, for the active life style that may no longer be possible, over possible disfigurements and after effects of surgery, for the relinquishment of cherished roles, and often for the crumbling illusion that death only happens to others. Finally, the grieving client becomes increasingly aware of the significance of loss: life itself.

Concurrent with the experience of anticipatory grieving, the client may experience profound loneliness and vulnerability. The client recognizes that, although others may be supportive, the trauma of this experience must be ultimately dealt with alone. There is no escape exit, thus the client frames and says goodbye to memories. A separation from people, with a concurrent desire for less social contact, may occur during this time.

Anticipatory grieving is normal and may be a productive experience in that the client recognizes the need to put things in order. Adaptive anticipatory grieving is not immobilizing, but rather gives the client incentive to complete unfinished business [1]. Maladaptive anticipatory grieving is an immobilizing experience and will result in perceived helplessness [1]. Professional interventions similar to those used in the problem of perceived helplessness may be effective with these clients.

DEPRESSION

During the dying process, depression may be intermittent or continuous, and is a lonely isolating experience. The health professional must differentiate between depression and normal grieving, since the latter may require only supportive intervention. The depressed client feels threatened, unable to cope, and is certain that others cannot help [43]. Depression may be manifested overtly by decreased verbal activity, insomnia, increased or decreased appetite, reduction in performance of self-care, reduction of interest in other people or external activities, lethargy, and easy fatigability [9, 57]. Depression may be manifested covertly by psychosomatic complaints, such as headaches, backaches, and stomachaches [9].

Depression may often be misinterpreted by others as rejection. The client seems to reject help when in fact he or she deeply needs to receive care and nurturing, so frequently a vicious cycle of the client refusing help and the caregiver complying with that refusal will result in isolation for the client.

If depression reduces the client's quality of life, professional intervention is needed. Continuous depression acts as an obstacle to emotional growth and sense of self-worth [9]. Interventions are based on the principle of "being there" for the client. Anticipation of client needs will facilitate his or her belief that the health team cares and that they can indeed help. Interpersonal contacts without a secondary purpose, such as vital signs, physical care, procedures, etc., will facilitate the client's sense of self-worth and value. Finally, allowing the client to express feelings of sadness will facilitate resolution of those feelings and a moving away from depression.

SUICIDE

It is possible that the fatally ill person may elect to commit suicide in order to control the manner of death. The vast majority of fatally ill persons with cancer do not attempt suicide [45]. If, however, a suicide attempt or suicidal ideation is rooted in despondency and helplessness, the health professional has a responsibility to intervene. If the client succeeds in a suicide attempt, the opportunity to complete unfinished business and to resolve the anguish is lost. If the attempt fails, the client must continue to exist in a world perceived to be full of despair, and, in addition, an already difficult clinical situation is worsened.

Clients at risk for suicide may hold certain characteristics in common. The suicidal client may be overinvolved in the treatment protocol, exhibiting controlling and demanding behavior. This client may be more likely to have other life stressors, such as marital difficulty, small children at home, or financial problems. The suicidal client may be less tolerant of pain and may be more likely to exhibit severe depression.

A suicide attempt may be precipitated by incidents interpreted by the client as rejection [16]. The suicidal individual commonly has few and limited emotional outlets [5], and the staff may determine that suicidal ideation is really a demand for attention and special treatment, thus overtly rejecting the client.

Signs indicative of a potentially suicidal client have been identified [45]. These signs include history of a previous suicide attempt; history of suicidal ideation; history of alcoholism; severe depression, anxiety, mood swings, or agitation; lack of a social support system; the presence of a major stress that could be interpreted as rejection, such as death of a spouse, discontinuation of active treatment, or transfer to a nursing home; severe or intractable pain; and/or marital or financial difficulties.

Intervention is based upon the principle of ensuring that the client has a reason to live until death. Social support systems must be maximized, pain controlled, and distressing symptoms eased. Professional assistance should be provided for the problems of depression, anxiety, and/or marital or financial difficulties.

COMMON FEARS

Dying clients often have common fears. Conscious fears of death represent underlying fears of dependency and helplessness, physical injury, or abandonment [1]. For many adults, fears of death are related to the process of dying rather than the death event itself [48]. These clients fear mutilation and deformity; isolation; pain; loss of control over body functions; loss of control over one's own life; the unknown; and/or permanent physiological and/or psychological disintegration. Uncertainty about a prognosis or the dying process frequently produces more intolerable fear than does the grimmest certainty.

Many dying clients are fearful of being alone or abandoned at the time of death [9]. Fear of aloneness is related to the fear of the unknown. Abandonment may be experienced if personal contacts with significant others ceases or if the client is not allowed to have objects of personal value nearby. Clients who are fearful of being alone may refuse sleeping medications despite insomnia and may even reverse sleeping patterns so that sleep occurs during the day. Contact with others during the night reduces the risk of dying at night and alone [9].

DIGNITY

Dignity is a special type of self-esteem, implying that one is regarded well in one's own eyes as well as in the eyes of others [61]. The opposite of dignity, shame, also carries the implication of being seen or regarded, so both dignity and shame are possible only when one is being seen by another person, either in reality or in the imagination.

Interventions enhancing the preservation of dignity are those aimed at reducing helplessness and increasing self-control over life events. Situations that destroy dignity are those in which the client loses positive regard in his or her own eyes or in the eyes of others. The situations that destroy dignity include physical helplessness; psychological helplessness; situations of being exposed, such as visitors or physicians rounds during the bath, presence of family or visitors during episodes of severe pain or vomiting, etc.; and situations in which the client is treated as a "case." Efforts to preserve the client's dignity will, in the end, preserve the nurse's dignity as well.

CONCEPT V:
Palliative care must include recognition and relief of social pain.

Social pain occurs when psychic or physical pain is experienced as a result of interpersonal relationships. It is crucial to maintain interpersonal relationships until death, for facing the unknown alone is frightening, and when a fatally ill person is an important part of a healthy social network, his or her sense of isolation decreases.

To alleviate social pain and maximize interpersonal relationships, the nurse could ask, "What would you like to do or see or go to if you had the chance?" [9]. Do not imply a guarantee that any request can be fulfilled, but keep in mind that usually wishes are simple and easily attained when once identified.

Social pain may result from the client's inability to sustain valued relationships. Hospital rules regarding visitation by children and/or pets should be bent. Additionally, facilitating a visit home or to a special event may ease social pain.

Social pain may result from the phenomenon of "premortem dying." Family and/or staff may unknowingly begin to treat the client as if he or she were already dead. Signs of this phenomenon may include fewer and shorter visits, discussion of the client in his or her presence without the client's participation, and/or assignment of care to less expert nursing personnel [9]. Recognition of the phenomenon of "premortem dying" and alteration of staff/family behavior will relieve this type of social pain.

As the client proceeds through the dying process, verbal interaction with others may decrease. Families often misunderstand this process of disengagement and may attempt to create verbal contact with "small talk." Explanation to the family about the process being observed and assisting family members to simply sit quietly with the client can ease this type of social pain.

When we do not abandon the dying person, we alleviate some of the social pain. We may not be able to prevent death, but what really counts to the person who is dying is that we care.

CONCEPT VI:
Palliative care must include recognition and relief of spiritual pain.

Spiritual pain is psychic or physical pain resulting from unresolved spiritual conflicts. Spiritual pain may be precipitated by various factors: challenge of the client's belief system by the disease condition, anger at God because of the situation, and/or desire to resolve spiritual conflicts with one's church before death occurs.

The nurse can facilitate spiritual comfort by provision of private time for religious or spiritual counseling. The nurse should assure the client that the priest, minister, or rabbi of his or her choice will be called upon request. For those clients who are Roman Catholic or Episcopalian, offer to call a priest of the client's choice for the Sacrament of Reconciliation or Sacrament of the Sick. If the nurse is comfortable with joining the client in prayer, this experience will ease spiritual pain and increase trust between nurse and client. It is important that the nurse not engage in religious debate or argument with the client or family, even though their belief system may be different from that of the nurse.

CONCEPT VII:
Families who have a dying member are families in crisis.

The family must not be viewed as the refuge for the dying member but rather as a unit facing assault and therefore the target of nursing care [24] (see Table 12.2).

The goal of nursing care for the family is to keep them involved in caring for the dying member. The health team must also provide the necessary support to help

Table 12.2.   Family's Response to Dying [24]

Main Stages	Family Experiences	Nurse Can Foster:
LIVING WITH CANCER The client learns diagnosis, tries to carry on as usual, undergoes treatment.	1. *Impact:*—Emotional shock, despair, disorganized behavior.	*Hope* as different treatment methods are used, communication, helpful resources.
	2. *Functional disruption*—much time spent at hospital, ignoring of home tasks and of emotional needs, weakening of family structure, emotional isolation.	*Family cohesiveness*
	3. *Search for meaning*—questioning why this happened; casting blame of various persons, deity, habits, institutions; realization that "someday I will die too."	*Security*
	4. *Informing others*—ascent from isolation, possible need to retreat again into emotional isolation.	*Courage,* reliable help, understanding why some people can't help.
	5. *Engaging emotions*—beginning of grieving, fearing loss of emotional control, assumption of roles once carried by dying person.	*Problem-Solving,* idea that life will change but will be ongoing.
LIVING-DYING INTERVAL Client ceases to perform family roles, is cared for either at home or hospital.	6. *Reorganization*—Firmer division of family tasks.	*Cooperation* instead of competition, analysis to see if new role distribution is workable.
	7. *Framing of memories*—reviewing life of dying person—what he has meant and accomplished, new sense of family history, relinquishment of dependency on dying member.	*Identity*—focus on life review rather than only on what client is now.
BEREAVEMENT Client death	8. *Separation*—absorption in loneliness of separation.	*Intimacy* among family members.
	9. *Mourning*—resolution of guilt: "Could I have done more?"	*Relief*—release of guilt as normal.
	10. *Expansion of social network*—overcoming feelings of alienation and guilt.	*Relatedness,* looking back with acceptance and forward to new growth and socialization with a reunited, normally functioning family.

Source: From B. Giacquinta, Helping Families Face the Crisis of Cancer, *American Journal of Nursing* 77 (October 1977): 1585. Copyright © 1977, American Journal of Nursing Company. Reprinted by permission.

the family cope with the stress of caring for a dying member. Equally important is assisting the family to adjust to the idea of life without the dying member.

Various preexisting factors may heighten the family's vulnerability to maladaptive responses to stress [62]:

1. loss of another immediate family member to cancer
2. diagnosis of cancer in another immediate family member
3. living at a distance from family members
4. lack of close friends nearby to help
5. moving to a new location within the last year
6. marital difficulties prior to this diagnosis of cancer in the family member
7. other forms of chronic illness in the immediate family
8. children having problems
9. change in work status necessitated by diagnosis of cancer
10. evidence of psychosomatic symptoms

Interventions for the family with a dying member are based on support and understanding of family needs (see Table 12.3). The nurse should provide opportunity for the family to express feelings and concerns, and daily information about the client's condition should be given to the family. Acknowledgement of the family's role in caregiving and support of the client is crucial.

The family that chooses to care for their dying member at home has special teaching needs regarding aspects of physical care [26]:

1. ambulation
2. bowel and bladder management
3. comfort care
4. dietary management
5. pain management
6. wound and skin care
7. injection techniques
8. tube feedings
9. suctioning
10. administration of oxygen
11. ostomy care

Various factors make home care difficult for families to manage without external support [62]:

1. care of the children living at home
2. lack of help with the client's physical care
3. necessity of preparing different meals
4. living a long distance from the medical center
5. lack of help with the client's emotional needs
6. fear of leaving the client alone
7. lack of knowledge about physical care for the client
8. trying to work concurrently

Table 12.3.   Needs of the Grieving Spouse in a Hospital Setting [31].

Need Identified by the Grieving Spouse	Percent Who Stated Need Was Met
To be with the dying person	63
To be helpful to the dying person	74[a]
For assurance of the emotional comfort of the dying person	7[c]
For assurance of the physical comfort of the dying person	33[b]
For assurance of the physical comfort of the dying person	
To be informed of the mate's medical condition by the M.D.	48
To be informed of the mate's daily condition by the R.N.	19[d]
To be informed of impending death of the mate	74[e]
To ventilate emotions	32
For comfort and support of family members	41
For acceptance, support, and comfort from health professionals	15[f]

[a]7% did not mention this as a need.
[b]18% were upset about lack of client cleanliness.
[c]41% did not mention this as a need.
[d]19% did not expect nurses to explain anything.
[e]19% were told their mate's diagnosis or that he/she was critically ill but not told the prognosis. 7% were informed in private, 11% insisted on privacy, and 81% were informed in hospital hallways.
[f]26% stated that the need was partially met by individuals.

Families unable to bring satisfactory closure to their relationships with the dying member are at risk physically and emotionally during bereavement.

> **CONCEPT VIII:**
> **When the dying person is a child, nursing attention to the special needs of the fatally ill child and the family unit is necessary (see Chapter 10).**

INFANTS' AND TODDLERS' CONCEPT OF DEATH

The very nature of wakefulness and sleeping establishes a cycle of being and nonbeing for the child. The fatally ill child in this age group will respond more to the pain and discomfort accompanying the condition than to the fatal prognosis. The greatest threats to these children are immobility, separation from significant others, intrusive and painful procedures, and alteration in ritualisitic routines.

Infants and toddlers may perceive the seriousness of their situation from parental reactions of anxiety, sadness, depression, or anger. Although the child is unaware of the reason behind such emotions, the child nevertheless is disturbed and upset by the parent's behavior. If the nurse helps the parents to deal with their own feelings, this will allow them to better meet the needs of their child. Encouraging them to stay in the hospital as much as possible and to participate in the child's care facilitates both the parent's and the child's adjustment to the situation [63].

PRESCHOOL CHILDREN'S CONCEPT OF DEATH

Children between the ages of three and five view death as a departure, a "going away," possibly as a kind of sleep. Death is viewed as temporary: the child may bury a dead puppy in the fall and be surprised that the puppy does not come back to life in the spring when the flowers come up [63].

A primary characteristic of preschool children's thinking is precausal thinking, a belief that all causality is psychological, willed, or intentional. The child of this age simply cognitively links one event with another and assumes a cause-and-effect relationship. Characteristically, the child believes that there exists a mutual influence and interaction between himself and the environment, and this egocentricity implies a tremendous sense of self-power. Thus, he believes that his thought is sufficient to cause events.

If a child of this age is fatally ill, the illness is perceived as a punishment for his or her thoughts. The usual painful diagnostic and treatment procedures, enforced hospitalization and immobility, and general feelings of being ill serve only to confirm the child's belief that he or she is being punished [63].

SCHOOL-AGE CHILDREN'S CONCEPT OF DEATH

School-age children have a deeper understanding of death in a concrete sense, and death is frequently personified as the devil, the bogeyman, etc. These children particularly fear the mutilation and punishment they associate with death, and they still associate misdeeds or "bad" thoughts as the cause of death and thus feel intense guilt and responsibility. However, because of their more advanced cognitive skills, they respond well to logical explanation. By age nine or ten, most children have formulated the adult concept of death as being universal, irreversible, and inevitable.

If a child of this age group is dying, he or she tends to fear the unknown more than the known. For this reason, preparation is very necessary and effective during all phases of treatment: explanation of disease, signs and symptoms, drugs, radiotherapy, etc. The nurse can help these children achieve independence, self-worth, and self-esteem by assisting them to maintain control over their own bodies. Because death represents the ultimate loss of control, the realization of impending death is a tremendous threat to the child's sense of security, and they are likely to communicate their fear through verbal means and uncooperative behavior. Encouraging the child to talk about feelings and providing an outlet for hostility through play therapy are effective means of dealing with these problems [14, 63].

ADOLESCENTS' CONCEPT OF DEATH

Adolescents have a tremendous difficulty dealing with their own impending death. Although they have reached the adult concept of death, they are not likely to accept the ending of their own lives [59, 63].

THE CHILD'S MODE OF COMMUNICATION

When asked direct questions and given the chance to discuss thoughts and feelings, the child often answers in a symbolic way that must be interpreted in view of the child's age and cognitive abilities. Children may also symbolically communicate their thoughts through writing or telling stories and through art and play [63]. Often, symbolic communication from a dying child contains direct references to death and disease [7].

EXPLAINING DEATH: TO TELL OR NOT TO TELL

Fatally ill children are aware of conspiracies of silence. They realize from the reactions of other people that something is very wrong; yet they also realize that no one wants to talk about it, so they silently comply with the "don't tell" game. However, this conspiracy of silence denies the child the opportunity to discuss fears, questions, or thoughts. The child is not given the truth, leaving him or her to fantasies that may be more bizarre and frightening than the grimmest truth.

To tell a child that the illness is incurable and death inevitable does dispel hope, and possibly even life. Yet, to tell the child the name of the illness, its effect on the body, and the reason for treatment instills hope and allows for open support and communication with others.

THE GRIEF WORK OF THE PARENTS

Grief work is defined as the behavioral reactions that result in resolution of the loss [44]. It is a normal process with these identifiable characteristics: (1) it has definite symptoms, (2) the syndrome usually appears immediately after the crisis, and (3) through intervention, abnormal reactions may be transformed into normal grief work with successful resolution. The grief work of the parents of a fatally ill child is anticipatory in nature until the actual death of the child.

During the terminal phase of illness, the parents' reactions are influenced by their previous acceptance or denial of the child's illness, and it is a period of intense anticipatory grieving. As the child's condition worsens, there is an intensification of many fears.

The parents may express fear of the death event itself: "What will he die from?" "How will he die?" "When will we know that he is actually dying?"

Fear of pain is prevalent in the minds of many parents at this time. Often parents will report that the child is in pain even when the child appears to be pain-free. The parents' pain of watching their child die is an immeasurable agony and subjectively affects the parents' perception of the child's condition.

The parents may fear loss of emotional control and may attempt to hide this fear by requesting that the child be heavily sedated. Supporting the parents by being physically present at the time of impending death, by making the child as comfortable and pain-free as possible, and by talking with the awake child will assist the parents to retain self-control without the need for sedation of the child.

Parents often fear that the child will die when they are not present. The nurse should assure the family that if death approaches sooner than expected, the parents will be notified at once and that the child will not be left alone [63].

CONCEPT IX:
A major nursing goal is facilitation of "a good death" within the context of the client's desires.

For most clients, there is a specific sequence of physiological events that occur during an extended dying process. Good terminal care starts with good nursing and good medicine, and if physiological needs are not met, a "good death" cannot occur.

Sensation, mobility, and reflexes are first lost in the lower extremities, progressing to the upper extremities. The nurse should use loose clothing, untucked bed sheets, and a bed cradle to reduce bothersome pressure on the lower extremities. The client should be turned frequently and gently, paying careful attention to comfortable positioning of the legs.

A cool skin surface belies a rising internal body temperature [28]. Disphoresis occurs as peripheral circulation fails, with the most profuse perspiration on the upper parts of the body and on the extensor rather than the flexor surfaces. Regardless of how cold their skin may feel to others, most dying persons are not aware of feeling cold. Internal body temperature rises; thus, a dying person's restlessness may be due to a subjective sense of being hot even though skin surfaces are cold to the touch. The nurse should use light clothing and ensure that there is fresh, circulating air. Heavy blankets should be removed, and the client covered with light sheets. The nurse should explain to significant others that the client has a high internal body temperature despite cool skin.

The sense of vision begins to fail, and the dying person sees only what is nearby and always turns his or her head toward the light. Although bright, direct light is irritating, do not draw the shades and dim the lights. Instead, the use of indirect light will increase the ability of the dying person to see. Significant others should be seated near the head of the bed.

As the dying process continues, the sense of touch is diminished yet the dying person can sense pressure [28]. Since touch may be an unwelcome intrusion, assess the client's desire for touch. Touch the dying person gently but firmly, since extremely light stroking can be an irritant. Adapt routine care to decrease unnecessary manipulation of the client's body at this time.

The sense of hearing diminishes during the dying experience. The staff and significant others should talk in a clear, distinct voice, not whispers. Ensure that significant others sit near the head of the bed, and encourage the family to continue talking to the client, even if he or she is comatose, until death has occurred. Save conversation about the client for areas other than the client's room.

Many dying persons report minimal or no pain during the death experience. If other needs have been met, the client may require little or no pain medication. However, if analgesics are required and the oral route is no longer feasible, analgesics should be given intravenously since intramuscular injections are not effective because of failing peripheral circulation.

Respiratory abnormalities may worsen during the death experience. Elevation of the head of the bed by 30 to 45 degrees will increase thoracic capacity through the force of gravity, facilitating easier expansion of the lungs. If oxygen is administered, a nasal cannula should be used since mask administration of oxygen increases the client's subjective sense of suffocation and impedes communication. Oral suctioning and gentle mouth care hourly will remove uncomfortable oral secretions. The "death rattle" results from accumulated oropharyngeal secretions and can be minimized or prevented by small doses of parenteral atrophine or scopalamine [41].

In conscious clients, an interval of peace followed by restlessness that is not controlled by medication often signals soon-impending death. If the family is not present, the nurse should notify the family if the phenomenon of peace followed by restlessness is observed.

CONCEPT X:
Nursing measures can facilitate the progression of normal grieving within the family after the client's death.

Immediately after the death, families experience shock and numbness. The nurse should validate that the family did all they could do for their dead family member and had loved him or her well. Assist the family to grieve by providing a private place immediately after the death. Sedatives for the family will usually delay the grieving process and thus should be used judiciously. Closure of this segment of the family's life can be facilitated if the nursing staff sends a sympathy card and/or attend the client's funeral.

REFERENCES

1. Atchley, M. W., Cohen, S. B., and Weinstein, L. Anticipatory Grief in a Cancer Hospital. In B. Schoenberg, et al. (Eds.). *Anticipatory Grief.* New York: Columbia University Press, 1974. Chapter 14.
2. Baldonado, A. A. and Stahl, D. A. *Cancer Nursing: A Holistic Multidisciplinary Approach.* Garden City, NY: Medical Examination Publishing Co., 1978. Chapter 11.
3. Barbus, A. J. The Dying Person's Bill of Rights. *Am J Nurs* 75:99, 1975.
4. Becker, E. *The Denial of Death.* New York: The Free Press, 1973.
5. Bennett, A. E. Recognizing the Potential Suicide. *Geriatrics* 22:175, 1967.
6. Biorck, G. How Do You Want to Die? *Arch Intern Med* 132:605, 1973.

7. Bluebond-Langer, M. *The Private Worlds of Dying Children.* Princeton, NJ: Princeton University Press, 1978.

8. Blumefield, M., Levy, N. B., and Kaufman, D. The Wish to be Informed of a Fatal Illness. *Omega* 9:323, 1978.

9. Burkhalter, P. K. Living Until Death: Caring for the Dying Cancer Patient. In P. K. Burkhalter and D. L. Donly (Eds.). *Dynamics of Oncology Nursing.* New York: McGraw-Hill, 1978. Pp. 275–308.

10. Carey, R. G. and Posavac, E. J. Attitudes of Physicians on Disclosing Information to and Maintaining Life for Terminal Patients. *Omega* 9:67, 1978.

11. Cassem, N. and Stewart, R. S. Management and Care of the Dying Patient. *Int J Psychiatry Med* 6:293, 1975.

12. Cassileth, B. R., et al. Information and Participation Preferences Among Cancer Patients. *Ann Intern Med* 92:832, 1980.

13. Craven, J. and Wald, F. S. Hospice Care for Dying Patients. *Am J Nurs* 75:1816, 1975.

14. Dezendorf, A., et al. *There is a Rainbow Behind Every Dark Cloud.* Millbrae, CA: Celestial Arts, 1978.

15. Evarts, C. M. and Rubin, P. Bone Tumors. In P. Rubin (Ed.). *Clinical Oncology for Medical Students and Physicians* (5th Ed.). Rochester, NY: American Cancer Society, 1978. Pp. 203–209.

16. Farberow, N. L. and Schneidman, E. S. *The Cry for Help.* New York: McGraw-Hill, 1961.

17. Feifel, H. Perception of Death. *Ann NY Acad Sci* 164:19, 1969.

18. Ferrari, N. A. Institutionalization and Attitude Change in the Aged Population: A Field Study in Dissonance Theory. Unpublished Ph.D. dissertation, Western Reserve University, 1962.

19. Fitzpatrick, J. J., Donovan, M. J., and Johnston, R. L. Experience of Time During the Crisis of Cancer. *Cancer Nurs* 3:191, 1980.

20. Foster, Z. Standards for Hospice Care. *Health Soc Work* 4:124, 1979.

21. Freidenbergs, I., Gordon, W., Ruckdeschel-Hibbard, M., and Diller, L. Assessment and Treatment of Psychosocial Problems of the Cancer Patient: A Case Study. *Cancer Nurs* 3:111, 1980.

22. Fulton, R. The Sacred and the Secular: Attitudes of the American Public Toward Death, Funerals and Funeral Directors. In R. Fulton (Ed.). *Death and Identity.* New York: John Wiley and Sons, 1965. Pp. 89–105.

23. Fulton, R. and Gilbert, G. Death and Social Values. In R. Fulton (Ed.). *Death and Identity.* New York: John Wiley and Sons, 1965. Pp. 65–75.

24. Giacquinta, B. Helping Families Face the Crisis of Cancer. *Am J Nurs* 77:1585, 1977.

25. Glaser, B. G. and Straus, A. L. *Awareness of Dying.* Chicago: Aldine, 1965. Part II.

26. Glaser, B. G. and Straus, A. L. *Time for Dying.* Chicago: Aldine, 1968.

27. Goth, A. Medical Pharmacology: Principles and Concepts (10th Ed.). St. Louis: C. V. Mosby, 1981. P. 250.

28. Gray, V. R. Some Physiological Needs. In P. S. Chaney (Ed.). *Dealing with Death and Dying* (2nd Ed.). Jenkintown, PA: Intermed Communications, 1976. Pp. 15–20.

29. Grobe, M. E., Ilstrup, D. M., and Ahmann, D. L. Skills Needed by Family Members to Maintain the Care of an Advanced Cancer Patient. *Cancer Nurs* 4:371, 1981.

30. Gullo, S. V., Cherico, D. J., and Shadick, R. Suggested Stages and Response Styles in Life-Threatening Illness: A Focus on the Cancer Patient. In B. Schoenberg, et al (Eds.) *Anticipatory Grief.* New York: Columbia University Press, 1974. Chapter 8.

31. Hampe, S. O. Needs of the Grieving Spouse in a Hospital Setting. *Nurs Res* 24:113, 1975.

32. Hiroto, D. S. Locus of Control and Learned Helplessness. *J Exp Psych* 102(2):187, 1974.

33. Hiroto, D. S. and Seligman, M. E. P. Generality of Learned Helplessness in Man. *J Per Soc Psychol* 31:311, 1975.

34. Hoggatt, L. and Spilka, B. The Nurse and the Terminally-Ill Patient: Some Perspectives and Projected Actions. *Omega* 9:255, 1978.
35. Holden, C. Hospices: For the Dying, Relief from Pain and Fear. *Science* 193:389, 1976.
36. Kassakian, M. G., Bailey, L. R., Stewart, C., and Rinker, M. A Revival of an Old Custom. *Onc Nurs Soc News* 4(3):15, 1977.
37. Klagsbrun, S. C. Cancer, Emotions, and Nurses. *Am J Psychiatry* 126:1237, 1970.
38. Krant, C. and Caldwell, J. The Dying Patient. *Psychosomatics* 10:293, 1969.
39. Krant, M. J. and Johnston, L. Family Members' Perceptions of Communications in Late Stage Cancer. *Int J Psychiatry Med* 8:203, 1978.
40. Kubler-Ross, E. *On Death and Dying.*, New York: Macmillan, 1969. Chapter 4.
41. Lamerton, R. *Care of the Dying* (Rev. Ed.). Middlesex, England: Penguin Books, 1980. Chapter 4.
42. Lerner, M. When, Why, and Where People Die. In O. Brim, et al. (Eds.). *The Dying Patient.* New York: Russell Sage Foundation, 1970. P. 22.
43. Liaschenko, J. M. Assessment of Anxiety and Depression in the Dying Patient. *Topics Clin Nurs* 2(4):39, 1981.
44. Lindemann, E. Symptomatology and Management of Acute Grief. *Am J Psychiatry* 101:141, 1944.
45. Maxwell, M. B. Cancer and Suicide. *Cancer Nurs* 3:33, 1980.
46. McCorkle, R. The Advanced Cancer Patient: How He Will Live—and Die. In L. Kruse, J. L. Reese, and L. R. Hart (Eds.) *Cancer: Pathophysiology, Etiology, and Management.* St. Louis: C. V. Mosby, 1979. Pp. 477–481.
47. Mundinger, M. O. Nursing Diagnosis for Cancer Patients. *Cancer Nurs* 1:221, 1978.
48. Murray, R. B. and Zentner, J. P. *Nursing Assessment and Health Promotion Through the Life Span* (2nd Ed.). Englewood Cliffs, NJ: Prentice-Hall, Inc. 1979. Chapter 10.
49. National Hospice Organization Standards and Accreditation Committee. *Standards of a Hospice Program of Care* (6th Rev.). McLean, VA: National Hospice Organization, 1979.
50. Oken, D. What to Tell Cancer Patients. *JAMA* 175:1120, 1968.
51. Rossman, P. *Hospice.* New York: Fawcett Columbine, 1977.
52. Ryder, C. F. and Ross, D. Terminal Care: Issues and Alternatives. *Public Health Rep* 92:20, 1977.
53. Saunders, C. The Last Stages of Life. *Am J Nurs* 65:70, 1965.
54. Schmale, A. H. Psychological Aspects of Anorexia. *Cancer* 43:2087, 1979.
55. Schulz, R. and Aderman, D. Effect of Residential Change on the Temporal Distance to Death of Terminal Cancer Patients. *Omega* 4:157, 1973.
56. Schulz, R. and Aderman, D. Physician's Death Anxiety and Patient Outcomes. *Omega* 9:327, 1978.
57. Seligman, M. E. P. *Helplessness of Depression, Development and Death.* San Francisco: W. H. Freeman and Co., 1975. Chapter 8.
58. Shands, H. C. Psychological Mechanisms in Patients with Cancer. *Cancer* 4:1159, 1951.
59. Sternberg, F. and Sternberg, B. *If I Die and When I Do.* Englewood Cliffs, NJ: Prentice-Hall, 1980.
60. United States General Accounting Office. *Report to the Congress of the United States by the Comptroller General.* HRD–79–50. March 6, 1979.
61. Verwoerdt, A. Some Aspects of Communication with the Fatally-Ill. In American Cancer Society. *Proceedings of the American Cancer Society Second National Conference on Human Values and Cancer.* New York: American Cancer Society, 1973. Pp. 61–68.
62. Welch, D. Planning Nursing Interventions for Family Members of Adult Cancer Patients. *Cancer Nurs* 4:365, 1981.
63. Whaley, L. F. and Wong, D. L. *Nursing Care of Infants and Children.* St. Louis: C. V. Mosby, 1979. Chapter 27.

Chapter 13

Oncologic Complications and Emergencies

CONCEPT I:
The malignant process may cause neurological complications and emergencies.

BRAIN METASTASES

Expanding metastatic mass lesions in the brain cause either insidious or rapid loss of neurological function. Metastatic brain lesions occur in 12 percent to 24 percent of persons with cancer [1, 25, 31]. The blood-brain barrier may actually act as a sanctuary for malignant cells, enabling them to proliferate even though the primary tumor is controlled by chemotherapy. Any malignant tumor can metastasize to the brain. Lung carcinomas account for approximately half of all metastatic brain lesions, and breast carcinoma is the second leading type of primary tumor involved in brain metastases. Other primary tumors that are commonly metastatic to the brain include melanoma and carcinomas of the kidney, gastrointestinal tract, pancreas, prostate, and testis.

The appearance of metastatic brain lesions is an ominous sign indicative of shortened survival time. If the brain lesions are not treated, median survival is only one month after the appearance of neurological signs and symptoms. Survival time seems to be only slightly influenced by antineoplastic treatment. Treatment with adrenocorticosteroid hormones may relieve many symptoms but median survival is prolonged to only two months. Whole brain irradiation relieves symptoms in about half of those people with metastatic brain cancer; however, survival time is extended to only three to six months. Surgical tumor resection also extends survival time to a median of five to six months [29, 32].

Metastatic spread of cancer to the brain is almost always by arterial circulation [30]. The most common site for a metastatic brain lesion is in the parietal lobe. Multiple brain metastases are more common than single tumors. Carcinomas of the lung and malignant melanoma most often produce multiple brain lesions, whereas breast and renal cancers generally result in a single metastatic tumor.

Generalized Signs and Symptoms

Generalized signs and symptoms of brain lesions are a direct result of increased intracranial pressure and/or obstruction to the normal flow of cerebrospinal fluid. *Altered mentation* may initially be very subtle, characterized by increased sleeping, difficulty in concentration, memory loss, increased irritability, or poor judgment in making decisions. *Headache* occurs in 30 percent to 50 percent of persons with brain tumors and are more common in persons with multiple lesions or with cerebellar masses [32]. The headaches are usually bioccipital or bifrontal. The pain is thought to be due to traction on pain-sensitive intracranial structures. It is characteristically worse upon awakening and usually disappears soon after the person arises. The headache may be intensified or precipitated by any activity that increases intracranial pressure, such as straining at stool, stooping, or coughing. *Vomiting* occurs in about one-third of persons with brain lesions and often accompanies headache. Vomiting may or may not be projectile, and may or may not be accompanied by nausea. Vomiting is more common in persons who have cerebellar or brainstem tumors. *Papilledema* is dependent upon tumor location and is a late sign if the tumor does not obstruct cerebrospinal fluid flow. *Pupillary changes* are an ominous late sign of increased intracranial pressure, indicating herniation of the cerebrum into the tentorial notch and subsequent compression of the third cranial nerve (oculomotor nerve) as it passes through the tentorial notch. *Changes in vital signs* are also a late sign of increased intracranial pressure. Changes include an elevated systolic blood pressure, bradycardia, and slow irregular respirations.

FOCAL MANIFESTATIONS

Focal manifestations of a space-occupying brain lesion are caused by the local compression or destruction of the brain tissue as well as compression secondary to edema. *Seizures* occur in approximately one-third of persons with metastatic brain tumors [21, 32]. Persons with cerebral hemisphere masses are more likely to exhibit seizure activity, as are persons with multiple lesions. Seizure activity may be generalized, focal, or a combination of both. Although the exact cause of the seizure activity is unknown, it is associated with neuronal hyperexcitability and abnormal electrical discharge patterns. Left, or dominant, hemisphere lesions may cause *aphasia* since the dominant hemisphere is responsible for language function, speech and reading comprehension, and other analytical functions. Right, or nondominant, hemisphere lesions may cause *memory impairment* or an *inability to dress oneself* since the nondominant hemisphere is responsible for spatial and visual perceptions. Frontal lobe tumors may result in *changes in affect* or *dementia* [28]. Temporal masses may cause *hallucinations*, whereas *visual abnormalities* occur with occipital tumors.

MEDICAL TREATMENT

Medical treatment of brain metastases may include surgical resection. Surgical resection is usually reserved for those individuals with a solitary lesion and a disease-free interval of at least twelve months since treatment of the primary neoplasm. A shunt may be inserted to decreased elevated intracranial pressure if hydrocephalus is present. Surgical intervention may also be considered if rapidly increasing intracranial pressure persists despite a previously placed shunt or high-dose steroid treatment.

External beam radiotherapy is often used to treat metastatic brain lesions. Postoperative irradiation is recommended for malignant metastatic tumors, and whole brain irradiation is used for multiple intracranial lesions.

Chemotherapy is not successful by the traditional intravenous route because of the presence of the blood-brain barrier. However, chemotherapeutic drugs may be administered intrathecally either by lumbar puncture or an Omaya reservoir. High-dose adrenocorticosteroids are commonly administered to reduce elevated intracranial pressure and thus provide symptomatic relief.

Nursing Measures

Nursing assessments not only provide baseline data but also allow for continued evaluation of the client's neurological status, the degree of treatment success, and progression of neurological dysfunction. The following indices are used:

1. Level of consciousness
2. Orientation
3. Judgment, insight, and memory
4. Mood, affect
5. Posture, gait, ambulatory ability, localized weakness
6. Ability to speak and comprehend verbal and written communication
7. Ability to dress oneself
8. Visual abnormalities
9. Presence of hallucinations
10. Signs and symptoms of increased intracranial pressure

Nursing measures will also prevent or minimize complications of brain metastases and/or the medical treatment. Identification of early signs and symptoms of neurological complications will allow earlier and thus more effective treatment. It is important that the nurse pay careful attention to family reports of any subtle differences in the client's behavior, mood, memory, or sleeping patterns. Assessment indices must be monitored regularly and at appropriate intervals to allow comparison and evaluation of the patterns of neurological function. Safety measures must be instituted as appropriate for those persons with deficits in ambulation, balance, judgment, level of consciousness, and visual acuity.

Seizure precautions should be instituted since a significant percentage of persons with metastatic brain lesions exhibit seizure activity. Persons at high risk for seizures are those with cerebellar lesions and/or multiple tumors. Accurate description of any seizure activity allows for possible localization of the intracranial disturbance and thus more specific treatment.

SPINAL CORD AND NERVE ROOT COMPRESSION

Spinal cord and nerve root compression cause either insidious or rapid loss of neurological function [28]. This phenomenon occurs in approximately 5 percent of persons with systemic cancer. It may be caused by primary spinal cord tumors that lie within the spinal cord (intramedullary), within the dura mater (extramedullary), or extradurally. Carcinomas of the lung, breast, prostate, and kidney may produce metastases that ultimately result in spinal cord and nerve root compression. Lymphoma and multiple myeloma may also produce this neurological complication. The spinal cord is most often compressed anteriorly by direct growth of a tumor.

Primary spinal cord tumors usually produce a slow onset of symptoms, whereas metastatic tumors are characterized by rapid development of symptoms. The characteristic initial symptom of both is pain. Discomfort may be thoracolumbar back pain in a belt-like distribution, and the pain may extend to the groin or legs. Pain often precedes the definitive diagnosis of spinal cord and nerve root compression by weeks or months.

Other characteristic symptoms include weakness, sensory changes, bladder dysfunction, and ataxia. If the condition progresses, the ultimate outcome will be paralysis.

Medical treatment includes the administration of adrenocorticosteroids with concurrent high-dose radiotherapy and decompressive laminectomy. High dosages of steroids may be started as soon as the diagnosis is confirmed and are usually continued for three days while concurrent high-dose radiotherapy is delivered. After this, the steroids are rapidly tapered as tolerated. Since compression of the spinal cord is usually located anteriorly, a decompressive posterior laminectomy is not always effective as the sole treatment. Persons who have previously received maximum irradiation to the site of the spinal cord compression usually receive decompressive laminectomy since adequate irradiation of the area is not possible. Persons who experience neurological deterioration during radiotherapy may also receive decompressive laminectomy.

Nursing assessments and interventions prevent or minimize further complications of spinal cord and nerve root compression. Neurological status must be assessed every two hours during the first three days. The individual's response to radiotherapy and corticosteroids must be monitored since further deterioration is an indication for decompressive laminectomy. Safety measures must be implemented for those persons whose ambulatory ability is compromised. Prevention or treatment of diarrhea may be necessary if the field of irradiation includes the abdomen.

HEPATIC ENCEPHALOPATHY

Hepatic encephalopathy is a potentially fatal condition characterized by failure of brain function secondary to the liver's inability to transform ammonia into urea [3]. Ingested protein is broken down into free amino acids in the stomach and small intestine. The amino acids are returned to the liver where they are degraded into carbon and ammonia. Since free ammonia is toxic to the human body, the liver then transforms it into urea. Urea is ultimately excreted in the urine, thus safely ridding the body of toxic waste.

Hepatic encephalopathy is caused directly or indirectly by a marked elevation of the serum ammonia level [22]. The basic mechanism seems to be cerebral intoxication secondary to impairment of the Krebs Cycle [33]. Interference in brain metabolism by toxic levels of serum ammonia results in the clinical manifestations of hepatic encephalopathy.

Any condition that results in a reduced ability of the liver to synthesize urea at a rate sufficient to prevent toxic levels of serum ammonia may precipitate hepatic encephalopathy. Hepatocellular demage, for example, decreases the liver's ability to transform ammonia into urea, thus increasing the serum ammonia level. Gastrointestinal bleeding increases the amount of ammonia absorbed from the intestine, also increasing serum levels. Increased ammonia retention may also occur secondary to the administration of diuretics.

Signs and Symptoms

Clinical signs and symptoms of hepatic encephalopathy are divided into four stages. Progression from the slight mental clouding characteristic of Stage I to the deep coma of Stage IV may occur rapidly.

Stage I manifestations are easily missed because they are characterized only by subtle changes in personality and behavior. Signs of Stage I include an unkempt appearance, a vacant stare, slurred speech, forgetfulness, slight confusion, increased lethargy, and changes in sleeping patterns.

Stage II manifestations are more easily detected because they are more marked. Asterixis (liver flap) commonly occurs, and there is an inability to write clearly (constructional apraxia). Stage I manifestations also become more pronounced.

Stage III manifestations include possible combative behavior and increased sleeping. During Stage III, definite electroencephalogram changes can be seen.

Stage IV is characterized by a markedly elevated serum ammonia and grave prognostic signs. The client lapses into a deep coma. Hyperactive reflexes and a positive Babinski sign are seen. There is a sweet, musty odor to the breath called hepatic fetor. Electroencephalogram abnormalities increase.

Nursing and Medical Treatment

Appropriate medical and nursing treatment may reverse the progression of hepatic encephalopathy and prevent death. Ammonia production secondary to the breakdown of exogenous protein must be reduced. Exclude all protein from the diet and discontinue infusions of total parenteral nutrition solutions that contain amino acids. It is equally as important to decrease ammonia production secondary to the breakdown of endogenous protein. In order to spare muscle from being used as the body's energy source, give nourishment that is high in carbohydrates or provide intravenous glucose solutions as prescribed. Any gastrointestinal bleeding must be medically corrected. Ammonia levels are also reduced by the appropriate administration of drugs. Neomycin, a nonabsorbable antibiotic, may be given orally or rectally to inhibit the activity of ammonia-producing bacteria in the intestine [22]. Magnesium sulfate may also be given to purge the bowel of protein contents if gastrointestinal bleeding has occurred [33]. Narcotics and barbiturates must be used cautiously because of their toxic effects on the liver.

The client should be monitored for signs and symptoms indicative of the progression or remission of hepatic encephalopathy. Assess the client's level of consciousness, orientation, and amount of time spent sleeping. Assess for asterixis (liver flap) by having the client raise both arms with the forearms fixed and fingers extended. Observe for an involuntary flapping tremor in the wrists and hands. Regularly compare samples of the client's handwriting, observing for deterioration and constructional apraxia. Monitor the client's serum ammonia level, and assess for hyperactive reflexes, a positive Babinski sign, and hepatic fetor in clients with a diminished level of consciousness.

MENINGEAL INFILTRATION

Meningeal infiltration by malignant tumor cells is occurring with increasing frequency as overall survival time lengthens [28]. In children with relapsing acute lymphoblastic leukemia, the incidence of meningeal infiltration is so high (about 50 percent) that effective prophylactic treatment to the central nervous system has become a routine part of initial medical management.

Meningeal carcinomatosis consists of a diffuse or multifocal spread from solid primary tumors to the cerebral, cerebellar, and spinal leptomeninges. The most common primary tumors identified in meningeal carcinomatosis are adenocarcinomas of the breast and lung [18]. There may be widespread multifocal malignant cell seeding and sheet-like tumor cell proliferation along the surfaces of the brain and spinal cord.

Signs and symptoms are reflective of intracranial, cranial nerve, and/or spinal nerve root dysfunction. Those signs that indicate intracranial dysfunction are the results of rising intracranial pressure: headache (usually diffuse and severe), vomiting with or without nausea, changes in mentation and level of consciousness, and seizure activity. Cranial nerve signs and symptoms are results of pressure on the cranial nerves. They may include visual loss or diplopia, deafness, facial paralysis, dysarthria, and dysphagia. Tumor or fluid pressure within the spinal column cause the symptomatology indicative of spinal root dysfunction: leg or low back pain, neck pain or stiffness, weakness, paresthesias, unsteady gait, sensory abnormalities, and autonomic dysfunction (e.g., loss of bowel or bladder control).

Although many of the clinical manifestations of meningeal infiltration are vague, this condition should be suspected when there are signs and symptoms of widespread neurological dysfunction reflective of involvement at more than one anatomical site. Diagnosis of meningeal infiltration by malignant cells is established by examination of cerebrospinal fluid. Typical findings are increased pressure, increased white blood cell count, and protein with decreased glucose levels. The cerebrospinal fluid examination is never completely normal, although elevated pressure may be the only abnormal finding. Initial cerebrospinal fluid cytology examinations are positive in less than half of the persons with this condition [10, 28]. Thus, several cytology examinations may be necessary to definitively establish the presence of malignant cell seeding.

Medical Treatment

Appropriate medical intervention may successfully induce remission and prevent death. Reduction of intracranial pressure and inflammation is achieved by the administration of hyperosmolar agents (e.g., mannitol) and corticosteroids. The malignant cell infiltrate may also be destroyed by craniospinal irradiation and/or chemotherapy. Since most chemotherapeutic drugs will not cross the blood-brain barrier, the agents must be given by the intrathecal or intraventricular route.

Nursing Treatment

Clients at risk must be identified. They include children with acute lymphoblastic leukemia and persons with adenocarcinomas of the breast or lung. Monitor the client for early signs and symptoms of meningeal infiltration. Assess for remission or progression of neurological signs and symptoms, and intervene into the adverse side effects of chemotherapy or external beam radiotherapy.

CONCEPT II:
Superior vena cava syndrome is a cardiovascular emergency that may result from malignant disease.

Superior vena cava syndrome results from the compression of the superior vena cava by a primary or metastatic mediastinal tumor. Venous drainage of the head, neck, and upper thorax is impaired. Approximately 75 percent of malignant superior vena cava obstructions are caused by lung cancer, with another 15 percent to 20 percent caused by diffuse histiocytic lymphoma. Superior vena cava obstruction is rarely seen in Hodgkin's disease or nodular non-Hodgkin's lymphoma [28].

The onset of signs and symptoms may be insidious. Impaired venous drainage of the head, neck, and upper thorax results in thoracic and neck vein distention and facial edema [26]. Laryngeal edema may produce stridor. Obstruction of the superior vena cava also causes diminished cardiac venous return, resulting in tachypnea, dyspnea, and fatigue. Headache, changes in level of consciousness, and blurring of vision may also accompany this condition.

MEDICAL TREATMENT

The medical treatment of choice for superior vena cava syndrome is external beam irradiation to the mediastinal mass. For carcinomas, initially high doses of radiation are given for three days, followed by a gradual reduction of the radiation dosage for the remainder of the treatment time. The radiotherapy usually lasts five to six weeks. This approach to radiotherapy seems to produce a more rapid regression of the tumor than does low-dose irradiation. Improvement of the client's condition is usually seen within seventy two hours after initiation of radiotherapy.

Medical treatment may include the administration of diuretics (e.g., furosemide or ethacrynic acid) or corticosteroids. Early administration of corticosteroids may be useful in severely symptomatic clients, but routine use is controversial. The emergency use of nitrogen mustard during the initial course of radiotherapy is no longer recommended [16, 28].

NURSING TREATMENT

Monitor for signs and symptoms of superior vena cava syndrome in clients at risk. Intervene into the adverse side effects of radiotherapy. If diuretics are used, monitor for signs indicative of developing inappropriate antidiuretic hormone secretion.

CONCEPT III:
Respiratory system complications and emergencies may result from the malignant disease process.

TRACHEAL OBSTRUCTION

Tracheal obstruction is an oncologic emergency requiring rapid medical and nursing intervention to prevent airway occlusion and death. Several etiological factors may be implicated in the development of tracheal obstruction. The obstruction may result from stenosis of the trachea following intubation, tracheotomy, or laryngeal trauma. Primary malignant neoplasms of the trachea may cause obstruction, or the trachea may be directly invaded by neoplasms originating in the esophagus, lung, or thyroid.

Signs and symptoms commonly associated with tracheal obstruction include hemoptysis, wheezing, cough, and progressive dyspnea. If a tracheoesophageal fistula has developed, aspiration and pneumonia accompanied by rapidly progressive dyspnea occur. Diagnosis is most often confirmed by X-ray and/or computerized axial tomography. In order to avoid edema and possible complete obstruction, bronchoscopy is deferred if the airway is significantly narrowed. Even slight manipulation of an occluding tumor may produce hemorrhage, increased edema, and death.

Medical treatment of tracheal obstruction is dependent upon the causative factors. Tracheal stenosis may be managed by endoscopic dilatation or surgical resection of the affected area. Obstructing tumors are most often surgically removed. Inoperable or incompletely resected tumors are usually treated with external beam radiotherapy; corticosteroids are sometimes administered at the same time.

Appropriate nursing assessment of clients at risk may allow earlier intervention into tracheal obstruction. The primary nursing intervention is to maximize oxygen supply to the client. Oxygen may be administered, and positioning of the client should promote optimal airway space.

PLEURAL EFFUSION

Pleural effusion restricts lung expansion, compromises the lung's capacity for gas exchange, and may cause atelectasis and/or infection. Pleural effusions are often caused by malignancies and may even be the initial diagnostic sign of cancer [15, 28]. Malignancies most often associated with pleural effusion are lung cancer, breast cancer, leukemia, and lymphoma. A malignant pleural effusion carries an ominous prognosis, with a mean survival of only three months [28].

Signs and symptoms indicative of pleural effusion depend upon its size, whether it is unilateral or bilateral, and the functional status of the lungs. Dyspnea, pleuritic pain, and deviation of the trachea away from the side of the effusion are common. If the effusion is large, the intercostal spaces may bulge. Delayed and diminished chest movement on the affected side is often noted. There are usually flat percussion sounds and diminished breath sounds over the affected area, and diminished vocal and tactile fremitus are often observed.

Since pleural effusion predisposes the client to atelectasis and pulmonary infection as well as causing unnecessary discomfort, proper medical and nursing measures will relieve distressing symptoms, will help to prevent recurrence, will enhance quality of life, and may prolong survival time. Medical treatment may be initiated by a thoracentesis to establish etiology of the effusion and to determine the recurrence of a pleural effusion. Cytological studies of the pleural fluid are diagnostic of underlying malignancy in a large proportion of cases [17, 35]. The average time interval for reaccumulation is only four days after a thoracentesis. Thus, repeated thoracenteses may provide temporary symptomatic relief but do not prevent fluid reaccumulation.

Approximately 50 percent of clients with malignant pleural effusion are successfully treated by draining the effusion with chest tubes, after which a drug is instilled through the chest tubes to sclerose pleural surfaces. After instillation of the drug, the client must be rolled side to side in order to distribute the drug over the pleural surface. The drug of choice is tetracycline because it is nonmyelosuppressive and has the least morbidity. Tetracycline causes fever and significant pleural pain during instillation. Nitrogen mustard, thio-TEPA, and 5-FU have been used as sclerosing agents but may result in myelosuppression. Chest tubes are removed only when no further fluid is draining.

Systemic chemotherapy may be used to attempt control of the pleural effusion prior to local treatment. In clients with mediastinal lymphoma, external beam radiation may resolve the effusion.

An important nursing consideration is the prevention of adverse effects of thoracentesis. Assess breath sounds and dyspnea every four hours after thoracentesis in order to monitor for the development of pneumothorax or fluid reaccumulation. Nursing measures may also prevent the adverse effects of drug instillation through chest tubes. Maintain a closed chest drainage system and chest tube patency. Treat the client for pain *prior* to the instillation of drugs, especially tetracycline. Monitor for and treat fever if tetracycline is administered, and monitor for the development of myelosuppression if nitrogen mustard, thio-TEPA, or 5-FU are given. Finally, intervene into the adverse effects of systemic chemotherapy or mediastinal irradiation as indicated.

CONCEPT IV:
The malignant process and/or antineoplastic treatment may cause blood component dysfunction.

LEUKOPENIA

Leukopenia is an oncologic complication that may become life-threatening. Since infection is the cause of death in nearly half of all persons with cancer [28], leukopenia must be treated as a grave condition necessitating aggressive care.

Normal bodily defenses against infection may be altered by the malignancy itself. Tumor infiltration of the bone marrow and/or hypersplenism causes neutropenia and compromised phagocyte function. Abnormal cellular (T-cell) immunity is common in persons with lymphoma or metastatic solid tumors. Hypogammaglobulinemia and decreased antibody responses often result from chronic lymphocytic leukemia, multiple myeloma, and lymphomas.

A variety of stressors compromise normal defenses against infection. Antineoplastic drugs and irradiation suppress bone marrow and lymph tissue function, causing leukopenia, phagocyte dysfunction, and immunoincompetence. Normal immune system function is suppressed by malnutrition, and advanced age is associated with altered host defenses against infection. The integrity of the skin and mucous membranes may be disrupted by surgical procedures, indwelling catheters, drug- or radiation-induced mucositis, decubitus ulcers, multiple intravenous punctures, invasive procedures, or tumor infiltration.

If serum levels of granulocytes (segmented and banded neutrophils, eosinophils, and basophils) fall below 1,500/mm^3, the risk of infection is approximately 12 percent. If the granulocyte level falls below 100/mm^3, nearly 100 percent of clients will develop serious infections [28]. The severity of infection and the mortality rate correlate with the level of granulocytopenia and its duration. Septic phenomena are associated with a total white cell count of less than 2,000/mm^3. A total white cell count of less than 1,000/mm^3 is considered to be life-threatening.

Bacteremia of undetermined origin and pneumonia are the most common infections among cancer clients. Over half of the cases of bacteremia are associated with gram-negative bacteria, especially *Escherichia coli, Pseudomonas aeruginosa,* and *Klebsiella pneumoniae.* Although fungal sepsis is much less common, fungal superinfections are found upon autopsy in approximately half of people with leukemia or lymphoma [28].

The prognosis of the leukopenic client with sepsis is dependent upon several factors. The causative organism itself influences prognosis. *Pseudomonas, Klebsiella, Candida,* and polymicrobial infections have a mortality rate greater than 50 percent. The source of the infection affects prognosis, with pulmonary infections being associated with at least a 70 percent mortality. Also important are the degree and duration of neutropenia. A granulocyte count less than 500/mm^3 is associated with a 40 percent mortality rate, and granulocytopenia persisting for more than ten days increases the mortality rate to more than 80 percent. If septic shock develops, mortality is approximately 70 percent [28].

The nursing and medical care provided to persons with significant leukopenia profoundly affects both prognosis and mortality. For a description of skillful nursing measures that can minimize or prevent the adverse complications of leukopenia, refer to Chapter 7.

THROMBOCYTOPENIA

Thrombocytopenia is an oncologic complication that may become life-threatening. Since uncontrolled bleeding is the direct cause of death in 7 percent of all persons with cancer [12], thrombocytopenia must be treated as a grave condition necessitating aggressive care.

Thrombocytopenia is most often caused by bone marrow invasion by malignant cells and/or marrow hypoplasia secondary to chemotherapy. Hemorrhage due to thrombocytopenia is particularly common in persons with leukemia. More than half of all clients with acute myelocytic leukemia exhibit an increased bleeding tendency at the time of diagnosis, and major hemorrhage is most likely to occur during uncontrolled leukemic proliferation (e.g., just after diagnosis or during relapse) [37]. However, since profound thrombocytopenia can result from antineoplastic drugs, hemorrhage is a potential threat to any cancer client undergoing chemotherapy. Delayed marrow suppression secondary to chemotherapy may result in thrombocytopenia even when there is little or no evidence of active disease. Thus, it is important to be aware of the nadir of the specific drugs in use (see Chapter 7). Thrombocytopenia may also result from high-dose external beam radiotherapy to large areas of functioning marrow.

Hemorrhage often occurs in thrombocytopenic clients who are also septic. Thrombocytopenia and leukopenia often occur simultaneously. Hemorrhage may be caused or aggravated by local tissue injury such as infection, trauma, and/or ulceration of mucous membranes. Necrosis and subsequent sloughing of tissue may also cause hemorrhage because of the interruption of vascular integrity.

Life-threatening hemorrhages occur, in descending order of frequency, in the gastrointestinal tract, brain, and lung [12]. If the platelet count is less than $50,000/mm^3$, hemorrhage may be induced by relatively mild trauma. If the platelet count is less than $20,000/mm^3$, hemorrhage may occur spontaneously. Factors that increase vulnerability to major hemorrhage in the thrombocytopenic client include mucosal ulceration, infection, peptic ulcer, surgery, and arteriosclerosis.

Manifestations of thrombocytopenia include markedly reduced levels of circulating platelets, petechiae, bruises, and ecchymoses. Platelet counts are the best indicators of bleeding tendencies. However, since many leukemic clients have platelets that do not function normally, serious bleeding may occur even if platelet levels are greater than $20,000/mm^3$.

Appropriate nursing and medical care significantly reduces the risk of major hemorrhage in thrombocytopenic clients. For a description of appropriate nursing measures that will minimize or prevent hemorrhage secondary to thrombocytopenia, refer to Chapter 7.

For gravely low platelet levels, platelet transfusions may be prescribed. One unit of infused platelets will increase the circulating platelet level by 12,000 to 15,000/mm^3 [37], thus minimizing risk of hemorrhage and prolonging survival. The life span of infused platelets, however, may be as low as one to three days. Thus, multiple infusions of platelets are frequently necessary to prevent hemorrhage in the client with profound thrombocytopenia, and it is not uncommon for these clients to receive daily transfusions until the underlying problem is corrected. Prophylactic transfusions may be used if the platelet count is less than 20,000/mm^3 even in the absence of bleeding.

If platelet transfusions fail to achieve higher levels of circulating platelets, the refractory state phenomenon should be suspected. Platelet concentrates for infusion are usually prepared from random donor blood without histocompatibility typing and cross-matching, and the presence of human leukocyte antigens (HLA) stimulate the client's immune system to destroy the foreign platelets. Development of the refractory state is almost inevitable in persons who receive multiple platelet transfusions. Ensuring that the transfusion is typed and cross-matched will minimize platelet destruction but will not prevent the refractory state from occurring.

DISSEMINATED INTRAVASCULAR COAGULATION (DIC)

Disseminated intravascular coagulation (DIC) is an oncologic emergency in which the paradox of concurrent thrombus and hemorrhage occurs [13, 23]. In normal homeostasis, there is a dynamic balance between coagulation, fibrinolysis, and reticuloendothelial system function. When normal homeostasis exists, damage to a blood vessel activates the Hagemen factor (factor XII) and coagulation begins. Platelets adhere to the damaged area and release platelet factors. In the presence of these platelet factors, six plasma proteins (factors V, VIII, IX, X, XI, and XII) activate the intrinsic coagulation system. The injured tissue itself releases thromboplastin, thus activating the extrinsic coagulation system and converting prothrombin to thrombin. Both the intrinsic and extrinsic coagulation systems liberate free thrombin into the circulatory system, producing clotting and maintaining vascular integrity at the damaged site. Formation of the fibrin clot then activates the fibrinolytic system. Fibrinolysis, also known as plasmin, is produced and the clot is eventually dissolved. End-products of the fibrinolytic system are called fibrin split products. These are anticoagulants and are removed from the circulation by the reticuloendothelial system.

DIC occurs as a result of abnormal acceleration of the normal clotting process. This acceleration results in a decrease in circulating clotting factors and platelets. Bleeding results from the depletion of coagulation factors by excessive intravascular clotting (see Figure 13.1). Thrombin is abnormally released into the circulatory system, fibrinogen is converted to fibrin, and platelet aggregation is accelerated. This ongoing process consumes excessive amounts of fibrinogen, prothrombin, platelets, and coagulation factors V and VIII. Fibrin strands are disseminated throughout the microcirculation [2], and large amounts of fibrin are found in areas of relative circulatory stasis. This phenomenon causes thrombus formation. Fibrin split products, which are anticoagulants, cause bleeding. This bleeding is further worsened by the depletion of fibrinogen, platelets, and procoagulants. As levels of fibrinogen, platelets, and factors V and VIII fall below that which is necessary for normal homeostasis, hemorrhage begins and normal adaptive clotting is not possible. Thus, DIC results in:

1. Fibrin thrombi in small vessels
2. Thrombosis in large arteries and veins, especially in areas surrounding indwelling catheters

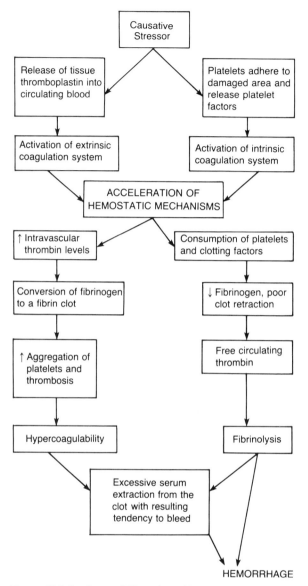

Figure 13.1. Syndrome of Disseminated Intravascular Coagulation.

3. Pulmonary emboli
4. Excessive consumption of plasma coagulation factors
5. Excessive aggregation and consumption of platelets
6. Activation of the fibrinolytic system
7. Hemorrhage

Three distinct forms of DIC have been documented in association with malignancies: hemorrhagic, thrombotic, and subclinical (asymptomatic). The common pathophysiological phenomenon is thought to be the release of thromboplastin-like material from the malignant tumor itself.

Hemorrhagic DIC

Hemorrhagic DIC is found in about 10 percent of all cancer clients and in a large percentage of persons with acute promyelocytic leukemia [28]. This condition is associated with sepsis, liver dysfunction, surgery, acute leukemia with very high leukocyte counts, and acute leukemia that is being actively treated. Hemorrhagic DIC has the most serious prognosis, with one study revealing that 75 percent of clients died within thirty days of diagnosis [28].

Thrombotic DIC

The thrombotic form of DIC is associated with thrombophlebitis, nonbacterial thrombotic endocarditis, and small vessel occlusions with micro-infarcts. The small vessel occlusions are most commonly found in the kidneys and/or brain. Thrombotic DIC is most often seen in persons with malignancies of the pancreas, lung, stomach, or ovary.

Most fibrin thrombi become lodged in small vessels, especially in the glomerular capillaries, dermal capillaries, venules, and the small vessels of the lung, myocardium, adrenal glands, testes, and/or the choroid plexus. Occluding fibrin thrombi may result in hemorrhage or bilateral renal cortical necrosis progressing to acute renal failure.

Subclinical DIC

Subclinical or asymptomatic DIC is the most common form of the syndrome and is defined as the laboratory confirmation of fibrinolysis in an asymptomatic client. Chronic subclinical DIC is more commonly found in clients with metastatic disease and in persons with cancers of the prostate, lung, breast, or pancreas.

Manifestations of DIC

Laboratory findings in DIC reveal common abnormalities (see Table 13.1). Clotting times are usually increased, and quantities of coagulation factors V, VII, VIII, and X are usually decreased. Fibrinogen and platelet levels are low, clot formation is poor, and hemolytic anemia is common. Fibrin split products are usually elevated; this is the most sensitive test for the diagnosis of DIC.

Clinical assessment of the cancer client with DIC will usually reveal a predisposition to hemorrhage associated with sepsis, hypotension, major thoracic surgical procedures, or acute promyelocytic leukemia. An early sign of DIC is abnormal bleeding from a venipuncture site. Organ failure resulting from infarction or bleeding is also common. For example, there may be renal insufficiency or failure, a sudden onset of heart failure, or sudden signs of central nervous system failure (e.g., stroke-like symptoms or seizure activity). Shock may follow organ failure.

Table 13.1.   Laboratory Findings in Disseminated Intravascular Coagulation

Test	Abnormality in DIC
Partial thromboplastin time (PTT)	↑ (>60–90 seconds)
Prothrombin time (PT)	↑ (>15 seconds)
Thrombin time	↑ (>15–20 seconds)
Coagulation Factor V	↓
Coagulation Factor VII	↓
Coagulation Factor VIII	↓
Coagulation Factor X	↓
Fibrinogen	↓ (<75 mg/100 ml)
Fibrin split products	↑ (>100 mcg %)
Platelets	↓ (20,000–75,000/mm³)
Clot formation	Poor

Medical Treatment

Since DIC is always a syndrome secondary to another pathological process, the primary medical treatment for acute disseminated intravascular coagulation is to treat the underlying disease. Underlying sepsis, hypovolemia and hypotension, hypoxia, and acidosis may be treated curatively. An underlying malignancy that is causing DIC may not be able to be treated curatively but supportive medical and nursing interventions may be life-saving.

Although the literature reveals much controversy, heparin is the most commonly recommended medical treatment for DIC [2]. Heparin prevents thrombin from converting fibrinogen into fibrin, thus inhibiting intravascular clotting and stopping hemorrhage. However, heparin therapy can be extremely hazardous if the client is thrombocytopenic and so is usually reserved for those individuals with severe clinical bleeding.

Nursing Treatment

Skillful nursing measures may minimize or prevent the adverse effects associated with DIC and allow for earlier medical intervention. Adverse effects of medical treatment with heparin must also be prevented.

Since a major manifestation of disseminated intravascular coagulation is hemorrhage, nursing assessments and interventions should be planned so as to prevent bleeding. Monitor the client for slow bleeding from a venipuncture site, which is an early sign of DIC. Assess daily for petechiae, ecchymoses, purpura, acral cyanosis (cyanosis of the extremities), subcutaneous hematomas following parenteral injections, hematuria, gastrointestinal bleeding, and bleeding of the mucous membranes. If DIC is suspected, institute protective hemorrhage precautions as specified for thrombocytopenia (see Chapter 7).

Failure of the kidneys, lungs, and central nervous system is a frequent sequelae of uncontrolled DIC. Monitor the client for renal insufficiency progressing to acute renal failure. Renal insufficiency may be manifested by oliguria or anuria accompanied by signs of fluid overload, but the laboratory abnormalities usually found in acute renal failure may or may not occur. Pulmonary failure resulting from DIC may be manifested by the sudden onset of rales, dyspnea, cyanosis, and hemoptysis. The chest X-ray usually reveals a characteristic "shock lung" appearance, and tachypnea and orthopnea may occur. Central nervous system failure may be manifested by stroke-like symptoms, a change in the level of consciousness, and/or seizures.

Shock can be both a cause and an effect of DIC. As the microcirculation becomes plugged with fibrin, blood return to the right side of the heart lessens and thus cardiac output is significantly reduced. The presence of shock, a high central venous pressure, and little or no pulmonary edema may indicate shock secondary to pulmonary intravascular coagulation. If signs and symptoms of shock are present and if DIC is suspected, institute emergency measures to combat shock and assist with medical treatment for DIC.

Anemia secondary to blood loss often occurs secondary to DIC. Monitor clients at risk for complaints of fatigue, weakness, and/or malaise. Assess the skin, conjunctivae, and mucous membranes daily for pallor or signs of bleeding. If DIC and resulting bleeding are suspected, institute nursing measures to decrease oxygen demand and increase oxygen supply until the bleeding has been corrected. Transfusion of erythrocytes and administration of oxygen may be prescribed.

Monitor the client's response to heparin therapy. Heparinization is usually continued as long as the acute underlying pathology is still active, which is usually between three and five days. Monitor serial coagulation studies through and beyond the period of heparin therapy to observe for and report continued improvement or exacerbation of the DIC syndrome.

HYPERCALCEMIA

Hypercalcemia is a common and potentially fatal metabolic complication of malignancy. The body's dynamic equilibrium between calcium intake, usage, and loss results from a sensitive regulatory mechanism involving parathyroid hormone (PTH), vitamin D, and calcitonin [11]. Activated vitamin D is necessary in order to absorb calcium from foods. PTH is normally secreted by the parathyroid glands in response to a decrease in serum calcium levels. PTH promotes resorption of bone, a process in which bone is broken down, thus releasing calcium into the serum. The presence of PTH is necessary for the activation of vitamin D. Calcitonin is a hormone secreted by the thyroid gland and causes a lowering of serum calcium levels.

Ninety-nine percent of the body's calcium is in the bones, and 1 percent is in the serum. Half of the serum calcium is ionized and is biologically active. The other half is bound to circulating proteins, primarily albumin, and is not biologically active. If the serum albumin level is low, the total serum calcium level reported by the laboratory will be falsely low.

Calcium maintains bones, teeth, normal clotting mechanisms, and cellular permeability. Changes in the serum calcium level will alter the excitability of nervous tissue and the contractility of cardiac, smooth, and skeletal muscles.

The most common cause of hypercalcemia in persons with cancer is metastatic involvement of bones. These metastatic tumors result in excessive bone breakdown and the mobilization of calcium into the serum [4]. The most common mechanism responsible for this phenomenon is direct invasion of the bone by tumor cells, and it is thought to be initially mediated by malignant cell release of prostaglandins. More than 80 percent of cancer clients with hypercalcemia have demonstrable bony metastases.

Another mechanism responsible for increased bone resorption and resulting hypercalcemia is the ectopic production of PTH or a PTH-like substance by the malignant tumor itself [6, 28]. This phenomenon probably accounts for most cases of hypercalcemia in which there are no demonstrable bony metastases. Renal cell carcinoma and squamous cell carcinomas of the lung, head, or neck are most commonly associated with ectopic PTH production.

Several factors have been identified that may aggravate and worsen the hypercalcemia of malignancy. Prolonged immobility, for example, may result in excessive bone resorption and subsequent aggravation of hypercalcemia. Normal muscular activity appears to be a requirement for normal bone resorption-accretion balance. This effect of immobility is very rapid, with increased bone resorption occurring within a few days and continuing for the duration of the immobility.

Hormonal treatment of breast cancer when bone metastases are present may stimulate the growth of bone tumors and subsequently worsen hypercalcemia [6, 36]. Dehydration and volume depletion in a hypercalcemic client may precipitate a life-threatening situation.

Signs and Symptoms of Hypercalcemia

Manifestations of hypercalcemia may include varying degrees of dysfunction in the neuromuscular, gastrointestinal, renal, and/or cardiac systems. Dysfunction may occur in one, a combination, or all of the systems.

Generalized muscle weakness is a result of decreased neuromuscular irritability and electrical changes in the cell membranes. Fatigue and headache may occur, and excessive sleepiness may progress to coma. Deep tendon reflexes, muscle tone, and muscle strength diminish. Deficits in visual and hearing acuity may be present.

Gastrointestinal signs and symptoms of hypercalcemia include anorexia, nausea, and constipation. Diminished bowel sounds and abdominal tenderness are common.

Polyuria secondary to the effects of a high calcium concentration in the renal tubules occurs, and polydipsia and dehydration resulting from the polyuria follow. The kidneys begin to excrete larger amounts of calcium into the urine, resulting in deposits of calcium salts throughout the tubules and collecting ducts. This will eventually cause kidney stones.

Cardiovascular symptoms may be produced both by deposits of calcium salts in the aorta and arterial walls and by changes in cardiac function resulting from the high serum calcium level. Deposits of calcium salts in arterial walls will cause increased total peripheral resistance to the flow of blood, resulting in hypertension. Changes in cardiac function include an increase in contractile strength, tachycardia, a depressed T-wave, and a shortened Q-T interval.

Medical Treatment

Medical management of the hypercalcemia of malignancy depends upon the clinical condition of the client and the degree of calcium elevation. If the total serum calcium level is less than 13 mg./100 ml., hydration with intravenous saline solution may be all that is necessary. Increased sodium delivery to the proximal tubules of the kidneys promotes excretion of calcium [8], and intravenous fluids will also correct dehydration and reduce the risk of kidney stone formation.

If the total serum calcium level is 13 to 15 mg./100 ml., concurrent administration of intravenous saline solution and furosemide (Lasix) may effectively reduce serum calcium levels [28]. Furosemide is commonly used because it acts by decreasing the renal reabsorption of both sodium and calcium. Thiazide diuretics, however, are contraindicated because they inhibit renal excretion of calcium.

Corticosteroids may be used to decrease the serum calcium level. Corticosteroids are particularly indicated for hypercalcemia associated with breast cancer, myeloma, and lymphoma. Although the precise mechanism is unknown, corticosteroids seem to decrease further bone resorption of calcium and have an antineoplastic effect on the tumor itself [24].

If hypercalcemia is unresponsive to treatment or if the serum calcium level is greater than 15 mg./100 ml., a single intravenous dose of mithramycin will usually reverse the hypercalcemic process within 24 to 48 hours. Since the cause of hypercalcemia in cancer clients is fundamentally the malignancy itself, control of subsequent hypercalcemia depends upon control of the cancer.

Nursing Treatment

Monitor clients at risk for symptoms indicative of hypercalcemia, realizing that many of the symptoms are vague and could be attributed to a number of other common conditions. An elevated serum calcium level is diagnostic, however, as is a high-normal serum calcium level with a concurrent low serum albumin level.

Intravenous hydration may result in fluid overload, so assessment of fluid, electrolyte, cardiac, and renal status is important. Weigh the client daily, monitoring for an unexplained increase in weight. Monitor intake and output records. Assess vital signs regularly for signs of fluid overload: hypertension and tachycardia. Auscultate breath sounds every eight hours for pulmonary congestion.

The administration of furosemide (Lasix) may result in electrolyte imbalance. Monitor for signs and symptoms of hypokalemia and hyponatremia. Clients who are also taking digitalis should be watched closely for signs of digitalis toxicity.

Reduce immobility as much as possible. Hospitalized clients should be ambulated as soon as possible and frequently. Outpatients must be taught the importance of frequent and regular exercise. Since the hypercalcemia of malignancy is primarily due to bone destruction by metastases, restriction of the dietary intake of calcium is usually not necessary.

CONCEPT V:
The syndrome of inappropriate antidiuretic hormone secretion (SIADH) is an endocrine complication of certain types of cancer and antineoplastic treatment [20].

The syndrome of inappropriate antidiuretic hormone secretion (SIADH) is defined as hyponatremia and hyposmolality secondary to the secretion of antidiuretic hormone (ADH) in the absence of normal physiological stimuli for ADH secretion. In other words, ADH is secreted inappropriately, and the client develops hyponatremia and hyposmolality as a result.

The primary role of ADH is to promote reabsorption of water by the kidney. In the absence of circulating ADH, the renal tubules and ducts are relatively impermeable to water. Little water is absorbed, urine flow rate is high, and urine osmolality is low. In the presence of circulating ADH, the renal tubules and ducts exhibit an increased permeability to water. Increased amounts of water are reabsorbed, urine flow rate is lower, and urine osmolality is higher. ADH has no significant effect on the rate of sodium reabsorption. ADH is synthesized in the hypothalamus and stored in the pituitary. Increased serum osmolality causes increased ADH release, resulting in water retention. Increased blood volume causes decreased ADH release, resulting in increased water excretion.

Several criteria have been established for the diagnosis of SIADH:

1. Hyponatremia and hyposmolality
2. Continuing sodium loss by the kidney
3. Inappropriately high urine osmolality
4. Absence of hypovolemia
5. Normal adrenal and renal function

SIADH may be caused by certain types of malignancies, intracranial complications of cancer, surgery, and the administration of vincristine (an antineoplastic drug). In clients with oat-cell bronchogenic cancer or with carcinomas of the pancreas or duodenum, it is thought that the tumor itself releases a high concentration of a substance that is physiologically identical to ADH. Meningitis, brain tumors, brain abscesses, and encephalitis are all associated with SIADH. Owing to the combination of hemorrhage and trauma, surgery may precipitate SIADH. Finally, vincristine administration may cause inappropriate release of antidiuretic hormone.

SIGNS AND SYMPTOMS OF SIADH

Manifestations of SIADH are identical to those of water intoxication. The client may be asymptomatic if the diagnosis is made early; but as osmolality falls, mild symptoms of anorexia and nausea appear. As hyponatremia becomes more severe (110–120 mEq/L.), changes in mentation and behavior develop. If serum sodium falls below 110 mEq/L., neurological signs such as decreased reflexes, marked weakness, a positive Babinski response, and stupor appear. At still lower sodium levels, seizure activity and death can occur.

A factor in symptom occurrence and severity is the rapidity with which SIADH develops. If the condition develops quickly, the guidelines listed above are generally true. If SIADH develops slowly, as in clients who experience tumor-caused SIADH, the body tends to adapt and symptoms appear later in the pathological process.

Hyponatremia is a result of fluid retention and is partially the result of hemodilution. The continuing urinary loss of sodium despite significant hyponatremia contributes to further reductions in serum sodium levels. Hyponatremia may also be partially due to sodium entering the cell where it becomes osmotically inactive.

The absence of decreased blood volume is an important diagnostic criterion since hypovolemia causes an *appropriate* release of ADH. Normal renal and adrenal functions are important to establish, since dysfunction of either organ can mimic SIADH but must be treated differently.

MEDICAL TREATMENT

The treatment of choice for the syndrome of inappropriate antidiuretic hormone release is simple fluid restriction since the inability to excrete water normally is central to the development of the condition. Fluid restriction causes a gradual fall in blood volume, and urinary sodium excretion will then decrease. Sodium that has abnormally entered the cell will tend to be released back into the serum, also raising serum sodium levels. Thus, the amount of sodium in the serum will gradually return to normal. Fluid restriction is the safest medical therapy and thus may be used prophylactically for clients at risk.

Intravenous infusion of hypertonic saline solution carries significant risk and thus is only appropriate for those clients whose serum sodium is so low that seizures or coma are present [10]. Hypertonic saline infusions are not generally useful for most clients with SIADH because of the already expanded intravascular blood volume. In addition, it further decreases renal reabsorption of sodium and makes the client vulnerable to fluid overload and congestive heart failure. In those clients for whom intravenous saline administration is appropriate, this treatment may be life-saving but should be immediately followed by strict fluid restriction.

The use of diuretics such as furosemide (Lasix) or ethacrynic acid (Edecrin) plus the concurrent fluid replacement of the amount of urine output has been recommended for treatment of symptomatic SIADH. The replacement fluid should be relatively hypertonic saline solution. Unlike larger amounts of intravenous hypertonic saline solution, this medical treatment protocol inhibits the formation of hypertonic urine. Instead, a large volume of nearly isotonic urine is formed and excreted. If this volume of urine is replaced with an intravenous saline solution, it is possible to rapidly increase the client's serum sodium level. This medical treatment protocol, however, carries with it the risk of severe fluid and electrolyte imbalances.

Ethanol may effectively reverse SIADH since it is a powerful inhibitor of ADH secretion. Oral or nasogastric tube administration of ethanol will often produce large volumes or hypotonic urine. Ethanol administration has few significant adverse side effects.

Lithium inhibits the effects of ADH and so may be used to treat SIADH. Lithium may produce prompt water diuresis with rapid correction of the hyponatremia. However, this is not a benign drug and carries with it significant risks. Signs of lithium toxicity include sluggishness, drowsiness, tremor, muscle twitching, and gastrointestinal disturbances. It is difficult to differentiate between lithium toxicity and severe hyponatremia since many of the signs and symptoms are identical.

NURSING TREATMENT

Identify clients at risk and monitor them carefully for signs and symptoms indicative of SIADH. These include anorexia and nausea, hyponatremia, fluid retention, behavior changes, diminished reflexes, muscle weakness, a positive Babinski response, stupor, seizures, and/or coma.

Prevent the adverse effects of medical treatment for SIADH. Monitor the client for the development of fluid overload. Assess carefully for electrolyte imbalances if diuretics are used. Monitor serum sodium levels for a rise to normal.

CONCEPT VI:
The malignant process may cause renal complications and emergencies.

URETERAL OBSTRUCTION

Ureteral obstruction can progressively destroy renal function. Obstructive uropathy causes dysfunction of all aspects of renal function but does not reduce the kidney's ability to actually produce urine. If infection does not occur, renal function may return even after fifty to seventy days of obstruction [28].

The most common cause of ureteral obstruction in persons with cancer include renal calculi, urinary tract injuries, abscesses, and extrinsic compression by neoplasms. The condition often has an insidious onset, with the first clinically detectable abnormality being acute renal failure. However, other abnormalities may occur, such as fever due to infection or flank pain, gastrointestinal disturbances, and microscopic hematuria due to renal calculi. Anorexia and subsequent weight loss secondary to the malignancy may be seen. Hypertension is a result of increased renin release, and urinary tract trauma in postsurgical clients is often reflected by prolonged ileus, abdominal pain, and fever.

Oliguria secondary to acute tubular necrosis, hypovolemia, or shock must be ruled out. It is rare for these conditions to cause the absolute anuria characteristic of bilateral ureteral obstruction.

If the obstruction is directly caused by the underlying malignancy, the physician may choose to perform a temporary nephrostomy in order to restore renal function until the obstruction is resolved. Malignant tumors that are extrinsically compressing the ureters may be treated by external beam radiotherapy and/or chemotherapy.

Appropriate nursing measures may prevent adverse complications until the ureteral obstruction is corrected. Monitor fluid and electrolyte balance to prevent the development of fluid overload, hyperkalamia, and hyponatremia. Monitor serum levels of uric acid to prevent the development of uric acid nephropathy.

URIC ACID NEPHROPATHY

Uric acid nephropathy may develop from the administration of chemotherapy and often results in oliguric acute renal failure [19, 27]. Hyperuricemia, or an elevated serum uric acid level, is often seen in clients with large tumor masses that have a high cell turnover. Clients with leukemia or lymphoma are particularly vulnerable to the development of hyperuricemia. Administration of chemotherapy to these clients may precipitate or worsen the hyperuricemia because of the large numbers of tumor cells that are killed. This high cell kill results in increased destruction of nucleoproteins and a subsequent increase in serum uric acid levels.

Hyperuricemia may progress to uric acid nephropathy and oliguric renal failure. Uric acid crystals may precipitate and deposit in the kidney, causing obstruction of urine flow. These crystals cause renal parenchymal damage. Interstitial inflammation and scarring occur in the kidney tissue.

The primary medical treatment for hyperuricemia is preventive in nature. Routine oral administration of allopurinol (Zyloprim) to clients at risk will inhibit uric acid formation. Prevention of hyperuricemia is particularly important for leukemia and lymphoma clients who are undergoing chemotherapy.

If hyperuricemia develops, medical treatment focuses on the prevention of uric acid nephropathy and renal damage. Allopurinol (Zyloprim) is administered to prevent further uric acid formation, and adequate hydration is maintained. Intravenous fluids are prescribed as appropriate. A high urine flow will dilute uric acid crystals in the kidneys and reduce the incidence of crystal deposits in renal tissue. Alkalinization of the urine is important to reduce the risk of uric acid stones. Sodium bicarbonate or acetazolamide (Diamox) may be administered to alkalinize the urine. Dialysis, especially hemodialysis, can be very effective in reducing extremely elevated serum uric acid levels.

Nursing treatment is focused on the maintenance of adequate hydration. The client's daily intake should consist of a minimum of three liters of oral or intravenous fluids. Intake and output records must be monitored for signs of oliguria and/or fluid overload. Assess vital signs every eight hours for hypertension and tachycardia that may be indicative of fluid overload. Weigh the client daily, monitoring for an unexplained increase in weight. Auscultate breath sounds daily for rales, and alkalinize the urine by administration of medications as prescribed.

ACUTE RENAL FAILURE

Acute renal failure may develop in persons with cancer as a result of either the disease or its treatment. The condition is characterized by a sudden deterioration in kidney function with concurrent rapidly progressive azotemia. Prerenal azotemia results from inadequate renal perfusion and often precedes and predisposes to the development of acute renal failure. Inadequate renal perfusion is caused by a decrease in renal perfusion pressure and/or marked renal vasoconstriction (see Table 13.2). Since the causative factors for prerenal azotemia and acute renal failure overlap, the development of the latter depends upon the outcome of medical and nursing therapy. If volume repletion and improvement of renal perfusion rapidly reverses the azotemia, then prerenal azotemia is diagnosed. If azotemia continues, however, postrenal azotemia or acute renal failure is suspected.

Postrenal azotemia results from obstruction to the flow of urine (see Table 13.3). Obstruction of urine flow may cause oliguria or anuria as well as acute azotemia. Diagnosis and treatment of the obstruction may restore normal renal function un-

Table 13.2.   Causative Stressors Resulting in Prerenal Azotemia [5]

Causative Stressor	Contributing Factors
Volume Depletion	Excessive diuresis
	Hemorrhage
	Excessive loss of gastrointestinal contents
	Third space fluid losses (burns, tissue trauma, peritonitis, pancreatitis)
Cardiovascular Dysfunction	Congestive heart failure
	Acute myocardial infarction
	Pericardial effusion with tamponade
	Acute pulmonary embolism
	Renal artery stenosis, embolus, or thrombus
Peripheral Vasodilation	Gram negative sepsis
	Antihypertensive drugs
Increased Renal Vascular Resistance	Surgery and anesthesia
	Hepatorenal syndrome
	Drugs inhibiting prostaglandin (e.g., aspirin, indomethacin)

less the obstruction has been prolonged to the point of irreversible damage to kidney tissue.

Acute renal failure is characterized by primary renal dysfunction in which azotemia cannot be resolved by the manipulation of factors external to the kidney (e.g., volume repletion, improvement of cardiac function, removal of obstruction, etc.). Acute renal failure in the cancer client may be caused by ischemia and necrosis of renal tissue and/or by nephrotoxic substances (see Table 13.4). The combination of two or more nephrotoxic drugs, such as antibiotics and chemotherapeutic agents, administered at the same time, is more likely to result in acute renal failure. This is especially true if poor renal perfusion is also present.

Table 13.3.   Causative Stressors Resulting in Postrenal Azotemia [5]

Causative Stressor	Contributing Factors
Urethral Obstruction	Urethral valve dysfunction
	Urethral strictures
Obstruction of Neck of Bladder	Prostatic hypertrophy
	Carcinoma of prostate or bladder
	Autonomic neuropathy
Intraureteral Obstruction	Calculi
	Blood clots
	Pyogenic debris
	Edema following surgery or diagnostic procedures
Extraureteral Obstruction	Carcinoma of prostate, bladder, or cervix
	Retroperitoneal fibrosis
	Accidental ureteral ligation or trauma during surgery

Table 13.4. Cancer-Related Stressors Resulting in Acute Renal Failure [9]

Causative Stressor	Contributing Factors
Ischemia and Necrosis of Renal Tissue	Tumor invasion of the kidney
	Radiation nephritis
	Nephrotic syndrome
	Vasomotor collapse and hypotension
Nephrotoxic Substances	Tumor breakdown products (hyperuricemia, hypercalcemia, abnormal proteins)
	Nephrotoxic antineoplastic drugs
	Nephrotoxic antibiotics

Signs and Symptoms of Acute Renal Failure

The kidneys largely control the body's fluid, electrolyte, and acid-base balance and are primarily responsible for the excretion of the body's metabolic wastes and excesses. Thus, manifestations of acute renal failure directly reflect the kidney's inability to carry out its normal functions.

Signs and symptoms that reflect tubular damage and loss of concentrating ability include *oliguria, a decreased urine specific gravity,* and *rising urine osmolality.* The urine osmolality eventually will reach a level near that of serum osmolality (280–320 mOsm.).

Fluid retention occurs secondary to the kidney's inability to excrete water normally. Dependent and/or periorbital edema is frequently seen, and the increased blood volume results in hypertension. The client often gains weight and displays shortness of breath and pulmonary congestion. Signs of *congestive heart failure* may appear, including heart murmur, tachycardia, tachypnea, pallor or cyanosis, and fatigue.

The retention of metabolic waste products results in the development of an *internal uremic environment.* Azotemia is present: increased blood urea nitrogen, increased serum creatinine, and increased serum uric acid. *Anemia* secondary to bleeding and/or reduced production of erythropoietin is common. Erythropoietin is a kidney-produced hormone that stimulates production of red blood cells. Since the damaged kidney is unable to produce normal amounts of this hormone, production of red blood cells falls. Complicating the deficit in erythrocyte production is the fact that the cell life of the erythrocyte is shortened in the uremic environment. *Defective platelet function* results in gastrointestinal bleeding, petechiae, and bruises; and the uremic environment causes a *nonspecific gastritis* with nausea, vomiting, anorexia, and diarrhea. *Central nervous system dysfunction* is common and is caused by acidosis, hypocalcemia, hyperphosphatemia, hyperkalemia, and hypernatremia. The client may exhibit lethargy, weakness, mental depression, tremors progressing to seizure activity, coma, and peripheral neuropathy (numbness and tingling in the fingers and toes). The *immune system* is suppressed by the uremic environment, predisposing the client to infection. *Metabolic acidosis* occurs secondary to the retention of acidotic nitrogenous waste products. *Electrolyte imbalances* commonly include hyperkalemia, hypocalcemia, hypernatremia, and hyperphosphatemia. *Precordial pain* and *pericarditis* may occur and result from pericardial irritation from the accumulated nitrogenous wastes in the bloodstream. *Pruritus* is caused by the precipitation of urate crystals on the skin, and *halitosis* is due both to acidosis and to the presence of urea in the saliva.

Medical Treatment

Medical management of acute renal failure includes the following goals: (1) restoration of fluid balance, (2) treatment of precipitating causes, (3) monitoring of drug usage, (4) restoration of normal electrolyte balance, and (5) restoration of normal acid-base balance [14].

Restoration of fluid balance is achieved by fluid restriction. Fluid intake should be limited to replacement of measured losses plus four hundred milliliters per day to compensate for insensible losses. The oliguric client should then lose about 0.5 kilograms of body weight per day. Fluid overload may precipitate pulmonary edema and/or congestive heart failure, so the fluid restriction must be monitored carefully.

Treatment of precipitating causes should include looking for and treating sepsis or covert infection. Since many drugs are dependent upon renal excretion, most antibiotics, chemotherapeutic agents, sedatives, and narcotics must be administered in decreased dosages to clients with acute renal failure.

Correction of electrolyte imbalances may be accomplished through diet, intravenous fluids, and/or drugs. Treatment of hyperkalemia includes correction of acidosis; if the hyperkalemia is severe, an intravenous glucose and insulin solution may be administered to drive serum potassium into the cells. Treatment of hyperphosphatemia includes the administration of phosphate-binding gels or, in severe cases, dialysis. Calcium is administered to clients who are hypocalcemic, and the restoration of normal acid-base balance may include the administration of sodium bicarbonate to correct acidosis.

Nursing Treatment

Appropriate nursing measures will help return the client with acute renal failure to physiological equilibrium and normal renal function. Clients who are particularly at risk for the development of acute renal failure should be identified and watched closely. Persons who have experienced tumor invasion of the kidney or who have received radiotherapy to the area of the kidneys carry a high risk of acute renal failure, and nephrotoxic drugs (especially if given in combination) predispose to the condition. Clients with the nephrotic syndrome, hypovolemia, hypotension, or high serum levels of tumor breakdown products are also at risk.

All clients at risk should be routinely assessed for the signs and symptoms indicative of renal insufficiency. Intake and output records must be monitored for oliguria progressing to anuria. Edema, rapid weight gain, hypertension, tachycardia, and other signs of congestive heart failure should be reported. Kussmaul respirations ("air hunger") is a compensatory mechanism for metabolic acidosis, and rales, pulmonary congestion, and shortness of breath indicate fluid overload. Neurological signs and symptoms may be vague and difficult to pinpoint. They include headache, blurred vision, personality changes, irritability, malaise, a decreased level of consciousness, tremors or seizure activity, and/or peripheral neuropathy. Fatigue, pallor, and weakness are often indicative of anemia, a condition that usually accompanies acute renal failure. Bruises, petechiae, and signs of gastrointestinal bleeding should make the nurse suspect thrombocytopenia. Infection often accompanies the abnormally low leukocyte level so frequently found in acute renal failure. Nausea, vomiting, anorexia, and diarrhea are signs of nonspecific gastritis but are often attributable to other stressors. Laboratory evidence of acute renal failure includes an increased blood urea nitrogen (BUN), increased serum creatinine, increased serum uric acid, anemia, and metabolic acidosis. Serum electrolytes show skewed values: increased serum potassium, increased serum sodium, hyperphosphatemia, and hypocalcemia.

When acute renal failure has been diagnosed, a primary nursing concern is to reduce the workload of the kidneys. Maintain adequate nutrition with a low-protein, low-sodium, low-potassium, high-carbohydrate diet. This diet reduces protein catabolism, thus reducing the amount of nitrogenous waste material that must be handled by the kidney. Restrict fluids as prescribed, encouraging the client to choose the distribution of allowed fluids. Teach the client to avoid salt substitutes and to read labels on processed foods. Salt substitutes are low in sodium but very high in potassium, and many processed foods are high in sodium. Restrict the client's activity in order to decrease the metabolic rate and thus reduce the kidney's workload; for the same reason, it is important that any infections be treated adequately and promptly.

When acute renal failure exists, there is a delicate balance between fluid overload and fluid deficit. The client requires fluids (oral or intravenous) in order to maintain this balance, but fluid overload and subsequent congestive heart failure are dangerous complications. Administer diuretics as prescribed, and maintain accurate intake and output records. If acute renal failure is due to stressors other than acute tubular necrosis, the kidney has not lost its ability to make urine and diuretics will be successful in increasing urine output and reestablishing renal function. However, diuretics will not be successful if acute tubular necrosis exists. Restrict fluids as prescribed, encouraging the client to choose the distribution of allowed fluids. Weigh the client daily and assess for changes in the client's weight indicative of fluid retention or fluid loss. Monitor for hypertension, and observe for distended neck veins and/or dependent edema. Auscultate the lungs at least daily, assessing for pulmonary rales and congestion. Observe for tachycardia and signs of poor perfusion of the skin, mucous membranes, and extremities.

Encourage self-care and independence as much as possible without inducing fatigue, and maintain environmental safety. Institute comfort measures as indicated. Give oral care every two to four hours and as needed, and give skin care without soap to decrease pruritus and skin dryness.

CONCEPT VII:
The malignant process may result in bone metastases, resulting in increased vulnerability to pathological fractures.

Bone metastases represent the initial sign of metastatic disease in many clients. Depending upon the primary site and the method of detection, the incidence of bone metastases ranges from 23 percent to 84 percent [34]. The primary symptom associated with bone metastases is pain. Pain may be chronic and debilitating, similar to a diffuse arthritic process; or it may be acute and severe when pathological fractures or vertebral collapse occur. Serum alkaline phosphatase is usually elevated in metastatic bone disease, and life-threatening hypercalcemia can result from bone destruction and the subsequent release of calcium into the serum. Bone lesions may be diagnosed by skeletal X-rays or bone scans. This destruction of normal bone by malignant lesions results in a fragile area of bone that is very vulnerable to fracture from even minor trauma.

MEDICAL TREATMENT

Appropriate medical treatment of bone metastases may shrink the lesions, thus reducing pain as well as decreasing vulnerability to fractures. External beam radiotherapy is the medical treatment of choice for clients with either painful localized bone lesions or with lytic vertebral or long bone metastases. Radiotherapy does not stabilize an already-impending fracture, but it will provide significant relief of pain. Pain relief occurs between two weeks and three months after initiation of radiotherapy. External beam radiotherapy produces permanent pain relief in about 85 percent of clients [7].

If a weight-bearing long bone demonstrates more than 25 percent involvement of the cortex, surgical fixation and stabilization of the affected bone is often the initial medical treatment [7, 28]. Fixation and stabilization may reduce pain, may avoid a pathological fracture, and allow the client to achieve increased mobility. This procedure can often be performed under local anesthesia, and it is associated with less morbidity than treatment of an accomplished fracture. If a pathological fracture has occurred in a long bone, medical treatment usually consists of fixation and stabilization followed by radiotherapy. Systemic chemotherapy and/or hormonal chemotherapy may be effective in reducing bone metastases.

NURSING TREATMENT

Appropriate nursing treatment for the client with metastatic bone lesions help to protect against pathological fractures. Protect the client from trauma. Turn the client carefully, applying pressure near the joints of the long bones rather than in the middle. Align the client properly in bed to reduce strain on ligaments and bones. Monitor for signs indicative of continuing osteolytic activity. These signs include increasing levels of serum alkaline phosphatase and calcium and X-rays or bone scans.

CONCEPT VIII:
The malignant process may cause gastrointestinal complications.

Bowel obstruction is a common gastrointestinal complication and may cause death. Approximately two-thirds of bowel obstructions involve the small intestine, and one-third involve the colorectum. Common causes of bowel obstruction include adhesions, hernias, intra-abdominal neoplasms, and constipation with impaction. The condition is always accompanied by varying degrees of abdominal pain, emesis, obstipation, and abdominal distention. In complete obstruction of the proximal small bowel, vomiting is the primary sign. Metabolic alkalosis occurs because of the loss of hydrogen ions in the massive emesis. Abdominal pain is poorly localized. Manifestations of complete obstruction of the distal small bowel include vomiting, colicky abdominal pain, distention, and constipation progressing to obstipation. Obstruction of the large bowel results in abdominal distention and obstipation. Vomiting and abdominal pain occur later. Hyperperistalsis may occur at first, but the ineffectiveness of the hyperperistalsis to resolve the obstruction results in smooth muscle fatigue and ileus. As smooth muscle fatigue progresses, bowel sounds become decreased or absent. If an ileus develops, the client is usually experiencing constant abdominal pain.

Medical and nursing measures may resolve bowel obstruction and prevent potentially fatal complications. Identify clients who are particularly at risk for this condition. The presence of an intra-abdominal tumor or a hernia makes the client vulnerable to the development of a bowel obstruction. Abdominal surgery or abdominal irradiation may result in adhesions that may cause obstruction. If constipation and impaction cause the obstruction, the client often has received treatment with routine narcotics but without concurrent routine stool softeners. Chemotherapy with the vinca alkaloids may also cause constipation and subsequent bowel obstruction.

Assess the frequency and characteristics of stools in clients at risk. The hyperperistalsis characteristic of early bowel obstruction often results in liquid feces escaping around the obstruction. Treatment of this seeming diarrhea will only worsen the client's condition. Obstipation is an early sign in complete obstruction of the colorectum but a later sign in small bowel obstruction.

Monitor for the development of abdominal pain accompanied by vomiting and abdominal distention. Routinely assess bowel sounds in all four quadrants of the abdomen, and monitor vital signs in clients who have a suspected or known obstruction. In early bowel obstruction, vital signs are usually normal, but fever and shock will result if infarction or perforation of the bowel occurs.

Initial therapy of bowel obstruction is usually focused upon allowing the obstructed bowel to rest. Intravenous fluids and electrolytes are administered, and the client must take nothing by mouth. Intestinal decompression by nasogastric tube is necessary to decrease vomiting, abdominal distention, and potential aspiration of emesis. Abdominal irradiation may be administered to those clients whose bowel obstructions are secondary to radiosensitive tumors, such as lymphoma, and surgery may be necessary if the obstruction has not been resolved by medical management or if strangulation is suspected.

REFERENCES

1. Abrams, R. D. and Victor, M. *Principles of Neurology.* New York: McGraw-Hill, 1977.
2. Bart, J. B. and Dear, C. B. Hematopoietic Disorders. In M. R. Kinney, C. B. Dear, D. R. Packa, and D. M. N. Voorman (Eds.). *AACN's Clinical Reference for Critical Care Nursing.* New York: McGraw-Hill, 1981. Pp. 593–596.
3. Bongiovanni, G. L. The Gastrointestinal Tract and the Liver. In M. R. Kinney, C. B. Dear,

D. R. Packa, and D. M. N. Voorman (Eds.). *AACN's Clinical Reference for Critical Care Nursing.* New York: McGraw-Hill, 1981. Pp. 200.

4. Burt, M. E. and Brennan, M. F. Hypercalcemia and Malignant Melanoma. *Am J Surg* 137:790, 1979.

5. Cronin, R. E. The Patient with Acute Azotemia. In R. W. Schrier (Ed.). *Manual of Nephrology: Diagnosis and Therapy.* Boston: Little, Brown and Co., 1981. Pp. 135–150.

6. Deftos, L. J. and Neer, R. Medical Management of the Hypercalcemia of Malignancy. In L. C. Kruse, J. L. Reese, and L. K. Hart (Eds.). *Cancer: Pathophysiology, Etiology and Management.* St. Louis. C. V. Mosby, 1979. Pp. 349–356.

7. Dewys, W. D. and Taylor, S. G. Metastases and Disseminated Cancer. In P. Rubin (Ed.). *Clinical Oncology for Medical Students and Physicians: A Multidisciplinary Approach* (5th Ed.). New York: American Cancer Society, 1978. Pp. 272–280.

8. Doogan, R. A. Hypercalcemia of Malignancy. *Cancer Nurs* 3:299, 1981.

9. Garnick, M. B. and Mayer, R. J. Acute Renal Failure Associated with Neoplastic Disease and Its Treatment. *Semin Oncol* 5:155, 1978.

10. Glass, J. P., Melamed, M., Chernik, N. L., and Posner, J. B. Malignant Cells in Cerebrospinal Fluid (CSF): The Meaning of a Positive CSF Cytology. *Neurology* 29:1369, 1979.

11. Groer, M. W. *Physiology and Pathophysiology of the Body Fluids.* St. Louis: C. V. Mosby, 1981. Pp. 196–201.

12. Inagaki, J., Rodriguez, V., and Bodey, G. P. Causes of Death in Cancer Patients. *Cancer* 33:568, 1974.

13. Jennings, B. M. DIC: Recognizing Impending Catastrophe. In H. Hamilton (Ed.). *Nursing Critically Ill Patients Confidently.* Horsham, PA: Intermed Communications, 1979. Pp. 167–180.

14. Leaf, A. and Cotran, R. S. *Renal Pathophysiology.* New York: Oxford University Press, 1976. P. 161.

15. Leuallen, E. C. and Carr, D. T. Pleural Effusion: A Statistical Study of 436 Patients. *N Engl J Med* 252:79, 1955.

16. Levitt, S., Jones, T., et al. Treatment of Malignant Superior Vena Caval Obstruction: A Randomized Study. *Cancer* 24:447, 1969.

17. Light, R. W., Erozan, Y. S., and Ball, W. C. Cells in Pleural Fluid: Their Value in Differential Diagnosis. *Arch Intern Med* 132:854, 1973.

18. Little, J. R., Dale, A. J. D., and Okazaki, M. S. Meningeal Carcinomatosis: Clinical Implications. *Arch Neurol* 30:138, 1974.

19. Martin, K. J. Renal Disease. In J. J. Freitag and L. W. Miller (Eds.). *Manual of Medical Therapeutics* (23rd Ed.). Boston: Little, Brown and Co., 1980. P. 51.

20. Mendoza, S. A. Syndrome of Inappropriate Antidiuretic Hormone Secretion (SIADH). *Pediatr Clin North Am* 23(1):681, 1976.

21. Merritt, H. H. *A Textbook of Neurology.* Philadelphia: Lea and Febiger, 1979.

22. Miller, F. N. *Pathology* (3rd Ed.). Boston: Little, Brown and Co., 1978. Pp. 42–43, 603.

23. Miller, R. B. The Patient with Chronic Azotemia, with Emphasis on Chronic Renal Failure. In R. W. Schier (Ed.). *Manual of Nephrology: Diagnosis and Therapy.* Boston: Little, Brown and Co., 1981. P. 164.

24. Nissenblatt, M. J. Oncologic Emergencies. *Am Fam Physician* 20:104, 1979.

25. Paillas, J. E. and Pellet, W. Brain Metastasis. In P. J. Vinken and G. W. Bruyn (Eds.). *Handbook of Clinical Neurology.* New York: American Elsevier, 1975. Pp. 201–232.

26. Perez, C. A., Presant, C. A., and Van Amburg, A. L. III. Management of Superior Vena Cava Syndrome. *Semin Oncol* 5:123, 1978.

27. Phillips, G. L. Chemotherapy in Malignant Disease. In J. J. Freitag and L. W. Miller (Eds.). *Manual of Medical Therapeutics* (23rd Ed.). Boston: Little, Brown and Co., 1980. P. 313.

28. Portlock, C. S. and Goffinet, D. R. *Manual of Clinical Problems in Oncology.* Boston: Little, Brown and Co., 1980.

29. Posner, J. B. Management of Central Nervous System Metastases. *Semin Oncol* 4:81, 1977.

30. Posner, J. B. Neurological Complications of Systemic Cancer. *Med Clin North Am* 63:783, 1979.

31. Posner, J. B. Brain Metastases: A Clinician's View. In L. Weiss, H. A. Gilbert, and J. B. Posner (Eds.). *Brain Metastasis.* Boston: G. K. Hall, 1980. Pp. 2–29.

32. Posner, J. B. Clinical Manifestations of Brain Metastases. In L. Weiss, H. A. Gilbert, and J. B. Posner (Eds.). *Brain Metastasis.* Boston: G. K. Hall, 1980. Pp. 189–207.

33. Price, S. A. and Wilson, L. M. *Pathophysiology: Clinical Concepts of Disease Processes* (2nd Ed.). New York: McGraw-Hill, 1982. Pp. 282–284.

34. Rubin, P. Introduction: Bone Metastases. In P. Rubin (Ed.). *Metastases and Disseminated Cancer.* New York: American Cancer Society, 1979. Pp. 131–132.

35. Salyer, W. R., Eggleston, J. C., and Erozan, Y. S. Efficacy of Pleural Needle Biopsy and Pleural Fluid Cytopathology in the Diagnosis of Malignant Neoplasms Involving the Pleura. *Chest* 67:536, 1975.

36. Tattersall, M. H. Hypercalcemia After Tamoxifen for Breast Cancer: A Sign of Tumour Response? *Br Med J* 24:132, 1979.

37. Welch, D. Thrombocytopenia in the Adult Patient with Acute Leukemia. *Cancer Nurs* 1:463, 1978.

Chapter 14

Nutritional Assessment and Management

CONCEPT I:
Malnutrition progressing to cachexia significantly contributes to the morbidity and mortality of cancer.

Most persons with cancer are not malnourished at the time of diagnosis and malnutrition need not be an inevitable consequence of malignancy. The common five- to ten-pound weight loss upon diagnosis is usually a result of anxiety, decreased oral intake, or a partial intestinal obstruction. The initial weight loss may also be associated with theoretical altered metabolic demand resulting from the malignant process. For example, persons with oat-cell (small cell) carcinoma of the lung lose weight rapidly and out of proportion to the extent of the tumor burden. On the other hand, persons with malignant melanoma or breast cancer often remain relatively well-nourished despite widespread disease [7]. Much controversy exists about the possibility of tumor-host competition for nutrients and its relationship to the development of malnutrition and cachexia.

Generally speaking, a decrease in nutritional status parallels an increase in tumor burden [7]. During starvation states, the body obtains its required energy by breaking down tissue protein. This process of protein breakdown is termed *protein catabolism*. Unless approximately 50 percent to 60 percent of a person's caloric requirement is obtained from ingested fats or carbohydrates, protein catabolism will occur [11]. When protein breakdown exceeds protein synthesis, a negative nitrogen balance exists. In the catabolic state, protein depletion in muscles and the liver is extensive. Minimizing protein catabolism is critically important since a rapid loss of approximately one-third of total body protein may be fatal [27]. It is estimated that 30 percent to 100 percent of all persons with advanced cancer have negative nitrogen balance secondary to protein breakdown [1].

Persons with cancer often encounter disease or treatment-related malnutrition, so that "normal" eating or a "regular" diet without supplementation is inadequate for their metabolic needs (see Figure 14.1). The side effects of antineoplastice treatment—nausea, anorexia, dysphagia, altered or diminished taste sensation (dysgeusia, hypogeusia), and early satiety—may be so severe that oral food intake ceases entirely. Cancer-related malnutrition is profoundly affected by diminished oral intake of nutrients, and malnutrition progresses rapidly to cachexia unless early and effective nursing and medical intervention is carried out. Cancer clients who ingest less than one thousand calories and thirty grams of protein daily will experience rapid malnutrition and progressive cachexia.

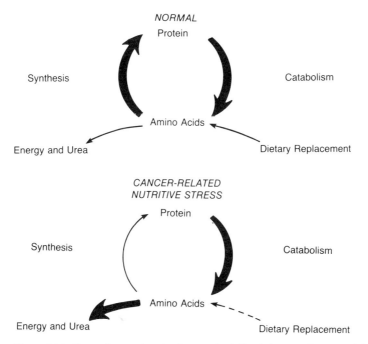

Figure 14.1 Comparison and contrast: normal nutritive balance and cancer-related nutritive stress.

Overt protein-calorie malnutrition is seen in about one-half to two-thirds of both adults and children with cancer [10, 22, 25, 34], and the condition must be diagnosed and treated as definitive problems separate from the malignancy. Malnutrition and cachexia are seen more frequently during relapses rather than at diagnosis or during periods of remission. Incidence may increase as survival times increasingly lengthen. Ewing's sarcoma and neuroblastoma (children) and oat-cell carcinoma of the lung seem to predispose to the development of malnutrition and cachexia. Malignant growths produce profound alterations in host organs, functions, and possibly metabolism. The overall result is malnutrition.

The etiology of cancer-related malnutrition is much more complex than a mere lack of food. Cancer-related cachexia seems to be somewhat different from the cachexia of starvation in that the life-saving physiological feedback mechanisms that occur in the starvation state appear to be impaired in persons with uncontrolled malignancy. The resting basal metabolic rate is decreased in the starvation state but is increased in clients with cancer. Thus, the resting energy expenditure is greater for malnourished persons with cancer. Host metabolism is thrown into chaos: metabolic reactions take place inappropriately and without normal controlling feedback mechanisms. The body burden of tumor does not account for the increased energy expenditure and increased basal metabolic rate [3, 24].

CHARACTERISTICS OF CANCER-RELATED MALNUTRITION

Oxidative Metabolism

In cancer-related mulnutrition and cachexia, oxidative metabolism is increased. The basal metabolic rate (BMR) and body energy expenditure is inappropriately high. One study revealed that cancer clients with large tumor burdens may require a caloric intake exceeding 100 percent of their normal requirements [31]. To adapt to the stressor of increased oxidative metabolism, body stores of fat and muscle protein are used for energy, thus putting the client into a state of protein catabolism.

Organ Function

Hepatomegaly is characteristic of cancer-related malnutrition and cachexia, and is due to the accelerated rate of protein catabolism [22, 24]. All other tissues and organs exhibit atrophy, and malabsorption of ingested nutrients may occur. Rapid depletion of body stores of protein, fat, vitamins, and trace elements occurs.

Weight Loss

An unintentional weight loss of 10 percent or more of the ideal body weight is nearly universal in cancer-related malnutrition and cachexia, although weight loss may be masked by third-space edema. This weight loss often begins early in the disease process and is the result of both reduced oral intake and subsequent protein catabolism.

Immune System Dysfunction

Depletion of body protein stores results in immunoincompetence in both the humoral and cell-mediated immune systems [6, 7, 15, 32, 33]. One study revealed a 100 percent mortality risk in clients who continued to exhibit anergy (inability to mount an immune response) and suppression of the immune system during antineoplastic treatment [15]. Decreased immunocompetence leads to a reduced tolerance for aggressive treatment and a shorter survival time, and there is abundant evidence that malnourished and cachectic cancer clients who are also experiencing anergy, infection, and impaired wound healing have a greatly increased morbidity and mortality.

Conversely, infection worsens the client's nutritional status by decreasing the appetite, increasing the basal metabolic rate, and decreasing gastrointestinal absorption of nutrients if infection affects the intestinal tract. Since there seems to be a synergistic relationship between malnutrition and infection, and since infection is a primary cause of death in the persons with cancer, then it may be said that increased survival correlates positively to the degree of nutritional health before and during anticancer therapy.

In one study, the effects of total parenteral nutrition on malnourished cancer clients was assessed. A positive response to chemotherapy and a clinical regression of metastatic disease was seen *only* in those clients who either had positive skin tests before total parenteral nutrition was begun or whose skin tests converted to positive during nutritional repletion. Surgical clients who displayed initial or converted positive skin tests and whose cellular immunity remained adequate after surgery had an uncomplicated postsurgical recovery. In contrast, 50 percent of those surgical clients whose skin tests remained negative died postoperatively. The investigators concluded that the absence of established cellular immunocompetence in cancer clients is probably secondary to generalized malnutrition and that cell-mediated immunity can be restored with adequate nutrition [8]. In another study, septic and immunoincompetent clients with cancer needed a 40 percent increase in dietary protein over that required by persons without cancer. It may safely be concluded that malnutrition-induced immunoincompetence plus antineoplastic treatment contribute significantly to mortal infections in cancer clients.

Muscle Wasting

Emaciation and muscle wasting are hallmark signs of cancer-related malnutrition and cachexia. Muscle wasting and emaciation are both directly reflective of protein catabolism and negative nitrogen balance. Muscle wasting in the respiratory muscles may result in atelectasis, pulmonary infection, and reduced respiratory capacity. Muscle weakness, easy fatigability, and reduced ambulatory ability commonly occur. This predisposes the client to skin breakdown and the other complications of immobility. The skin of cachectic clients becomes pale and atrophic owing to hypoxia and protein catabolism.

Behavioral Aberrations

The severe protein-calorie malnutrition and cachexia of cancer often results in behavioral changes. These changes commonly include a flat affect (apathy, listlessness), irritability, and detachment from the external environment.

Laboratory Abnormalities

The malnutrition and cachexia of cancer is biochemically manifested by decreased serum levels of lymphocytes and other white blood cells, albumin, calcium, folate, vitamins A and C, magnesium, phosphorus, and potassium. Serum creatinine is increased secondary to excessive protein breakdown. There is also a decreased level of urobilinogen in the feces. Cellular immunoincompetence is characterized by negative delayed hypersensitivity skin tests.

Physiological Alterations in Metabolism

The degree of malnutrition and cachexia has a complex correlation with tumor burden, tumor cell type, and anatomical site of involvement [9]. Significant loss of body fat and protein, alterations in metabolism, and fluid/electrolyte imbalances are common although the exact pathogenesis of these abnormalities is unknown.

Alterations in Protein Metabolism

Alterations in protein metabolism consist primarily of protein catabolism (which has been discussed previously) and hypoalbuminemia. Hypoalbuminemia occurs in most persons with cancer even when the malignant disease is well-localized. It is theorized that there might be a positive correlation between the extent of the hypoalbuminemia and the extent of the tumor burden, since hypoalbuminemia is more marked with extensive disease [10, 33]. Even when dietary protein is increased, serum albumin usually remains depressed in persons with cancer [15]. This may be because of either a deficit in albumin synthesis or an abnormal distribution of albumin within the body. Evidence for either hypothesis has not been conclusive.

Alterations in Fat Metabolism

Alterations in fat metabolism revolve around abnormal mobilization of fat stores, the overloading of the blood with lipids, and the loss of adipose tissue. The abnormal mobilization of lipids may be an adaptive mechanism to meet increased caloric requirements. Profound and sometimes early loss of adipose tissue is a common nutritive finding in persons with cancer. For example, muscle biopsies taken at the time of initial surgery for breast or colon cancer revealed a muscle fat content approximately half of normal [9].

Alterations in Carbohydrate Metabolism

Cancer clients commonly exhibit an abnormally high glucose tolerance curve and a slower than normal disappearance rate of intravenous glucose. These abnormalities may be the result of either a decreased sensitivity to insulin or an impairment of insulin response to glucose. Evidence for either of these two hypotheses has been inconclusive.

Fluid/Electrolyte Imbalances

The most common electrolyte imbalance in persons with advanced cancer is hyponatremia. This condition may be the result of hypoalbuminemia and water retention, which cause hemodilution.

The most common fluid imbalance in persons with advanced cancer is dehydration, a potentially fatal condition since a loss of only 20 percent to 22 percent of body water is lethal. Extracellular fluids comprise about 17 percent of the total body fluid, and intracellular fluid and third-space fluid account for about 43 percent and 40 percent respectively [2]. Rapid, acute dehydration with concurrent weight loss is almost entirely an extracellular fluid loss, whereas chronic dehydration tends to be evenly distributed among the body's fluid compartments.

Body water is required for (1) the transport of nutrients and electrolytes into cells, (2) the transport of waste material away from the cells, (3) the excretion of urea, mineral salts, and the waste products of metabolism, and (4) as a catalyst in a number of biochemical reactions within the body. Fluid intake may be exogenous (preformed water in liquids and foods) or endogenous (from the products of metabolism). In stress or wasting diseases such as cancer, endogenous water is retained by the body. Basic water requirements are 35ml/kg/day for adults and 50 to 60 ml/kg/day for children. Water requirements are increased when extrarenal losses arc high, such as in vomiting, fistulous drainage, fever, and increased diaphoresis.

Dehydration can develop if water intake is less than what is needed for fluid requirements. Daily weight comparisons can give an extremely accurate indication of dehydration in that water losses as little as 2 percent can be detected [28, 29]. Other signs and symptoms of dehydration include dry skin, parched oral mucous membranes, oliguria with a urinary output of less than five hundred milliters per day, and a urine specific gravity greater than 1.030. Dehydration is treated with an immediate increase in fluid intake, either by oral, enteral, or intravenous routes.

CONCEPT II:
The causative stressors of cancer-related malnutrition and cachexia include the disease process itself, antineoplastic treatment, and the client's behavioral responses. See Figure 14.2.

DISEASE-RELATED STRESSORS

Since most fatal tumors constitute less than 5 percent of the host's total body mass, true tumor-host competition for nutrients is probably rare. However, certain disease-related stressors causing malnutrition have been identified.

Mechanical obstruction of strategic organs is a major cause of malnutrition in the person with cancer [5, 25], and malabsorption or maldigestion of certain ingested nutrients may cause malnutrition. Bile salts may be deficient or the small bowel may be infiltrated by carcinoma or lymphoma cells. Fistulous bypass of the small bowel will result in malabsorption, as will an intestinal blind loop secondary to partial upper small bowel obstruction. There may be gastric hypersecretion inhibiting the production and release of pancreatic enzymes (Zollinger-Ellison Syndrome), resulting in malabsorption and maldigestion.

Protein-losing enteropathies, such as those commonly seen with gastric carcinoma, lymphoma, or lymphatic obstruction, contribute to malnutrition and cachexia. Persistent vomiting secondary to intestinal obstruction or increased intracranial pressure caused by brain lesions will predispose the client to malnutrition. Diarrhea may lead to nutrient malabsorption and is often caused by small bowel dysfunction, villous adenoma of the colon, or hormone-secreting tumors (e.g., carcinoid tumors, medullary thyroid carcinoma).

Although tumor toxins have not been absolutely identified, tumors may secrete a number of potent ectopic hormones and other toxic substances that cause malnutrition. In addition, hyperadrenalism secondary to increased corticotropin or corticosteroid production and the syndrome of inappropriate antidiuretic hormone secretion (SIADH) have both been associated with the development of malnutrition.

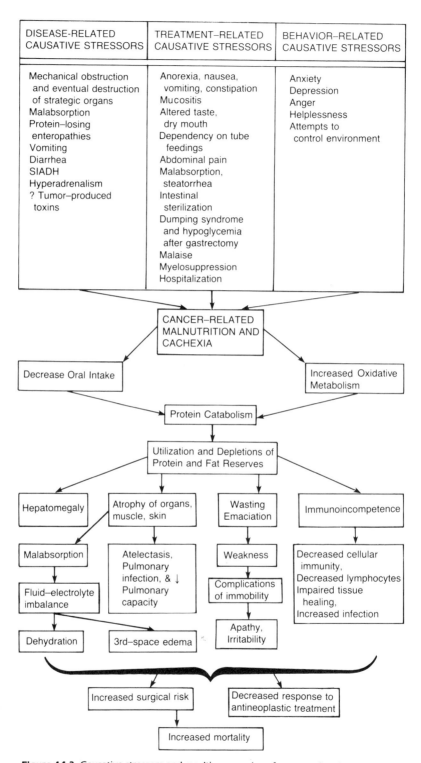

DISEASE-RELATED CAUSATIVE STRESSORS	TREATMENT–RELATED CAUSATIVE STRESSORS	BEHAVIOR–RELATED CAUSATIVE STRESSORS
Mechanical obstruction and eventual destruction of strategic organs Malabsorption Protein–losing enteropathies Vomiting Diarrhea SIADH Hyperadrenalism ? Tumor–produced toxins	Anorexia, nausea, vomiting, constipation Mucositis Altered taste, dry mouth Dependency on tube feedings Abdominal pain Malabsorption, steatorrhea Intestinal sterilization Dumping syndrome and hypoglycemia after gastrectomy Malaise Myelosuppression Hospitalization	Anxiety Depression Anger Helplessness Attempts to control environment

CANCER–RELATED MALNUTRITION AND CACHEXIA

Decrease Oral Intake

Increased Oxidative Metabolism

Protein Catabolism

Utilization and Depletions of Protein and Fat Reserves

Hepatomegaly

Atrophy of organs, muscle, skin

Wasting Emaciation

Immunoincompetence

Malabsorption

Atelectasis, Pulmonary infection, & ↓ Pulmonary capacity

Weakness

Decreased cellular immunity,
Decreased lymphocytes
Impaired tissue healing,
Increased infection

Fluid–electrolyte imbalance

Complications of immobility

Dehydration

3rd–space edema

Apathy, Irritability

Increased surgical risk

Decreased response to antineoplastic treatment

Increased mortality

Figure 14.2. Causative stressors and resulting sequelae of cancer-related malnutrition.

TREATMENT-RELATED STRESSORS

All antineoplastic treatment modalities have profound negative effects on nutritional status. Anorexia, nausea, vomiting, and diarrhea are common adverse effects of both chemotherapy and radiotherapy, and the associated reduced oral intake and malabsorption certainly predispose the client to malnutrition. Constipation secondary to the use of the vinca alkaloids or opiate analgesics also causes anorexia and possible malnutrition. Stomatitis or mucositis commonly occurs after chemotherapy and may be so severe and painful as to cause the client to stop eating completely.

Altered taste sensation and dry mouth are commonly seen after radiotherapy to the head and neck, and these treatment side effects result in an aversion to food, dysphagia, and a subsequent decrease in food intake. Head and neck surgeries result in a prolonged dependency on tube (enteral) feedings and the possible eventual development of an esophageal fistula or stenosis. Reduced oral intake may also occur secondary to abdominal pain, which may be due to constipation, diarrhea, intestinal obstruction, or abdominal surgery.

Radiotherapy of the abdomen and pelvis may result in bowel damage and the possible development of diarrhea, malabsorption, stenosis, or obstruction. Radiotherapy-induced bowel damage is a major cause of malnutrition in persons with cancer. The small bowel is extremely radiosensitive and postradiation malabsorption syndrome is common. Steatorrhea and protein-losing enteropathy result. Of all persons receiving high-dose abdominal or pelvic irradiation, 88 percent to 92 percent experience severe weight loss secondary to induced malnutrition [25].

Intestinal sterilization by oral antibiotics (e.g., neomycin) is often carried out in order to decrease infection in the person with cancer. However, sterilization of the intestine also results in the malabsorption of fats, nitrogen, sodium, potassium, calcium, lactose, sucrose, and vitamin B-12 [5].

Gastrectomy, a surgical procedure, predisposes the client to malnutrition because of the accompanying dumping syndrome and hypoglycemia that commonly occurs. Malaise, a response in which the client feels generally unwell and listless, is commonly observed in persons undergoing anticancer treatment and tends to reduce food intake. Anemia secondary to myelosuppression tends to worsen malnutrition by causing further hypoxia of already energy-starved cells. Hospitalization itself seems to have a negative effect on nutritional status. One study revealed some degree of protein-calorie malnutrition in 33 percent to 50 percent of *all* medical or surgical clients whose illnesses required hospitalization for two weeks or more [6].

BEHAVIOR-RELATED STRESSORS

Behavior-related stressors causing malnutrition in persons with cancer include anxiety, anger, helplessness, and attempts to maintain control of the external environment. All of these behavioral responses tend to result in anorexia and/or decreased food intake.

CONCEPT III:

The client's nutritional status before and during antineoplastic therapy has a profound effect on response to treatment, although the effect of nutritional support on overall outcome is unknown.

Nutritional intervention by oral, enteral, or intravenous routes generally results in an improved sense of well-being, weight gain, an increased immune response, and an improved response to antineoplastic treatment (see Figure 14.3). Nutritional repletion reduces gastrointestinal toxicity and pain, and increases ambulatory ability and mental alertness. Even if the malignancy continues to progress, appropriate nutritional intervention improves quality of life and enhances the client's sense of well-being.

Malnutrition and cachexia need not be an inevitable condition for all persons with cancer. Approximately two-thirds of malnourished cancer clients can receive adequate nutritional replenishment with oral supplementation or enteral hyperalimentation (tube feedings). The remaining one-third require intravenous hyperalimentation to meet their metabolic needs [26].

Dietary counseling and nutritional monitoring are necessary for all persons with cancer. Supplemental formulas taken by mouth are indicated for those clients who need decreased bulk while meeting their caloric demands. Supplements are also needed by those who cannot mechanically manage solid foods and so need a liquid diet, and by those who are receiving tube or gastrostomy feedings.

Elemental or other adjusted diets are indicated for clients with specific malabsorption problems. The transition periods between intravenous hyperalimentation and oral feedings after a prolonged bowel rest or a recent bowel trauma also require an adjusted diet. Enteral feedings, whether supplemental or elemental formulas, are contraindicated in clients who are experiencing gastrointestinal bleeding, intestinal obstruction, or intractable vomiting.

Intravenous hyperalimentation, sometimes called total parenteral nutrition (TPN), is indicated for clients who need bowel rest or for whom oral or enteral feedings are not possible. Clients who require supplementation beyond what is possible with oral or enteral feedings are also candidates for intravenous hyperalimentation, and this mode of nutritional repletion is also indicated for those clients whose absorption of nutrients is adequate for their caloric demands.

There is no conclusive evidence that any form of nutritional intervention has anticancer activity in itself. Although nutritive deficiencies may produce biochemical alterations within the body that promote cancer growth, there is no indication that replenishment of those deficiencies would prevent or eradicate cancer. There is insufficient evidence that either megadoses or decreased amounts of any nutrient prevents cancer or has a useful role as a direct antineoplastic treatment [25].

CONCEPT IV:

Often the decision regarding a client's nutritional status is determined by a quick glance rather than by assessment of data.

Nutritional assessment is necessary before effective intervention can be made. A working definition of malnutrition has three criteria: (1) a recent, unin-

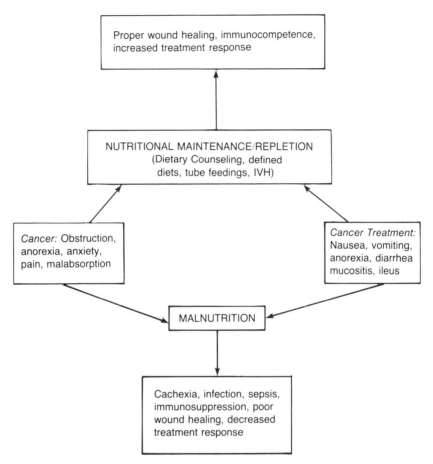

Figure 14.3. Significance of Nutritional Status.

tentional weight loss of 10 percent or more of ideal body weight, (2) a serum albumin less than 3.4 grams, and (3) negative delayed hypersensitivity skin tests. A weight loss of 4.5 kilograms (ten pounds) during antineoplastic therapy should alert caregivers to carefully scrutinize the client's nutritional status.

Supportive nutritional therapy has as its goal to maintain or rehabilitate the previously good nutritional status of the client. *Adjunctive* nutritional therapy is a vital part of the entire therapy program. Its goals are (1) to improve the client's immune status, (2) to allow a better and faster response to anticancer therapy, and (3) to enhance the client's sense of well-being. *Definitive* nutritional therapy exists when nutritional intervention becomes the primary therapy modality upon which the person's life depends. Special oral, enteral, or intravenous nutritional therapy permits the survival of clients who have had a massive bowel resection, severe intestinal radiation enteritis, or some other serious intestinal dysfunction. For these clients, neglecting to give definitive nutritional therapy will result in progressive debilitation and death.

Table 14.1. Working Definition of Malnutrition

Criterium	Malnutrition
Weight loss	Recent, unintentional weight loss of 10% or more of ideal body weight
Serum albumin	< 3.4 grams
Status of cellular immunity	Negative delayed hypersensitivity skin tests

NUTRITIONAL ASSESSMENT CRITERIA

Nutritional assessment includes the assessment of general clinical status, ambulatory ability, anthropometric measurements, and specific laboratory data. This information is synthesized to give an in-depth evaluation of the client's nutritional status.

General Clinical Status and Ambulatory Ability

General clinical status is assessed by the Karnowsky Scale Placement (see Table 14.2) and is a good way to monitor the client's overall improvement or decline. Ambulatory ability assessment provides basic information about the client's improvement or decline in strength and endurance (see Table 14.3).

A comparison of the person's preillness weight and current weight will give the nurse basic data about the extent and rapidity of weight loss. A comparison of current weight with ideal weight gives valuable information about the extent of weight loss.

Anthropometric Measurements

Anthropometric measurements are designed to estimate the client's muscle mass as well as protein and fat stores. The measurements are taken on the non-

Table 14.2. Karnowsky Scale Placement

Scale Placement	Description
0	Fully active, able to carry on all predisease performances without restriction.
1	Restricted in physically strenuous activity but ambulatory and able to carry out work of a light or sedentary nature, e.g., light housework, office work.
2	Ambulatory and capable of all self-care but unable to carry out any work activities. Up and about more than 50% of waking hours.
3	Capable of only limited self-care. Confined to bed or chair more than 50% of waking hours.
4	Completely disabled. Cannot carry on any self-care. Totally confined to bed or chair.
5	Dead.

Source: Copyright (c) Southwest Oncology Group. Used with permission.

Table 14.3.   Assessment of Ambulatory Ability

Classification	Performance
Good	Walks 200 feet without help.
Fair	Walks 200 feet with help.
Poor	Cannot walk 200 feet even with help.

dominant arm, and findings less than the fifteenth percentile are considered to be indicative of malnutrition [26, 30].

The *Triceps-skinfold measurement* (TSF) is an estimation of available fat stores. For this test, the skinfold thickness over the triceps muscle is measured using Lange or Harpenden calipers. Find the midpoint on the client's freely hanging, nondominant arm. The midpoint lies halfway between the acromial process and the olecranon process. Lightly mark the midpoint with a pen (see Figure 14.4). Lift the skinfold and measure at the midpoint with the calipers as shown in Figure 14.5. Make sure that skin—not muscle—is being measured, and then record the reading from the

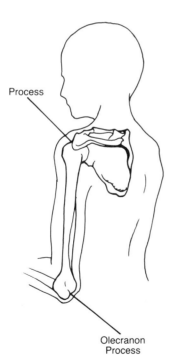

Process

Olecranon
Process

Figure 14.4. Finding the Midpoint
for Anthropometric Measurements.

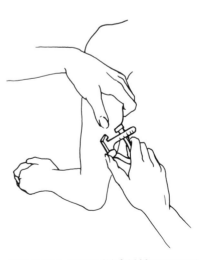

Figure 14.5. Triceps Skinfold Measurement.

calipers. Determine in which column of the Nutritional Assessment Summary (Figure 14.7) the client's measurement falls. The Triceps Skinfold Measurement is reflective of the body's caloric reserve and is decreased when malnutrition is present.

The *Mid-Arm Circumference* (MAC) is a measurement of available fat and protein stores. To find the Mid-Arm Circumference, measure the circumference of the client's freely hanging, nondominant arm at the previously marked midpoint as shown in Figure 14.6. Record the reading from the measuring tape, and then determine in which column of the Nutritional Assessment Summary (Figure 14.7) the client's measurement falls. The Mid-Arm Circumference is frequently inaccurate because depletion of fat and protein stores is often masked by edema. Thus, its primary use is to calculate the Mid-Arm Muscle Circumference.

The *Mid-Arm Muscle Circumference* (MAMC) is an accurate measurement of muscle protein stores. It is calculated with a formula using the client's Triceps Skinfold Measurement and the Mid-Arm Circumference. Begin by transforming the client's Triceps Skinfold Measurement from millimeters to centimeters by moving the decimal point one space to the left. Multiply the Triceps Skinfold Measurement (in centimeters) by 3.14, and then subtract this value from the Mid-Arm Circumference to obtain the Mid-Arm Muscle Circumference. Record the calculated Mid-Arm Muscle Circumference, and then determine in which column of the Nutritional Assessment Summary (Figure 14.7) the client's measurement falls. The Mid-Arm Muscle Circumference is the most accurate and the most important of the anthropometric measurements. It is decreased when protein malnutrition exists and indicates that muscle protein has been used to meet energy needs. The complete formula is MAMC = MAC − (3.14 × TSF in centimeters).

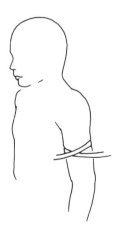

Figure 14.6. Mid-Arm Circumference.

Serum Albumin and Transferrin

Whereas muscle stores of protein are measured by anthropometric measurements, estimations of visceral protein stores are determined by comparing the client's serum levels of albumin and transferrin to normal values. Since albumin is synthesized in the liver, hypoalbuminemia of less than 3.4 grams reflects a depletion in liver protein stores. Few hospitals and clinics have the facilities to directly measure serum transferrin levels, but it may be easily calculated with a formula using the more common laboratory test of total iron-binding capacity (TIBC). The complete formula is: serum transferrin = $(0.8 \times \text{TIBC}) - 43$. A value less than the fifteenth percentile is indicative of depletion of visceral protein stores and malnutrition.

Creatinine-Height Index

A twenty-four hour urine collection for the determination of urine creatinine is necessary for a thorough nutritional assessment. The urine creatinine level is used only to calculate the Creatinine-Height Index (CHI). This is an extremely accurate measurement of lean body mass and degrees of protein depletion. If protein malnutrition is present, the Creatinine-Height Index will be decreased. The formula to calculate the Creatinine-Height Index is:

$$\text{CHI} = \frac{\text{Actual urine creatinine}}{\text{Ideal urine creatinine}} \times 100.$$

A value less than the fifteenth percentile is indicative of muscle protein depletion and malnutrition.

Nitrogen Balance

The twenty-four hour urine collection is also assessed to determine the twenty-four hour urine urea nitrogen level. During the same twenty-four hour period of time, a calorie and protein count is done, and these two measurements will determine whether the client is in positive or negative nitrogen balance. The formula is:

$$\text{Nitrogen Balance} = \frac{(\text{Protein intake})}{6.25} - (\text{Urinary Urea Nitrogen} + 4)$$

If the final result of the calculation is a positive number, the client is in positive nitrogen balance. If the final result is a negative number, the client is in negative nitrogen balance.

Nutritional Assessment Summary Sheet

Patient _____ Room _____   Diagnosis _____

Physician _____ Date _____   Admission Weight _____ Preferred Weight _____

Service _____   Height _____

Parameters:	Patient Values:	Assessment:			
		Above 50th Percentile*	50-15th Percentile*	15-5th Percentile*	Below 5th Percentile*
Weight for height	lb in				
Triceps skinfold (TSF)	mm				
Midarm circumference (MAC)	cm				
Midarm muscle circumference (MAMC) MAMC (cm) = MAC (cm) − [3.14 × TSF (cm)]**	cm				
		>90% Standard* Not Depleted	60-90% Standard* Moderately Depleted	<60% Standard* Severely Depleted	
Lymphocytes, total count	/mm³				
Albumin, serum	g/100 ml				
Total iron-binding capacity (TIBC)	mcg/100 ml				
Transferrin Serum transferrin = (0.8 × TIBC) − 43**	mg/100 ml				
Urinary creatinine	mg				
Creatinine height index (CHI) CHI = $\dfrac{\text{Actual urinary creatinine}}{\text{Ideal urinary creatinine}} \times 100$**	%				

*see reference data

Dietary Intake Evaluation:

Calories _____ Cal/24 hr   Protein _____ g/24 hr

Nitrogen Balance = $\dfrac{\text{Protein Intake}}{6.25}$ − (Urinary Urea Nitrogen + 4)**

☐ Positive   ☐ Negative

Hematocrit _____ %   Hemoglobin _____ g/100 ml

Antigen _____ Induration

	24 hrs	48 hrs
_____	mm	mm
_____	mm	mm
_____	mm	mm

☐ Abnormal reactivity (anergy)   ☐ Normal reactivity

Nutritional Status:

☐ Marasmus (M)   ☐ Kwashiorkor (K)

☐ Combination M-K   ☐ Normal

Proposed Nutritional Therapy:

_____
_____
_____
_____
_____
_____
_____
_____
_____
_____
_____
_____

**Blackburn GL, et al: Nutritional and metabolic assessment of the hospitalized patient. JPEN 1:11-22, 1977

Figure 14.7. Nutritional Assessment Summary Sheet.

Serial Nutritional Assessment

Anthropometric Measurement

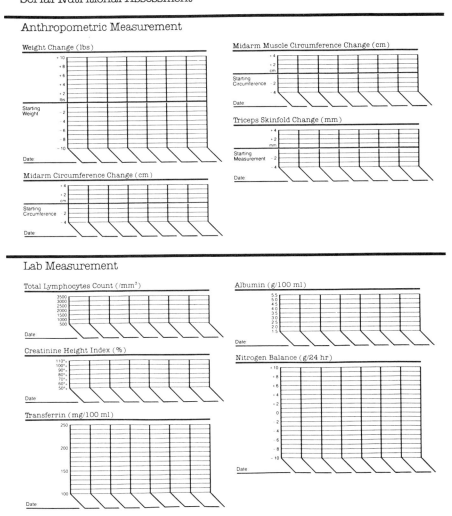

Lab Measurement

Figure 14.7. Cont'd.

Table 1.
Weight (lb) For Height (in), Males[1]

Height in inches	Percentile	Age group in years					
		18-24	25-34	35-44	45-54	55-64	65-74
62 inches	50	130	141	143	147	143	143
	15	102	109	115	118	113	116
	5	85	91	98	100	96	100
63 inches	50	135	145	148	152	147	147
	15	107	113	120	123	117	120
	5	90	95	103	105	100	104
64 inches	50	140	150	153	156	153	151
	15	112	118	125	127	123	124
	5	95	100	108	109	106	108
65 inches	50	145	156	158	160	158	156
	15	117	124	130	131	128	129
	5	100	106	113	113	111	113
66 inches	50	150	160	163	164	163	160
	15	122	128	135	135	133	133
	5	105	110	118	117	116	117
67 inches	50	154	165	169	169	168	164
	15	126	133	141	140	138	137
	5	109	115	124	122	121	121
68 inches	50	159	170	174	173	173	169
	15	131	138	146	144	143	142
	5	114	120	129	126	126	126
69 inches	50	164	174	179	177	178	173
	15	136	142	151	148	148	146
	5	119	124	134	130	131	130
70 inches	50	168	179	184	182	183	177
	15	140	147	156	153	153	150
	5	123	129	139	135	136	134
71 inches	50	173	184	190	187	189	182
	15	145	152	162	158	159	155
	5	128	134	145	140	142	139
72 inches	50	178	189	194	191	193	186
	15	150	157	166	162	163	159
	5	133	139	149	144	146	143
73 inches	50	183	194	200	196	197	190
	15	155	162	172	167	167	163
	5	138	144	155	149	150	147
74 inches	50	188	199	205	200	203	194
	15	160	167	177	171	173	167
	5	143	149	160	153	156	151

15th Percentile values computed from reference 1 data by Ross Laboratories

Table 2.
Weight (lb) For Height (in), Females[1]

Height in inches	Percentile	Age group in years					
		18-24	25-34	35-44	45-54	55-64	65-74
57 inches	50	114	118	125	129	132	130
	15	85	85	89	94	97	100
	5	68	65	67	73	77	82
58 inches	50	117	121	129	133	136	134
	15	88	88	93	98	101	104
	5	71	68	71	77	81	86
59 inches	50	120	125	133	136	140	137
	15	91	92	97	101	105	107
	5	74	72	75	80	85	89
60 inches	50	123	128	137	140	143	140
	15	94	95	101	105	108	110
	5	77	75	79	84	88	92
61 inches	50	126	132	141	143	147	144
	15	97	99	105	108	112	114
	5	80	79	83	87	92	96
62 inches	50	129	136	144	147	150	147
	15	100	103	108	112	115	117
	5	83	83	86	91	95	99
63 inches	50	132	139	148	150	153	151
	15	103	106	112	115	118	121
	5	86	86	90	94	98	103
64 inches	50	135	142	152	154	157	154
	15	106	109	116	119	122	124
	5	89	89	94	98	102	106
65 inches	50	138	146	156	158	160	158
	15	109	113	120	123	125	128
	5	92	93	98	102	105	110
66 inches	50	141	150	159	161	164	161
	15	112	117	123	126	129	131
	5	95	97	101	105	109	113
67 inches	50	144	153	163	165	167	165
	15	115	120	127	130	132	135
	5	98	100	105	109	112	117
68 inches	50	147	157	167	168	171	169
	15	118	124	131	133	136	139
	5	101	104	109	112	116	121

15th Percentile values computed from reference 1 data by Ross Laboratories.

Table 3.
Triceps Skinfold (mm), Males[2]

Age (years)	Percentile		
	50th	15th	5th
18-19	8.5	6.0	4.5
20-24	10.0	6.0	4.0
25-34	12.0	6.0	4.5
35-44	12.0	7.0	5.0
45-54	11.0	7.0	5.0
55-64	11.0	6.5	5.0
65-74	11.0	6.5	4.5

Table 4.
Triceps Skinfold (mm), Females[2]

Age (years)	Percentile		
	50th	15th	5th
18-19	17.5	12.0	9.0
20-24	18.0	12.0	10.0
25-34	21.0	13.5	10.5
35-44	23.0	16.0	12.0
45-54	25.0	17.0	13.0
55-64	25.0	16.0	11.0
65-74	23.0	16.0	11.5

Table 5.
Midarm Circumference (cm), Males[2]

Age (years)	Percentile		
	50th	15th	5th
18-19	30.1	27.4	25.3
20-24	31.0	27.7	26.1
25-34	32.0	28.9	27.0
35-44	32.7	29.6	27.8
45-54	32.1	28.9	26.7
55-64	31.7	28.2	25.6
65-74	30.7	27.3	25.3

Table 6.
Midarm Circumference (cm), Females[2]

Age (years)	Percentile		
	50th	15th	5th
18-19	26.2	23.2	22.1
20-24	26.5	23.6	22.2
25-34	27.8	24.8	23.3
35-44	29.2	25.8	24.1
45-54	30.3	26.6	24.3
55-64	30.2	26.1	23.9
65-74	29.9	26.2	23.8

Figure 14.7. Cont'd.

Table 7.
Midarm Muscle Circumference (cm), Males*

Age (years)	Percentile		
	50th	15th	5th
18-19	27.4	25.5	23.9
20-24	27.9	25.8	24.8
25-34	28.2	27.0	25.6
35-44	28.9	27.4	26.2
45-54	28.7	26.7	25.1
55-64	28.3	26.2	24.0
65-74	27.2	25.3	23.9

*Values computed using MAMC (cm) = MAC (cm) − [3.14 × TSF (cm)] from data in Tables 3 and 5 by Ross Laboratories.

Table 8.
Midarm Muscle Circumference (cm), Females**

Age (years)	Percentile		
	50th	15th	5th
18-19	20.7	19.4	19.3
20-24	20.8	19.8	19.1
25-34	21.2	20.6	20.0
35-44	22.0	20.8	20.3
45-54	22.5	21.3	20.2
55-64	22.4	21.1	20.5
65-74	22.7	21.2	20.2

**Values computed using MAMC (cm) = MAC (cm) − [3.14 × TSF (cm)] from data in Tables 4 and 6 by Ross Laboratories.

Table 9.
Selected Normal Values For Adults[3]

(a) Hematocrit (vol % red cells)
    Male   40%-54%
    Female   37%-47%

(b) Hemoglobin
    Male   *14-17 g/100 ml*
    Female   *12-15 g/100 ml*

(c) Lymphocytes, total count   *1500-3000/mm³*

(d) Albumin, serum   *4.0-5.5 g/100 ml*

(e) Iron-binding capacity
    total, serum   *250-410 mcg/100 ml*
    % saturation   *20%-50%*

(f) Transferrin   *170-250 mg/100 ml*

(g) Creatinine   *1.0-1.5 g/24 hr*

Table 10.
Ideal Urinary Creatinine Value (mg), Adults[4]

Male*		Female**	
Height (cm)	Ideal Creatinine (mg)	Height (cm)	Ideal Creatinine (mg)
157.5	1288	147.3	830
160.0	1325	149.9	851
162.6	1359	152.4	875
165.1	1386	154.9	900
167.6	1426	157.5	925
170.2	1467	160.0	949
172.7	1513	162.6	977
175.3	1555	165.1	1006
177.8	1596	167.6	1044
180.3	1642	170.2	1076
182.9	1691	172.7	1109
185.4	1739	175.3	1141
188.0	1785	177.8	1174
190.5	1831	180.3	1206
193.0	1891	182.9	1240

*Creatinine coefficient (males) = 23 mg/kg of ideal body weight.
**Creatinine coefficient (females) = 18 mg/kg of ideal body weight.

Table 11.
Estimated Caloric Expenditure (ECE)[5]

$$ECE\ (men) = (66.47 + 13.75W + 5.0H - 6.76A) \times (activity\ factor) \times (injury\ factor)$$

$$ECE\ (women) = (655.10 + 9.56W + 1.85H - 4.68A) \times (activity\ factor) \times (injury\ factor)$$

W = weight in kg
H = height in cm
A = age in years

Activity factor:
Confined to bed, use 1.20
Out of bed, use 1.30

Injury factor:
Minor operation, use 1.20
Skeletal trauma, use 1.35
Major sepsis, use 1.60
Severe thermal burn, use 2.10

1. Abraham S, Johnson CL, Najjar MF: Weight by height and age of adults 18-74 years: United States, 1971-74. *Advancedata*, 14:7-8, 1977.

2. Basic data on anthropometric measurements and angular measurements of the hip and knee joints for selected age groups 1-74 years of age, United States, 1971-1975. National Health Survey, Vital and Health Statistics Series No. 219. US Dept of Health and Human Services, Public Health Service, 1981, pp 20, 26.

3. Lagua RT, Claudio VS, Thiele VF: *Nutrition and Diet Therapy Reference Dictionary*. ed 2. St Louis: CV Mosby Co, 1974.

4. Bistrian BR, Blackburn GL, Sherman M, Scrimshaw NS: Therapeutic index of nutritional depletion in hospitalized patients. *Surg Gynecol Obstetr*, 141:512-516, 1975.

5. Long CL, Schaffel N, Geiger JW, Schiller WR, et al: Metabolic response to injury and illness: Estimation of energy and protein needs from indirect calorimetry and nitrogen balance. *JPEN*, 3:452-456, 1979.

**The Ross
Medical Nutritional
System**

A total commitment
to enteral nutrition.

ROSS LABORATORIES
COLUMBUS, OHIO 43216
Division of Abbott Laboratories USA

G636 JANUARY 1982

LITHO IN USA

Figure 14.7. Cont'd.

Immune Status

Since malnutrition significantly affects immune status, assessment of the immune system is important. Humoral immune status can be evaluated by a simple lymphocyte count, and a value less than the fifteenth percentile indicates malnutrition. Lymphocyte production is particularly sensitive to depleted protein stores.

Cellular immunity is evaluated by the administration and assessment of delayed hypersensitivity skin tests. Six antigens commonly encountered in the environment are injected intradermally into the client's forearms: mumps, PPD, *Candida Albicans*, streptokinase, streptodornase, and a normal saline control. At twenty-four and forty-eight hours after administration, the sites are observed for a positive response of erythema and induration at least five millimeters in diameter. Erythema alone does not constitute a positive response. If the client is immunocompetent and able to mount an immune response, a positive response to the injected antigens will usually occur in twenty-four hours and certainly in forty-eight hours. At least two injected sites must have a positive response in order to judge the person as immunocompetent. In malnourished clients, there will be minimal or no response, and whatever response occurs is often delayed.

CONCEPT V:
Analysis of assessment data will yield information about the client's nutritional status.

VISCERAL ATTRITION STATE

The visceral attrition state often occurs in an apparently well-nourished or even over-nourished person who has been exposed to a sudden catabolic stressor [30]. This condition is characterized by decreased levels of visceral protein (serum albumin and transferrin) and immunoincompetence. Anthropometric measurements and body weight remain normal. This type of malnutrition is often overlooked until the serious consequences of negative nitrogen balance become apparent.

ADULT MARASMUS

Adult marasmus is the type of malnutrition associated with chronically ill persons who have maintained an inadequate diet for an extended period of time [30]. Anthropometric measurements and body weight are markedly decreased, although serum proteins (albumin, transferrin, and lymphocytes) and the immune response remain normal.

PROTEIN-CALORIE MALNUTRITION

Protein-calorie malnutrition is typically the type of malnutrition seen in persons with cancer, severe wasting disease, and/or sepsis. All visceral protein levels are decreased and anthropometric measurements and body weight are significantly reduced. Immunosuppression is also evident. This type of malnutrition progresses rapidly to cachexia.

CONCEPT VI:
After the initial in-depth nutritional assessment, analysis of data must continue as an ongoing process in order to provide adequate nutritional monitoring and repletion.

The initial in-depth assessment should dictate the type and extent of nutritional therapy necessary for the individual client. Daily assessment factors include weight, fluid intake and output, calorie and protein intake, and ambulatory ability. Weekly assessment factors include a summary of all daily factors for the week, serum albumin level, total lymphocyte count, and Karnowsky Scale placement. The need for additional in-depth assessment must be determined by each individual's unique clinical condition, prognosis, and the appearance of any other stressors that might affect nutritional status.

Determination of the type and extent of nutritional therapy is based on the client's nutritive status and clinical condition (see Figure 14.8). The overall goal is to restore or maintain a positive nitrogen balance.

CONCEPT VII:
Oral or enteral (tube feeding) supplementation is safe, uses the gastrointestinal system in a normal way, and is relatively inexpensive.

A general rule for nutritional therapy is: if the gut works, use it. Oral nutritive intake is necessary to maintain the structural and functional integrity of the small intestine [14, 19, 21]. Oral or enteral feedings use the gut in a normal way, resulting in less atrophy of gastrointestinal mucosa. Thus, proper gastrointestinal function is maintained for absorption of nutrients and water and for excretion of solid waste. Even if the gastrointestinal tract has been damaged by the disease process or by treatment, manipulation of the oral or enteral diet may preclude the necessity of intravenous hyperalimentation.

A major cause of protein-calorie malnutrition and cachexia is anorexia—often the cancer client simply cannot willingly eat enough. To determine how many calories per day is "enough," the nurse must calculate the basal energy expenditure (BEE) which, for adults, is a fairly constant function of height, weight, age, and sex (see Table 14.4). If the cancer client has complications, such as a pathological fracture or sepsis, further increases in calories are necessary (see Tables 14.4 and 14.5). It must be remembered that cancer causes an increase in oxidative metabolism, so it is wise to add an extra 50 percent to the number of calories needed daily by the client.

Most people associate eating with feeling well, and persons with cancer quite often simply do not feel well, particularly if they are receiving chemotherapy or radiotherapy. To motivate these people who do not feel well enough to eat, main-

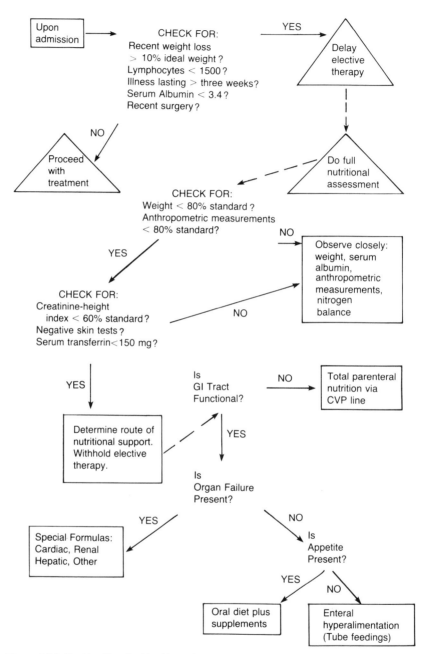

Figure 14.8. Decision Tree for Nutritional Support.

Table 14.4. Calculating Basal Energy Expenditure [18]

Sex	Calculation
Males	BEE = 66 + (13.7 × W) + (5 × H) − (6.8 × A)
Females	BEE = 665 + (9.6 × W) + (1.7 × H) − (4.7 × A)

BEE = Basal Energy Expenditure
W   = Weight in kg
H   ▬ Height in cm
A   = Age in years

Table 14.5. Calories Necessary to Adapt to Certain Stressors

Stressor	Increase Over Basal Caloric Needs (BEE)
Fever	BEE × 1.1
Minor surgery	BEE × 1.2
Fractures	BEE × 1.35
Sepsis	BEE × 1.6
Confined to bed	BEE × 1.2

tain an attitude of gentle, persistent encouragement. *Forcing* food or fluids usually does not succeed. Instead, coax them to eat with the objective of feeling better *today*. The nurse may make a contract with the client, in which the nurse promises to furnish foods that the client wants, and the client promises to eat. Appropriate teaching about the role of adequate nutrition in tissue healing and enhancement of well-being is often effective with anorexic clients, since it gives them reason to eat. Clients receiving enteral hyperalimentation at home may find this intervention more acceptable if the tube feedings are given at night and the tube withdrawn during the day. Finally, families need to understand clearly that anorexia, changes in taste, and aversion to food are common responses to both the disease and the treatment, not just "picky" behavior or whims.

Oral or enteral hyperalimentation is also more economical and more convenient than intravenous hyperalimentation. In 1979, three liters of intravenous hyperalimentation solution cost approximately $135; at that same time, three liters of enteral hyperalimentation formula cost $5 to $20 [16]. Enteral hyperalimentation does not require aseptic technique, whereas intravenous hyperalimentation does. Thus, enteral hyperalimentation can be carried out easily and safely by the client, family, or nurses in the home environment. Intravenous hyperalimentation, however, requires much more extensive teaching, equipment, and supplies.

Therefore, for several reasons, oral or enteral hyperalimentation is the treatment of choice for malnourished cancer clients. If an oral diet plus supplemental nutrients is selected as the treatment of choice, the diet and supplements must be selected carefully. A high-protein, high-calorie diet is the minimal nutritional inter-

Figure 14.9.

Brooke Army Milkshake Recipe

2 eggs
¼ cup liquid polycose
1¼ cups ice cream
3 Tablespoons chocolate syrup
¼ cup milk
1½ teaspoons medium-chain triglyceride (MCT) oil

Mix all ingredients well. Serve immediately, or store in freezer for later use. Yield: 470 cc + 860 calories

Table 14.6.   Nutritional Management with Radiotherapy

Irradiated Area	Problems	Foods Encouraged	Foods Discouraged
HEAD, NECK	Dry mouth Change in or loss of taste Mucositis Nausea (occasional) Indigestion (occasional)	Supplementary feedings Small frequent meals Bland foods Increased fluid intake Foods served at room temperature Chewing sugar-free gum or sucking hard candy to aid dry mouth Use a straw if mucositis is present	Alcohol Carbonated beverages Extremely hot or cold foods Spicy or highly seasoned foods Acidic foods Foods with sharp, rough edges Sweets Gas-forming foods
UPPER ABDOMEN	Nausea, vomiting	Carbonated drinks Small frequent meals A light meal 1½–2 hours before treatment Cold, nonodorous foods Cold, clear liquids Relaxation, chewing foods well, eating slowly Dry crackers or toast after rest or sleep	Alcohol Fried, greasy foods Foods with high fat content Cooked foods with strong odor Not eating for long periods of time
PELVIS, LOWER ABDOMEN	Diarrhea Malabsorption	Low residue diet Small frequent meals High protein diet High fluid intake Low residue or elemental supplement to increase protein calories	Alcohol Foods with "roughage" Spicy or highly seasoned foods Fried, greasy foods Gas-forming foods Foods with a high fat content Milk, milk products, milk-based formulas unless well tolerated

vention. A "regular" or "general" diet without supplementation is simply not adequate for the increased caloric needs of cancer clients. If the gastrointestinal tract is undamaged, the high-protein, high-calorie diet can be further supplemented with snacks that are also high in calories and protein, such as the "Brooke Army Milkshake" (see Figure 14.9) or a variety of homemade or commercially prepared supplements. If the gastrointestinal tract is damaged, manipulation of oral dietary intake will help to meet the caloric needs of the client without further damaging intestinal mucosa (see Table 14.6 and 14.7).

Table 14.7. Nutritional Management with Chemotherapy

Problems	Foods Encouraged	Foods Discouraged
Nausea, Vomiting	Small frequent meals Carbonated drinks A light meal 1½–2 hours before treatment Cold, nonodorus foods Cold, clear liquids Relaxation, chewing foods well, eating slowly Dry crackers or toast after rest or sleep	Alcohol Fried, greasy foods Foods with high fat content Cooked foods with strong odor Not eating for long periods of time Gas-forming foods
Diarrhea	Low residue diet Small frequent meals High protein diet High fluid intake Low residue or elemental supplement	Alcohol Foods with "roughage" Spicy or highly seasoned foods Fried, greasy foods Gas-forming foods Foods with a high fat content Milk products unless well tolerated
Constipation	Increase fiber or roughage in diet Chew food thoroughly Increase fluids	Low residue diets
Stomatitis	Cold, soft, nonacidic foods Use a straw to make swallowing easier Topical anesthesia as prescribed	Overly spicy, highly seasoned foods Very cold or very hot foods Foods with sharp, rough edges
Dysgeusia	Meat substitutes (eggs, cheese, beans, peanut butter) Extra seasonings if tolerated Acidic foods if tolerated to stimulate taste buds	Red meat

ENTERAL HYPERALIMENTATION

Indications and Administration

Enteral (tube) feedings are indicated when two conditions are present: (1) voluntary oral intake is inadequate and (2) gastrointestinal function remains unimpaired. If enteral, rather than oral, feeding is selected, use a small-bore, flexible nasogastric tube with a mercury-weighted tip if possible. The small-bore, flexible tubes cause less nasal and esophageal erosion than do larger, stiffer tubes. Thus, they are safer, more comfortable, and more appropriate if long-term enteral feeding is anticipated. Two types of small-bore, flexible tubes commonly used for enteral hyperalimentation include the Dobbhoff Enteric Feeding Tube™ (Biosearch Medical Products, Inc.) and the Keofeed Feeding Tube™ (Hedeco Corporation). If small-bore, flexible feeding tubes of this type are not available, a #8 French pediatric feeding tube may be substituted. However, it is tolerated less well because of its stiffer composition and is more likely to cause discomfort and nasal/esophageal erosion. Gastrostomy tubes may also be used to deliver enteral hyperalimentation.

Small-bore, flexible feeding tubes can easily provide the slow, constant rate of formula infusion that is recommended. Initiate the feedings at a rate of no more than fifty milliliters per hour, and increase the flow rate by twenty five milliliters per day until the prescribed volume per twenty-four (24) hours is reached [16]. A slow, constant rate of infusion will minimize the occurrence of abdominal cramps and diarrhea, and a common intravenous infusion setup can be used to regulate the rate of formula flow. The risk of gastric reflux and aspiration is minimized if the client is enterally fed with the head of the bed elevated and if the formula is infused slowly and continuously. Intolerance to enteral feedings (nausea, vomiting, abdominal cramps, diarrhea) is usually the result of uncontrolled changes in the formula flow rate, so a steady flow must be maintained.

If continuous feedings are not prescribed, specific nursing measures will help to prevent both mechanical and client problems. Flush the tubing with approximately ten milliliters of normal saline solution to avoid clogging of the tube while it is not in use. Do not interrupt the feeding for more than six hours at a time [16] to minimize risk of client hypoglycemia. Infuse the formula at a rate of not more than fifty to seventy five milliliters per hour to avoid reflux, nausea, and diarrhea. Keep the head of the bed raised during and for a short time after the feeding. Label the enteral formula clearly in order to avoid inadvertent intravenous administration with subsequent catastrophic results.

Initially begin formula feedings with diluted solutions. Standard dilution schedules are to begin enteral feeding with ¼ formula and ¾ water. If no complications or signs of intolerance develop within the first few days, increase the formula strength to fifty (50) percent formula and fifty (50) percent water. Again, if no complications develop after a few days, the client will probably be able to tolerate full-strength feedings. If, at any time during the escalation of formula concentration, signs of intolerance occur, revert to the previous formula strength for a few more days. This type of dilution schedule allows the small intestine to maximally adapt to the change in dietary content.

The increased length and mercury-weighted tips found in these tubes allow for passage of the tube into the distal duodenum or upper jejunum if it is determined that the formula must bypass the stomach. Mercury-weighted tips allow for radiological determination of tube placement. Although the stomach is generally able to tolerate formulas in a wide range of volumes and osmolalities, the small intestine is unable to tolerate rapid feedings of large volumes or extremely hypertonic solutions [12]. Thus, it is especially important to administer isotonic solutions at a slow, constant rate when the formula is directly delivered to the distal duodenum or upper jejunum. See Table 14.8.

Selection of Formula

Commercially prepared formulas for enteral feedings vary widely in amount and source of protein, carbohydrate and fat content, osmolality, viscosity, mineral content, and cost (see Table 14.9). For enteral hyperalimentation, 2.5 liters or more of formula are needed daily. However, some clients, especially those with

Table 14.8. Complications and Management of Enteral Hyperalimentation [16]

Type of Complication	Frequency	Management
Pulmonary aspiration of stomach contents	Rare	Discontinue if aspiration occurs. Prevent by elevating head of bed.
Esophageal erosion	Rare	Discontinue tube.
Hyperosmolar coma	Rare	Discontinue feeding. Other nursing and medical management as prescribed.
Hypernatremia	Infrequent	Adjust electrolyte content of formula.
Congestive heart failure	Infrequent	Prevent by slow feeding. If symptoms occur, administer diuretics and digoxin as prescribed.
Mechanical tube lumen clogged by solution	Infrequent	Flush tube with water. Replace tube if necessary.
Vomiting and bloating	Frequent	Reduce flow rate.
Hyperglycemia, glucosuria	Frequent	Reduce flow rate. Administer insulin as prescribed.
Diarrhea, cramping	Frequent	Reduce flow rate. Dilute solution. Try different type of solution. Administer antidiarrheal medication as prescribed.
Essential fatty acid deficit	Common if formula lacks linoleic acid	Administer linoleic acid supplement orally or IV as prescribed.

malabsorption, cannot tolerate this much fluid [16, 17]. If only partial dietary requirements are tolerated by enteral feedings, the rest may be given intravenously. One to one and a half liters (1.0–1.5) liters per day of an appropriate peripheral intravenous solution will supply the needed extra nutrients without overloading the gastrointestinal tract.

Since the enteral formula must be nutritionally adequate for the individual client, the selection of formula must be made carefully, with attention to the client's clinical condition [16]. If the gastrointestinal tract is functioning normally, suggested enteral formulas include Isocal (Mead-Johnson), Isocal plus Polycose (Ross), Ensure Plus (Ross), and Precision HN (Doyle). If the gastrointestinal tract is damaged and not functioning normally, Vivonex (Eaton), Vivonex HN (Eaton), and Flexical (Mead-Johnson) are suggested. If the client has a normal basal metabolic rate, a suggested enteral formula is Ensure (Ross). If the basal metabolic rate is elevated, Ensure Plus (Ross) or increased amounts of Ensure (Ross) are recommended. If the client is unable to eat at all, a suggested enteral formula is Precision Isotonic (Ross). Since the protein-calorie malnourished client is often deficient in lactase, milk products or enteral formulas containing milk are not suitable because of their lactose content [4]. Finally, solutions using meat as the source of protein are frequently too thick to easily pass through the small-bore tubes.

Formula Osmolality

A major factor in tolerance to enteral hyperalimentation is osmolality of the formula in use [13]. The human body is composed of approximately 50 percent to 69 percent water. The body attempts to keep the concentration of bodily fluids nearly equal between the intracellular and extracellular compartments by moving water through the semipermeable membrane from a dilute solution to a more concentrated one. Thus, the solutions are of a nearly equal osmolality. "Osmolality" refers to the number of osmoles of particulate matter that is found in one kilogram of solvent, and expressed in terms of milli-Osmoles (mOsm) per kilogram of water. Movement of water between the intracellular and extracellular compartments is achieved by osmosis. Since there are only small clinical differences between the phenomena of "osmolality" and "osmolarity," the former is the generally accepted terminology. The osmolality of a solution is related to the number of dissolved particles contained within one kilogram of the solution. The higher the proportion of particulate matter within the solution, the higher the osmolality. Small peptides and individual (free) amino acids have a significant effect on osmolality.

Carbohydrates of a high molecular weight are large particles whereas carbohydrates of a lower molecular weight are smaller particles. The size of the individual particle is inversely proportional to the osmolality of the solution. Thus, a solution of high molecular-weight carbohydrates has a lower osmolality than does a solution of equal caloric value that contains low molecular-weight carbohydrates.

In general, fats do not have a major effect on osmolality of a solution. The solubility of fats depends upon the length of the fatty-acid chain. Fats with greater proportions of high molecular-weight chains are virtually insoluble in water and thus have little effect on the solution's osmolality. Fats with high proportions of

Table 14.9. Survey of Common Oral/Enteral Supplements*

Product	Cal/cc	Cal	g Pro	g CHO	g Fat	mOsm/kg	Lactose
Ensure (Ross)	1.06	254	8.8	34.3	8.8	450	−
Ensure-Plus (Ross)	1.5	354	13.0	47.3	12.6	600	−
Osmolite (Ross)	1.06	254	8.8	34.3	9.1	300	−
Vital (Ross)	1.0	240	12.5	55.5	3.1	450	−
Isocal (Mead-Johnson)	1.06	254	8.1	31.6	10.5	350	−
Sustecal Pudding 5oz. (Mead-Johnson)	1.6	240	6.8	32.0	9.5	640	+
Magnacal (Organon)	2.0	500	17.5	62.5	20.0	590	−
Vivonex (Norwich-Eaton)	1.0	240	5.0	55.2	0.4	645	−
Precision Isotonic (Doyle)	0.96	230	6.9	34.5	7.2	300	−
Precision LR (Doyle)	1.1	266	6.2	59.7	0.2	520	−
Meritine Powder (whole milk) (Doyle)	1.2	277	18.0	31.0	9.0	560	+
Meritine Powder (skim milk) (Doyle)	0.85	203	18.3	31.6	0.6	560	+
Meritine Liquid (Doyle)	1.0	240	14.4	27.6	8.0	560	+
Citrotein (Doyle)	0.53	127	7.67	23.3	0.33	496	−
Nutri-1000 (Cutter)	1.06	254	4.0	10.1	5.5	500	+
Nutri-1000 LF (Cutter)	1.06	254	4.0	10.1	5.5	380	−
Vipep (Cutter)	1.1	333	8.3	58.5	8.3	520	−

*Values based on standard dilution and per 8 fl. oz. (240 cc.) serving.

lower molecular-weight chains are more water-soluble and thus effect a greater osmotic effect.

Electrolytes such as sodium and potassium are relatively small particles. Thus, elevated levels of electrolytes increase the solution's osmolality.

Therefore, formulas or intravenous solutions that are high in concentrations of simple sugars, water-soluble fats, small peptides and free amino acids, sodium, and potassium have the highest osmolality. When taken in large amounts or in concentrated solutions, those solutions with high osmolality can cause major upset in the body's normal water balance. When a concentrated solution of high osmolality enters the gastrointestinal tract, large volumes of water will transfer from the intracellular and intravascular fluid compartments into the stomach and intestines in the attempt to rapidly dilute the solution concentration. In other words, the higher the osmolality of the formula, the more water will be transferred from other body compartments into the gastrointestinal tract. Formulas with high osmolality capable of causing this water shift are those containing large amounts of simple sugars (e.g., 25%–50% dextrose, glucose), sodium, potassium, and free amino acids.

This adaptive water shift causes maladaptive bodily responses: nausea, increased gastrointestinal activity, a feeling of fullness, and increased peristalsis. Diarrhea also occurs due because of the now-diluted formula moving too rapidly through the gastrointestinal tract for the water to be adequately reabsorbed. Additional problems arise for the debilitated client who has not had adequate oral intake for extended periods of time and thus is even more sensitive to formula osmolality. The client who has a history of gastric distress secondary to administration of hypertonic formula is also osmotically sensitive, and clients who exhibit malabsorption may also be unable to tolerate formulas with a high osmolality. Osmolality-induced intolerance to feedings is worsened when the formula is administered rapidly or by bolus rather than slow, continuous infusion.

Formulas that are isotonic or that have low osmolality are better tolerated at least initially by most clients. Isotonic formulas may not need to be initially diluted unless the client shows symptoms of intolerance since the isotonic formula is equal in osmolality to body fluids. Movement of water into the gastrointestinal tract does not usually occur when isotonic formulas are administered. Thus, the gastrointestinal tract does not have to adapt to high formula osmolality. To compare oral/enteral formulas with common oral dietary substances, see Tables 14.9 and 14.10.

Other Tolerance Factors [12]

Although oral and enteral hyperalimentation do not require the use of aseptic technique for preparation and administration, use of clean technique will further increase the client's tolerance to feedings. Commercially prepared products are clean and ready to use when first opened. After opening the commercial formula, refrigerate any that is left in the can or bottle, and discard unused formula after twenty-four (24) hours. This will minimize bacterial contamination. When giving slow, continuous feedings, avoid keeping the formula at room temperature for long periods of time because of the danger of bacterial contamination. Keeping the container of formula in a second container with ice will minimize risk of bac-

Table 14.10. Osmolality of Common Oral Dietary Substances [13]

Oral Substance	mOsm/kg water
Sherbet	1225
Grape juice	1170
Ice cream	1150
Malted milkshake	940
Orange juice	935
Apple juice	870
Egg nog	695
7-Up™	640
Tomato juice	595
Gelatin dessert	535
Ginger ale	510
Whole milk	275

terial infection. By the very fact of the slow infusion, the formula will warm up by the time it travels through the tube and enters the client's body.

The temperature of the formula will affect client tolerance. If the formula is administered cold, the client will likely experience nausea and vomiting, diarrhea, and abdominal cramps. It is best that the formula be at or near room temperature when it enters the client's body.

Postoperative oral or enteral formulas must not be given until peristalsis has returned. Auscultate bowel sounds every four hours postoperatively for the return of peristalsis, and monitor for the appearance of flatus and/or stools. When peristalsis has returned, initiate postoperative oral and enteral feedings very slowly (25–50 milliliters per hour) and closely monitor the client for signs of intolerance. If intolerance occurs, the nurse may dilute the formula, slow the rate of infusion, or consult the physician about temporary discontinuation of the formula feeding for a few days. Continue to monitor bowel sounds and signs of intolerance until the client is tolerating full strength formula well. Clients whose gastrointestinal tracts have not been challenged by feedings for an extended period of time, whether because of surgery or prolonged intravenous feedings, may require an especially slow rate of formula infusion and/or an extended dilution schedule in order to allow the gastrointestinal tract to adapt.

Rate of administration affects client tolerance to feedings. If the formula is administered too fast for the gastrointestinal system to adapt, signs of intolerance will occur. If signs of intolerance occur, decrease the rate of formula administration.

Modification of oral or enteric formulas may be necessary. Clients with diabetes mellitus, cardiac or renal insufficiency, or liver dysfunction will require modified formulas.

Hyperglycemic hyperosmolar nonketotic coma (HHNK) may occur with enteral hyperalimentation if the formula contains very high carbohydrate concentrations. HHNK is most likely to occur in dehydrated or septic clients who are intolerant of high concentrations of glucose. This condition is characterized by coma, extremely elevated serum glucose levels, the absence of ketones in the urine, and an extremely high mortality rate despite emergency medical and nursing interventions. Closely monitor clients at risk for rapid elevations of serum glucose levels, and carefully scrutinize and record urine ketones four times daily, looking for the combination of a decreased level of consciousness, dehydration, extreme hyperglycemia, and the absence of ketones in the urine. If HHNK occurs, restore fluid balance as quickly as possible by prescribed intravenous infusions, give insulin as prescribed, and modify the formula as indicated.

Client tolerance of oral or enteral feedings is also affected by the daily fluid intake. Daily fluid intake is determined by the addition of oral intake, the amount of fluid in the formula, and intravenous fluid intake. Although fluid requirements vary from person to person, the average daily fluid requirement for adults is 2.0 to 2.5 liters per day.

Evaluation of Feedings

If the oral or enteral formula fails to provide adequate amounts of essential nutrients, deficiencies will quickly develop. Daily monitoring indices include watching for fluctuations in weight and observation of daily intake of both nutrients and fluids. If the client gains more than 0.7 kilograms per day (approximately ½–¼ pounds), this is probably reflective of fluid retention rather than true nutritional repletion. In this event, the client is predisposed to congestive heart failure, edema, or ascites. If the client becomes oliguric, this may be reflective of dehydration or organ failure and needs to be evaluated promptly.

Weekly monitoring indices include anthropometric measurements, serum albumin, and the creatinine-height index. Electrolytes, urine urea nitrogen, and serum glucose levels should be monitored every two days during at least the first week of therapy. This provides information about electrolyte status, positive or negative nitrogen balance, and hyperglycemia. If the client has adapted uneventfully to the feeding, these indices can be evaluated at longer intervals.

CONCEPT VIII:
Intravenous hyperalimentation (total parenteral nutrition) is indicated if voluntary oral intake is grossly inadequate and gastrointestinal function is significantly impaired.

Intravenous hyperalimentation is indicated for prevention of malnutrition and cachexia and for nutritional rehabilitation of those clients whose gastrointestinal tract is seriously dysfunctional. Clients who are experiencing gastrointestinal dysfunction secondary to ileus, bowel obstruction, severe malabsorption states, and/or high bowel fistulas will benefit from intravenous hyperalimentation. Clients who are likely to experience pulmonary aspiration of formula or who have severe dehydration are also candidates for this form of nutritional repletion. Intravenous hyperalimentation is also recommended for clients who must rest their gastrointestinal systems because of active, severe inflammatory disease. In one study in which all malnourished clients exhibited immunosuppression, immunocompetence was regained after just a relatively short time of intravenous hyperalimentation [20].

Central venous catheters (Hickman, subclavian, and jugular, in descending order of preference) are preferred over peripheral vein catheters for administration of intravenous hyperalimentation. Ensuring proper placement of a central venous line may be done by X-ray, whereas this is impractical for peripheral lines. Extremely hypertonic solutions of high osmolality, such as 50 percent dextrose, can safely be given by a central line because the rapid flow of blood in the large vein almost instantaneously dilutes the hypertonic solution. Conversely, 10 percent dextrose is usually the maximum osmolality tolerated by peripheral veins. Solutions of greater concentration are associated with an increased incidence of vein destruction and phlebitis. Placement of central venous catheters must be followed by X-ray examination to ensure proper placement and to assess for inadvertent pneumothorax.

Complications of intravenous hyperalimentation are more frequent and dangerous than those associated with enteral hyperalimentation. Placement of a catheter into one of the large veins leading directly to the heart is much more hazardous than slipping down a small-bore, flexible nasogastric tube. Pneumothorax may occur after placement of a central venous line. The needle and stylet may inadvertently puncture the pleural surface, resulting in some degree of pneumothorax. The nurse should mark the point of maximal intensity of the heart with a pen prior to insertion of the catheter. If a pneumothorax occurs, it can be detected by a shift in the PMI toward the deflated lung. Assessment of the point of maximal intensity should be assessed every two hours for the first twelve hours after insertion of the catheter. If a shift in the point of maximal intensity occurs, even without other common signs and symptoms of pneumothorax, the physician should be notified at once. In addition, the client should be kept in a semi-Fowler's position in bed to increase thoracic expansion. The nurse should auscultate breath sounds of both sides every two hours for the first twelve hours after catheter insertion, monitoring for diminished or absent breath sounds of one side. Other signs and symptoms of pneumothorax include dyspnea, shortness of breath, pain upon respiration, and shock-like symptoms if the pneumothorax is extensive. Medical treatment for pneumothorax includes: auscultation of breath sounds every four hours and as needed, monitoring for improvement or decline in breath sounds, and assessment of the location of diminished breath sounds. Keep the client in bed and in a semi-Fowler's position to increase thoracic expansion. Administer oxygen as prescribed.

Sepsis is a complication of central venous hyperalimentation. Sepsis is more likely to occur with intravenous rather than enteral hyperalimentation because of the direct port of entry into the circulatory system. The nurse must continually monitor for signs of localized inflammation at the site of entry as well as for signs of systemic infection. If sepsis is suspected, the central venous catheter should be removed and cultures performed on the catheter tip as well as on blood samples. After cultures have been performed, broad spectrum antibiotics are usually prescribed. The incidence of sepsis in intravenous hyperalimentation is relatively low, being documented in less than 3 percent of cases when aseptic technique is used for insertion and follow-up care [26].

Fluid overload may result from inadequately controlled intravenous hyperalimentation. The primary causative stressor of fluid overload resulting from intravenous hyperalimentation is too rapid an infusion of the solution. All intravenous hyperalimentation must be administered by a controlled-rate machine. The nurse must nevertheless closely monitor the infusion rate and not merely depend on a piece of equipment to accurately deliver the prescribed rate. If the amount infused is behind schedule, the nurse must not try to "catch up" by increasing the infusion rate over the prescribed levels. Instead, simply adjust the machine to the proper drip factor. The nurse must routinely assess for signs of fluid overload.

Hypoglycemia may occur when an intravenous infusion of hypertonic glucose is rapidly discontinued. If intravenous hyperalimentation must be discontinued, gradually reduce the rate of infusion over thirty to forty minutes in order to allow the body to adapt. If the intravenous hyperalimentation infusion discontinues suddenly and cannot be immediately resumed, maintain the client on bedrest and notify the physician. Usually, an infusion of 10 percent dextrose is prescribed to prevent hypoglycemia.

Because of the continuous infusion of hypertonic glucose, the client is at risk for hyperglycemia, diabetic ketoacidosis, or hyperglycemic hyperosmolar nonketotic coma (HHNK). Hyperglycemia hyperosmolar nonketotic coma has a much higher mortality rate than does diabetic ketoacidosis. Hyperglycemic hyperosmolar nonketotic coma develops most often in clients who are hyperglycemic, febrile, and dehydrated. Simple hyperglycemia may also occur with intravenous hyperalimentation. Blood and urine samples of glucose and acetone must be evaluated regularly to provide early detection of hyperglycemia. Insulin is not usually prescribed unless the glucosuria exceeds 3 + .

Since most persons receiving intravenous hyperalimentation are relatively immobile, either passive or active range of motion exercises to all extremities four times daily is necessary for restoration of atrophied muscle mass. Arterial puncture (an iatrogenic condition) and catheter embolus (a spontaneous condition) are uncommon life-threatening emergencies that require immediate, aggressive nursing and medical treatment.

CONCEPT IX:
Solutions of total parenteral nutrition have varying degrees of glucose, protein, fat, sodium, nitrogen, potassium, chloride, and zinc, as well as other minerals.

Although the minimal daily requirement of various nutrients has been determined for enteral hyperalimentation, it is not known if intravenous requirements are the same. Muscle and organ repletion by enteral or intravenous hyperalimentation will occur only if adequate amounts of calories, amino acids, carbohydrates, fats, and other essential nutrients are administered for a sufficient period of time and if positive nitrogen balance is restored.

CONCEPT X:
In cases of fatally ill persons with cancer, aggressive nutritional therapy is replete with ethical dilemmas.

When does intravenous hyperalimentation become a heroic measure? When does enteral hyperalimentation for a comatose, dying client becomes an extraordinary means to prolong life?

It is difficult to determine how aggressive nutritional intervention should be for the person dying from cancer. Although it is possible to put some clients with advanced, fatal disease into positive nitrogen balance through forced feedings or intravenous hyperalimentation, such measures have not been demonstrated to prolong life [32]. In addition, not all fatally ill persons desire aggressive nutritional intervention. For many clients, food tastes and smells terrible and makes them nauseated. Early satiety is very common. Mealtime for these clients often becomes a dismal and draining chore because of their aversion for food.

Nursing interventions in these cases are not specific and clear-cut. The nurse can help the client to optimally deal with this ordeal by supplying supplements of the client's preference, providing advice and counseling regarding ways to make food more palatable, and administering medications for nausea, pain, and mucositis appropriately. Refer the client to psychological counseling as appropriate. Beyond the above interventions, badgering and coercion by the nurse usually only serves to further alienate the client at a time when trust and confidence in the caregiver is of crucial importance. Aggressive coercion usually only increases the client's suffering and forced feedings will often exacerbate the client's depression and sense of helplessness.

REFERENCES

1. Blackburn, G. L. The Effects of Cancer on Nitrogen, Electrolyte, and Mineral Metabolism. *Cancer Res* 37:2348, 1977.
2. Bogert, L. J., Briggs, G. M., and Calloway, D. H. *Nutrition and Physical Fitness* (9th Ed.). Philadelphia: W. B. Saunders Co., 1973. Pp. 224–229.
3. Brennan, M. F. Uncomplicated Starvation versus Cancer Cachexia. *Cancer Res* 37:2359, 1977.
4. Bury, K. D. Elemental Diets. In J. E. Fischer (Ed.). *Total Parenteral Nutrition.* Boston: Little, Brown and Co., 1976. Pp. 395–411.
5. Butler, J. H. Nutrition and Cancer: A Review of the Literature. *Cancer Nurs* 3:131, 1980.
6. Butterfield, C. and Blackburn, G. Hospital Malnutrition. *Nutr Today* 10:8, 1975.
7. Copeland, E. M. III, Daly, J. M., and Stanley, J. D. Nutrition as an Adjunct to Cancer Treatment in the Adult. *Cancer Res* 37:2451, 1977.
8. Copeland, F. and Dundrick, S. Intravenous Hyperalimentation as an Adjunct to Cancer Chemotherapy. *Am J Surg* 2:129, 167, 1975.
9. Costa, G. Cachexia and the Systemic Effects of Tumors. In J. F. Holland and E. Frei (Eds.). *Cancer Medicine.* Philadelphia: Lea and Febiger, 1973. Pp. 1035–1043.
10. Costa, G. Cachexia, the Metabolic Component of Neoplastic Diseases. *Cancer Res* 37:2327, 1977.
11. Doyle Pharmaceutical Company. *The Importance of Nutrition in the Catabolic State.* Minneapolis: Doyle Pharmaceutical Co., 1976.
12. Doyle Pharmaceutical Company. *Factors Affecting Tolerance to Tube Feedings.* Minneapolis: Doyle Pharmaceutical Co. 1979.
13. Doyle Pharmaceutical Company. *A Critical Factor Affecting Tolerance to Tube Feedings . . . Osmolality.* Minneapolis: Doyle Pharmaceutical Co., 1980.
14. Eastwood, G. I. Small Bowel Morphology and Epithelial Proliferation in Intravenously Alimented Rabbits. *Surg* 82:613, 1977.

15. Harvey, K., Both, A., and Blackburn, G. L. Nutritional Assessment and Patient Outcome During Oncological Therapy. *Cancer* 43:2065, May Supplement, 1979.
16. Heymsfield, S. B., Bethel, R. A., Ansley, J. D., Nixon, D. W., and Rudman, D. Enteral Hyperalimentation: An Alternative to Central Venous Alimentation. *Ann Intern Med* 90:63, 1979.
17. Isaacs, J. W., Millikan, W. J., Siackhoust, J., Hirsh, T., and Rudman, D. Parenteral Nutrition of Adults with a 900 MilliOsmolar Solution via Peripheral Veins. *Am J Clin Nutr* 30:552, 1977.
18. Kinney, J. M. Energy Requirements for Parenteral Nutrition. In J. E. Rischer (Ed.). *Total Parenteral Nutrition.* Boston: Little, Brown and Co., 1976.
19. Koga, Y., Ikeda, K., Inokuchi, K., Waianahi, H., and Hashimoto, M. The Digestive Tract in Total Parenteral Nutrition. *Arch Surg* 110:742, 1975.
20. Law, D. Immunocompetence of Patients with Protein-Calorie Malnutrition. *Ann Intern Med* 72:545, 1973.
21. Levine, G. M., Deren, J. J., Steiger, E., and Zinno, R. Role of Oral Intake in Maintenance of Gut Mass and Disaccharidase Activity. *Gastroenterology* 67:975, 1974.
22. Lindsey, A. M., Piper, B. F., and Stotts, N. A. The Phenomenon of Cancer Cachexia: A Review. *Oncology Nurs Forum* 9(2):38, 1982.
23. Long, C. L. Parenteral Nutrition in the Septic Patient. *Am J Clin Nutr* 29:380, 1976.
24. Maxwell, M. B. Cancer, Hypoalbuminemia, and Nutrition. *Cancer Nurs* 4:451, 1981.
25. National Dairy Council. An Update on Nutrition, Diet, and Cancer. *Dairy Council Dig* 51 (5):25, 1980.
26. Portlock, C. S. and Goffinet, D. R. *Manual of Clinical Problems in Oncology.* Boston: Little, Brown and Co., 1980. Pp. 265–269.
27. Randall, H. T. Surgical Nutrition: Parenteral and Oral. In Committee on Preoperative and Postoperative Care, American College of Surgeons. *Manual of Preoperative and Postoperative Care.* Philadelphia: W. B. Saunders Co., 1971. Pp. 75–93.
28. Randall, H. T. Water, Electrolytes, and Acid-Base Balance. In R. S. Goodhart and M. E. Shils (Eds.). *Modern Nutrition in Health and Disease* (5th Ed.). Philadelphia: Lea and Febiger, 1973. Pp. 324–361.
29. Randall, H. T. Diet and Nutrition in the Care of the Surgical Patient. In R. S. Goodhart and M. E. Shils (Eds.). *Modern Nutrition in Health and Disease* (5th Ed.). Philadelphia: Lea and Febiger, 1973. Pp. 950–965.
30. Salmond, S. W. How to Assess the Nutritional Status of Acutely Ill Patients. *Am J Nurs* 80:922, 1980.
31. Steffee, W. P. Malnutrition in Hospitalized Patients. *JAMA* 244:2630, 1980.
32. Theologides, A. Cancer Cachexia. In M. Wineck (Ed.). *Nutrition and Cancer.* New York: John Wiley and Sons, 1977. Pp. 75–94.
33. Theologides, A. Pathogenesis of Cachexia in Cancer: A Review and A Hypothesis. In L. C. Kruse, J. L. Reese, and L. K. Hart (Eds.). *Cancer: Pathophysiology, Etiology, and Management.* St. Louis: C. V. Mosby., 1979. Pp. 357–363.
34. Van Eys, J. Nutritional Management as Adjuvant in Pediatric Cancer Therapy. In American Cancer Society. *Proceedings of the National Conference on the Care of the Child with Cancer.* New York: American Cancer Society, 1979. Pp. 86–92.

Chapter 15

Professional Survival: Care of the Caregiver

CONCEPT I:
A commitment to high-quality cancer nursing may produce profound emotional exhaustion and burnout.

The phenomenon of burnout and its accompanying emotional exhaustion can be better understood by examining the philosophical concept of the absurd. The basic confrontation of the absurd is the recognition of and personal struggle with the gap between human needs and the unreasonably unresponsive world [2]. When this philosophical concept is applied to the world of health professionals, it is often represented by the question, "What can I say to this dying person to give hope?" when, at the same time, the nurse or physician may realize that there is indeed nothing to say. Since nurses and physicians are unprepared by education for this inevitable philosophical confrontation and since nursing and medical education are heavily oriented toward cure, nurses and physicians may feel helpless and embarrassed when faced with a dying client for whom there is no future. Hope is almost always endogenous; in other words, even realistic hope must be internalized by the client before it becomes real [6]. Health professionals cannot "give" hope. They can combat despair and hopelessness with honesty, realism, teaching, and caring. But hope springs from within the ill person—it cannot be "given" like a medicine or a treatment, regardless of the health professional's desire to do so. Therein lies the conflict of the absurd.

The danger for nurses and physicians in this conflict of the absurd is that they may buy into the attitude of omnipotence, believing that it is within their power to alter the course of the client's life and to struggle mightily to defeat death. For these nurses and physicians, success is measured by cure rate, and a "No Code" written on the chart is an admission of failure. Because of the relative power held by nurses, and especially physicians, an attempt to resuscitate clients who could not possibly be restored to a meaningful existence is the common response of these health professionals—nurses and physicians who shout "*I* will not give up . . . *I* will not be defeated" even when the client has made it known that she or he does not desire extraordinary, heroic attempts to "save" his or her life. The sad result that is all too often seen in this situation is a client resuscitated to a brief extension of a life filled with suffering and pain, or, even worse, the absurd result of a dead mind in a "live" body. Nurses and physicians who respond to the confrontation of the absurd in this way have a relationship with the client characterized by an attitude of "I-It."

Nurses and physicians will hopefully eventually realize that they are *not* omnipotent and that death cannot always be defeated. Indeed, death is a normal part of life and is not always an enemy. A potentially healthy death can so easily be made into a painful, distressing, unhealthy death by the attitude of "I-It." Nurses and physicians must learn a better and more adaptive response to this confrontation with the absurd. For someone who is dying, presence without words is as helpful as listening and talking were earlier. By simply and compassionately sharing human existence with the client, "I-It" becomes "I-Thou."

Nurses and physicians face the unavoidable dilemma of the choice between avoidance and involvement in this confrontation with the absurd. There are both positive and negative aspects of cancer care that can create serious personal conflict within the caregiver. Most oncology nurses and physicians realize the importance of giving emotional support, counseling, and compassionate care to *all* clients and their families. Yet, as a result of this very involvement, the caregiver is extremely vulnerable to private, personal psychic distress. Although there are many rewards in cancer care, it must be realistically recognized that disease, pain, and suffering occupy a very large portion of the caregiver's daily life.

The phenomenon of burnout is a syndrome of physical and personal exhaustion accompanied by the development of a negative self-concept, negative job attitudes, and a loss of concern and feeling for ill clients [8]. The risk of developing burnout is not equal in all areas of nursing. Highly specialized nursing areas, which require that the nurse constantly deal with intense, emotionally charged situations (e.g., oncology, terminal care, intensive care) seem to carry an increased risk for burnout [7]. These types of nursing areas are characterized by a heavier workload of sicker clients, as well as the necessity for nurses to be assertive, independent, and possess advanced skills. Areas with these types of nurses predispose to the confrontation with the absurd. The nurse's skills, resources, and spirit are pitted against intractable circumstances, a confrontation that must take place before burnout can ever develop [11]. If burnout does come to be, the nurse experiences disillusionment and a sense of personal defeat in the face of the job's external realities. Because cancer nurses experience more enduring stress than do nurses in other high-stress areas [10], cancer nursing carries a high risk of burnout; cancer nursing is usually a more emotionally and physically depleting nursing experience. The end result of burnout is a self-reinforcing cycle of frustration, helplessness, and cynicism.

Besides the actual area of nursing practice, certain personal traits have been associated with a high risk for burnout. These include dedicated and committed nurses who take on too much for too long or the overly committed nurse who substitutes work for social life. Also at high risk for burnout are authoritarian nurses, those who view themselves to be indispensable, nurses who tend to personally overidentify with clients [4], and nurses who set unrealistically high standards for themselves, their peers, and their clients [12]. Conversely, nurses who seem to have a low risk for burnout include those who have (1) an internal locus of control, (2) a reasonable amount of personal flexibility, (3) the ability to voice disagreement or frustration, (4) a support system outside of the work situation, and (5) lower and perhaps more reasonable expectations of themselves and their jobs [12].

It is neither good nor bad to have a high or low risk for burnout. Although idealistic nurses with high levels of expectations may be at greater risk for burnout, these same nurses are the very ones who continuously work toward the goals of better client care and increased professionalism among nurses. Having lower expectations of themselves and their jobs—and thus a lower risk for burnout—might mean that the nurse recognizes his or her own human limitations. On the other hand, it might also mean that he or she is complacently satisfied to give mediocre nursing care. Thus, it is not necessarily "bad" to be at high risk for burnout or "good" to be at low risk. What is most important is to identify the stressors that are causing the burnout so that knowledgeable, skillful nurses with high ideals continue to provide high-quality cancer care.

CONCEPT II:
Like any other maladaptive condition, burnout has identifiable causative stressors that can be altered or eliminated.

SOCIAL STRESSORS

Our society is characterized as being highly competitive, individualistic, and oriented toward achievement and success. During the last two decades, the nursing profession has increasingly delineated areas of specialty practice and has become more and more concerned with professional and personal merit. Many nurses today are motivated toward high levels of self-actualization, wanting more out of nursing than merely a paycheck. Even the salaries of nurses with years of education and high levels of expertise, however, are not commensurate with the rapidly increasing health care costs and physicians' fees. Thus, the social reward of material success is withheld from even highly skilled, dedicated, and knowledgeable nurses.

PERSONAL STRESSORS

Because of the motivation toward self-actualization as well as the rapid and painful growth being experienced in nursing as a whole, nurses tend to have ever-increasing expectations of themselves. Nursing education, by and large, presents idealism along with college diplomas; and thus the nurse often expects herself or himself to always be a source of strength for clients, to have unlimited energy, and to be equipped to solve any and all problems. These expectations inevitably clash with hospital reality and lead to feelings of impotence and frustration, thus predisposing the nurse to burnout.

PROFESSIONAL STRESSORS

Health professionals have been taught that their ultimate goal is to save lives, which is a good and true goal *unless* the concept of a healthy death as a normal part of life is not included in that goal. In cancer care, many clients *are* cured of their disease process and so the reward of knowing that they helped to save a life is given to the caregivers. However, a large proportion of persons with cancer have a chronic disease course with both extended periods of quality life and acute exacerbations of disease-related problems, eventually culminating in death. Still other clients experience a rapid downhill course from diagnosis to death. It is usually not possible for the oncology nurse or oncologist to predict that trajectory of the client's disease process, and this very uncertainty about the kind of support or what meassage to give to the client and family can cause significant distress to the caregiver. If aggressive antineoplastic treatment is given, the morbidity experienced by the client in terms of painful, sometimes intractable side effects may make the nurse feel ambivalent or cynical about the efficacy of anticancer treatment and about the value of aggressive or investigational medical treatment. If the nurse is unable to prevent or control distressing side effects, feelings of impotence and anger increase. Finally—despite all of the skills, despite all of the knowledge, despite all of the compassionate human support that the nurses and physicians can give— many, many persons with cancer die from their disease. This situation may leave the caregivers with a sense of repeated failure. Dying persons and mourning families are not able to provide much gratification to their caregivers. The nurse who gives postmortem care to a client-become-friend must also then immediately walk into the room of yet another client-become-friend and give caring, support, and help.

Cancer nursing is filled with difficult decisions, ethical conflicts, and physically demanding work that can substantially decrease the nurse's energy and coping abilities. In teaching hospitals, highly knowledgeable and skilled oncology nurses often find themselves in the difficult situation of working with resident physicians who have much less expertise in the unique problems presented by cancer clients; yet these resident physicians may not seek or accept problem-solving advice from the nurses. This further increases any anger or frustration that the nurse might hold.

The advanced skills and knowledge held by cancer nurses provides increased satisfaction with their professional roles, yet may simultaneously engender serious conflict with physicians and other health care professionals who may perceive that the cancer nurse is impinging upon their territory. This often leads to internal "turf battles," damaging cohesion within the treatment team and placing the nurse in a position of defending his or her role and decisions.

INSTITUTIONAL STRESSORS

Stressors within the health care agency itself also contribute to the phenomenon of burnout. Heavy caseloads, the struggle with bureaucratic red tape, and large quantities of "necessary" paperwork deplete the nurse's physical and personal energy. The lack of strong leadership and good management, inadequate communication and supervision, and poorly defined job descriptions are also possible stressors that predispose nurses to burnout.

CONCEPT III:
If the nurse responds in maladaptive ways to these stressors, burnout is likely to occur.

PHYSICAL SYMPTOMS OF BURNOUT

The most common symptom of burnout is physical/emotional exhaustion and fatigue [7]. The nurse's own body is neglected rather than replenished and the result is a body that is distressed, diseased, and vulnerable to dysfunction [3, 7, 9]. This physical exhaustion and decreased resistance to disease is cumulative and progressive. Common complaints of physical distress include headaches, epigastric distress, insomnia, a decreased resistance to infection, and a general feeling of unwellness. The nurse experiencing burnout may increase his or her use of cigarettes, alcohol, or drugs.

PERSONAL SYMPTOMS OF BURNOUT

As burnout progresses, the caregiver may experience crippling anxiety that results in severe depression and disabled thinking processes. Problem-solving skills decline, the ability to make decisions is impaired, and the nurse may have difficulty controlling emotions. The nurse experiencing burnout may become excessively cynical, displaying rigid and stubborn behavior. He or she may seem determined to block change and progress [1, 5, 7].

Anger and denial are common defense mechanisms observed in nurses and physicians in the attempt to cope with this crippling anxiety. Since the nurse usually becomes the client advocate for the client, anger is especially common when the course of medical treatment is ambiguous or experimental. If the nurse is put in the position of carrying out painful, distressing treatments that are antithetical to nurturing, the nurse's anger is often directed toward the physicians and/or the family. The nurse may view himself or herself as the token torturer, with the physician prescribing the treatments and then being able to walk away from the situation. The nurse, then, is left to carry out treatment measures that he or she may not agree with and that cause more pain and suffering to the client. As a result, the nurse becomes angry and vulnerable to ever-increasing burnout.

Denial is most commonly exhibited by an increasing involvement in the more technical aspects of nursing. This increased orientation toward task performance puts a comforting shield of distance between the nurse and the client. One study revealed that the more chronic and intractable the client's disease was perceived to be, the greater the share of the nurse's time spent with administrative tasks. The nurse wanted pharmaceutical interventions rather than personal contact with the client [8].

SOCIAL AND PROFESSIONAL SYMPTOMS

As burnout progresses, the nurse's relationships with other people decrease in importance, and there is often a sense of detachment from coworkers, family, and friends. Negative feelings are often expressed at home rather than at work, and thus the nurse alienates those people outside of the work setting who could provide support.

CONCEPT IV:
Although burnout can be effectively and positively resolved, the best treatment is prevention.

The most important preventive measure for burnout is that the nurse must accept responsibility for his or her own health and well-being. Nurses must first attend to their own needs: a nutritious diet, adequate sleep, and regular physical exercise. Nurses should take time for "after-work decompression." A walk outside, a shower or bath, etc. after work allows the nurse to separate the worlds of work and home, thus making it easier to release the problems, the pain, the diseases that have filled the previous several hours. Nurses need to assess themselves for the prodromal signs of distress and inappropriate coping behaviors. If insomnia, anger, increased smoking or drinking, or feelings of depression are noted, the nurse needs to look for the source of the problem and deal with it openly before it becomes worse.

Cancer nurses, in particular, need effective support systems both at home and at work. By the very nature of the work involved in oncology nursing, cancer nurses may eventually feel surrounded by death, disease, and pain; and they may succumb to the frustration and feelings of impotence that lead to burnout. Adequate support systems allow the nurse to share problems, feelings, and struggles. The cancer nurse who does not get emotional support cannot give emotional support: one cannot give if one's own bucket is empty.

Health care agencies can implement special solutions to show special regard for cancer nurses in their employ. A pay differential, flexible work schedules, and innovative staffing patterns can provide special rewards for cancer nurses. It is important that the nurse in danger of burnout be able to temporarily withdraw from stressful job situations. Time off for educational experiences or rotation to a non-oncology unit reinforces the idea that not everyone in the world has cancer.

The oncology unit itself must provide adequate orientation instead of having a "sink-or-swim" attitude toward nurses new to the unit. The cancer nursing staff should collaboratively develop a strong unit philosophy, and this philosophy should be printed and posted in a highly visible place on the unit. Supervisors, head nurses, and other nurse-managers need to realize that rules and policies are necessary but that they must also be flexible.

In summary, to prevent burnout, nurses must first be true to themselves. By acknowledging their own human limitations and by having reasonable and realistic self-expectations, cancer nurses are less likely to perceive themselves as helpless and are thus less vulnerable to the debilitating ruin of burnout.

REFERENCES

1. Alexander, C. J. Counteracting Burnout. AORN J 3:597, 1980.
2. Camus, A. *The Myth of Sisyphus and Other Essays.* (Translated by J. O'Brien). New York: Vintage Books, 1955.
3. Clark, C. C. Burnout: Assessment and Intervention. *J Nurs Adm* 10:39, 1980.

 4. Freudenberger, H. J. Staff Burn-Out. *J Soc Issues* 30:159, 1974.
 5. Levine, A. S. The Doctor's Dilemma: "I-It" or "I-Thou"? In American Cancer Society. *Proceedings of the American Cancer Society Second National Conference on Human Values and Cancer.* New York: American Cancer Society, 1978. Pp. 29–35.
 6. Levine, A. S., Artiss, K. L., and Susman, E. J. The Impact of Childhood Cancer on Doctors and Nurses. In American Cancer Society. *Proceedings of the National Conference on the Care of the Child with Cancer.* New York: American Cancer Society, 1979. Pp. 137–143.
 7. McElroy, A. M. Burnout: A Review of the Literature with Application to Cancer Nursing. *Cancer Nurs* 5:211, 1982.
 8. Pines, A. and Maslach, C. Characteristics of Staff Burnout in Mental Health Settings. *Hosp Community Psychiatry* 29:233, 1978.
 9. Skinner, K. Burn-Out: Is Nursing Dangerous to Your Health? *J Nurs Care* 12:8, 1979.
10. Stewart, B. E., Meyerowitz, B. E., Jackson, L. E., Yarkin, K. L., and Harvey, J. H. Psychological Stress Associated with Outpatient Oncology Nursing. *Cancer Nurs* 5:383, 1982.
11. Storlie, F. J. Burnout: The Elaboration of a Concept. *Am J Nurs* 79:2108, 1979.
12. Vachon, M. L. S. Motivation and Stress Experienced by Staff Working with the Terminally Ill. *Death Ed* 2:113, 1978.

Concluding Remarks

There is an old story about how God took a man to two doors and showed him glimpses of Heaven and Hell. God opened the first door and the man looked inside. He saw a large table in the center of the room. In the middle of the table was a large pot of stew, and it smelled so good that it made the man's mouth water. There were many people sitting around the table and each person had a long-handled spoon, but all of the people were emaciated, pallid, and ill-looking. The man saw the problem at once: the handles on the spoons were longer than the arms of the people and so, although they could get a spoonful of delicious stew, they could not then get the spoonful of food into their mouths. Thus, they were starving in the midst of plenty. God closed the door and said to the man, "You have seen Hell." Then God opened the next door and said, "Now you shall see Heaven." The man look in and saw the same large table, the same pot of delicious stew, and the same long-handled spoons in the hands of each person. But in this room, the people were plump and well-fed, happy and laughing. The man was puzzled and turned to God, saying, "I don't understand." "It is simple," said God. "You see, here the people are feeding each other."

It is the author's sincere hope that, within the realm of cancer care, all of us—nurses, physicians, other caregivers, clients, and families—will begin to acknowledge our own struggles with the issues of pain, disease, suffering, life, and death. By doing so, we can perhaps begin to remove the old barriers between us and start to nurture one another, being bound together by what has been called the Fellowship of the Broken.

Glossary

Adaptation Successful change in one's internal or external environment in response to an aversive stressor, resulting in optimal wellness despite the stressor.

Adenocarcinoma A carcinoma with glandular elements.

Agglutinin See *lectin.*

Agonal Pertaining to death or extreme suffering.

Alkylating antineoplastic drugs Antineoplastic drugs that act by inserting an "alkyl" chemical group into a critical cellular component, such as DNA. This disrupts the molecular function of the cell and the cell cannot survive.

Alopecia Loss of hair resulting from destruction of or damage to the hair follicle.

Alpha-fetoprotein (AFP) An antigen tumor marker associated with testicular germ-cell tumors, liver cancer, and gastric malignancies.

Anabolism The constructive phase of metabolism in which body cells synthesize protoplasm for growth and repair.

Anaplasia Malignant, irreversible alteration in which the structural patterns of adult cells regress to more primitive levels.

Anemia Reduced quantity of erythrocytes and/or reduced hemoglobin in the circulating erythrocytes. Results in overall reduction of bodily oxygenation.

Anisocytosis Erythrocytes in the circulating blood that show abnormal variation in size.

Anorexia Lack of appetite.

Anthropometric Measurements of the size, weight, and proportions of the human body; used in nutritional assessment.

Antibody A protein that is produced in the body in response to invasion by a foreign antigen and that reacts specifically with it, neutralizing or destroying the foreign invader. Almost all antibodies are produced in lymph nodes, spleen, bone marrow, and lymphoid tissue.

Antigen Any substance, almost always a protein, not normally found in the body which, when present, stimulates production of an antibody that reacts specifically with the antigen.

Antimetabolite antineoplastic drugs Antineoplastic drugs that kill cells by interfering with specific metabolic steps critical to cell division.

Antineoplastic Anticancer, such as in antineoplastic drugs.

Antineoplastic antibiotic drugs Anticancer antibiotic drugs that have a variety of mechanisms of action, the most important of which is probably their ability to directly disrupt the function of the cell's DNA.

Asterixis "Liver flap"; a symptom of hepatic encephalopathy; a motor disturbance marked by intermittent sustained contraction of groups of muscles.

Bacteremia A serious pathological condition in which there is the presence of bacteria in the circulating blood.

Basal energy expenditure (BEE)   The minimum amount of calories and protein necessary for the person's survival; the minimum amount of calories and protein necessary to prevent catabolism.

Basophil   A medium-sized leukocyte with large granules; part of the group of leukocytes termed granulocytes; normally constituting 0.5% of the leukocytes in the circulating blood.

B-cell Immunity   See *Humoral immunity.*

Benign   Nonmalignant; noncancerous.

"Blast"   Immature leukocyte without the development of the definitive characteristics of the mature leukocyte.

-blastic   Suffix used in classification of leukemia, denoting the presence of immature "blast" leukocyte cells.

Blood/brain barrier   The barrier that prevents or delays certain substances in the blood from entering the brain tissue.

Body image   The perception that one has of one's own body (e.g., intact or damaged, whole or incomplete, pretty or ugly, etc.).

Body surface area   A calculation of the quantity of surface area of an individual's body; expressed in square meters.

Breast-cyst Fluid Proteins (BCFP)   Tissue-associated antigens thought to be tumor markers associated with breast carcinoma.

Cachexia   A condition of severe malnutrition, emaciation, and debility, usually seen in the course of a chronic illness.

Calorie   The amount of energy (heat) required to raise the temperature of one kilogram of water by one degree Celsius (C.).

Carcinoembryonic Antigen (CEA)   A tumor marker associated with malignancies of the gastrointestinal tract.

Carcinogen   A physical, chemical, or biological stressor that causes neoplastic change in normal cells.

Carcinogenesis   The development of cancer.

Carcinogenic   Having an effect on cells that results in malignant transformation of the normal cell; causing cancer.

Carcinoma   A solid malignant tumor composed of epithelial tissues (derived from primitive ectoderm or endoderm).
  Carcinoma in situ   A lesion with all the histological characteristics of malignancies except invasion.

Carcinomatosis   The development of multiple carcinomas throughout the body; commonly used to refer to widespread metastatic malignant disease.

Catabolism   The destructive phase of metabolism in which the body stores of calories, fat, and protein are used to maintain the basal energy requirements of the individual.

Cell cycle   The reproductive cycle of all cells.
  G_0 **phase**   Resting phase without reproductive activity; normal cells enter the next phase only by specific stimuli.
  G_1 **phase**   Reproductive activity begins with protein and RNA synthesis.
  S phase   Reproductive activity continues with synthesis of DNA.
  G_2 **phase**   Reproductive activity continues with additional synthesis of protein and RNA.
  M phase   Reproductive activity concludes with mitosis and cell division. The daughter cells either return to G_0 or G_1.

Cellular Immunity   One of three forms of immunological activity in which sensitized lymphocytes (T-cells) mature in the thymus and are stored in lymphoid tissue; upon stimulation by an antigen, the sensitized lymphocytes are released into the circulating blood and either destroy the antigens on contact or prepare the antigen for destruction by macrophages. Also known as *T-Cell Immunity.*

Chalone   Thought to be a glycoprotein that inhibits growth and proliferation of normal cells.

Chemotherapy   The use of chemicals and drugs to combat disease; most commonly used as a referral to anticancer drug therapy.
>   **Cell-cycle Dependent**   Refers to antineoplastic chemotherapeutic drugs that exert their anticancer effect only upon those cells that are in a certain stage of the reproductive cell cycle.
>   **Cell-cycle Independent**   Refers to antineoplastic chemotherapeutic drugs that will exert their anticancer effect on cells in any stage of the reproductive cell cycle.

Chromatin   The DNA-containing chromosomal substance of the nucleus of a cell.

Clonogenic   A cell that has the ability to clone (to reproduce itself asexually).

Colon mucoprotein antigen (CMA)   An investigational tumor marker that is apparently specific for cancer of the colon.

Colostomy   A surgical procedure in which an artificial opening is made on the surface of the abdomen for the purpose of evacuating the bowels and to act as a substitute for the rectum and anus. May be temporary or permanent.

-cytic   Suffix used in the classification of leukemia, denoting the presence of relatively mature leukocyte cells.

Cytocidal   An agent, such as a drug, that destroys cells.

Cytostatic   An agent, such as a drug, that prevents the reproduction of cells.

Cytotoxic   Having a deleterious effect on cells.

Death   The end of physical life as we know it, usually defined by the lack of brain activity.
>   **Healthy death**   A death in which the individual dies in the manner he/she desires, with a minimum of pain and suffering, and with the personal and social components of his/her life intact and functioning at optimal wellness.
>   **Unhealthy death**   A death in which the individual does not die in the manner he/she desires, without optimal control of pain and suffering, and without intact, optimally functional personal and social life components.

Death trajectory   The course of dying, unique to each person. There are four defined death trajectories: (1) certain death at a known time, (2) certain death at an unknown time, (3) certain death at an unknown time but a known time when a prognosis will be able to be made, and (4) uncertain death and an unknown time when a certain prognosis may be made.

Differentiated cells   Cells with recognizable specialized structures and functions.

Diffuse tumors   The leukemias, the diffuse lymphomas, and multiple myeloma.

Distress   Unhealthy, uncomfortable stress.

Drug addiction   An often-used but vague term, representing the extreme of a combination of physical/psychological dependence on a drug; a behavioral pattern of compulsive drug use, such as compulsive use of a narcotic without a pain experience.

Drug dependence   An abnormal physiological state resulting from repeated administration of a drug which then makes it necessary to continue to use that drug to prevent a withdrawal syndrome. *NOT* synonymous with "drug addiction." In clients with chronic cancer pain, the need for an increased drug dosage probably indicates a change in disease status rather than a problem with physical dependence.

Drug tolerance   A reduced responsiveness to *any* effect of *any* drug as a consequence of prior administration of that drug, necessitating larger doses of the drug to produce an equivalent effect to that of the initial dose. *NOT* synonymous with "drug addiction."

Dukes' criteria   Method for staging large-bowel malignant tumors.
  Stage A   Primary tumor restricted to bowel wall. Five-year survival approximately 90%.
  Stage B   Primary tumor has invaded through the bowel wall and into peritoneum or perirectal fat. Five-year survival approximately 65%.
  Stage C   Evidence of distant metastases. Five-year survival approximately 20%.

Dysplasia   A benign change in which an adult cell varies from its normal size, shape, or organization. Often due to chronic irritation. May reverse itself or may progress to malignancy.

Endorphins   Endogenous "natural morphines" released from the pituitary gland.

Enkephalins   Endogenous morphine-like analgesic hormones.

Enteral hyperalimentation   Nutritional hyperalimentation administered by nasogastric tube or gastrostomy.

Eosinophil   A medium-sized leukocyte normally constituting 1–2% of the leukocytes in the circulating blood.

Eosinophilia   An abnormal increase in the quantity of eosinophils in the circulating blood; usually associated with allergic conditions.

Epidermoid   A malignant tumor formed by epidermal cells.

Epistaxis   Nosebleed.

Epstein-Barr virus   A virus thought to be an etiological factor in the development of Burkitt's lymphoma, nasopharyngeal carcinoma, and Hodgkin's disease.

Erythrocyte   Red blood cell.

Etiology   The science of dealing with causes of disease.

Exacerbate   To make worse.

External environment   Any condition, stressor, or component (biological, personal, or social) outside of and capable of affecting the individual.

Extravasation   Escape of intravenous fluid from the blood vessel into surrounding tissue; intravenous infiltration.

Familial   Occurring in or affecting members of the same family.

Fibronectin   A substance occurring in greatly reduced amounts of the membranes of rapidly dividing cells (both normal and malignant).

Galactosyl transferase isoenzyme-II (GT-II)   An antigen thought to be a tumor marker associated with malignancies of the pancreas, stomach, and colon.

Genome   The total gene complement of the chromosomes of a cell.

Grade, grading   A method of classifying malignancies on a scale of I to IV based upon the degree of cellular anaplasia observed under the microscope.
  Grade I   Well-differentiated malignant cells closely resembling normal cells.
  Grade II   Moderately differentiated cells.
  Grade III   Poorly differentiated cells.
  Grade IV   Undifferentiated cells; may even be difficult to determine the tissue of origin.

Granulocyte   A leukocyte containing neutrophilic, basophilic, or eosinophilic granules in its cytoplasm. The first leukocyte to react to a foreign agent or pathogen in the body.
   Banded granulocyte   An immature granulocyte.

Granulocytopenia   An abnormally low number of granulocytes in the circulating blood.

Granulocytosis   An abnormally high number of granulocytes in the circulating blood.

Growth fraction   Tumor growth fraction is the ratio of proliferating to nonproliferating malignant cells.

Helplessness   A subjective feeling in which the individual believes that he/she cannot control his/her own life events.

Hematemesis   Vomiting of blood or blood-containing stomach contents.

Hepatomegaly   Enlargement of the liver.

Hepatosplenomegaly   Enlargement of the liver and the spleen.

Hickman catheter (Hickman-Broviac catheter)   A semipermanent intravenous line that is operatively placed by tunneling under the skin and entering the subclavian vein, with the tip of the catheter resting in the right atrium; useful for clients requiring frequent venipunctures.

Hodgkin's disease   A specific type of lymphoma, differing from all other lymphomas in its predictability of spread, microscopic characteristics, and occurrence of extranodal tumors.

Holistic   Pertaining to the whole person, inclusive of physiological, psychological, social, and spiritual aspects.

Homeostasis   A state of adaptive balance in the internal environment.

Hopelessness   A subjective feeling in which the client feels unable to believe that a desired outcome to an aversive situation is possible.

Hospice   A concept of care for fatally ill persons that includes the concepts of intensive caring rather than intensive care; the extensive therapeutic use of self rather than extensive use of technology and equipment; the family as the target of nursing care; and the broad goal being to relieve pain in its broadest sense and to facilitate optimal quality of life and a healthy death.

Human chorionic gonadotropin (HCG)   A placental antigen known to be a tumor marker for choriocarcinoma; may also be a tumor marker for testicular cancer.

Humoral immunity   One of three forms of immunological activity, known also as "B-Cell Immunity" and the "Antibody Response." B-cells are produced in the bone marrow and then differentiate into plasma cells that produce the antibody as a result of direct or indirect stimulation by the circulating antigen. The antibody response is highly specific for each antigen.

Hyperalimentation   Nutritional supplementation of calories, protein, and other nutritional elements.
   Enteral hyperalimentation   Nutritional supplementation by nasogastric tube or gastrostomy tube.
   Intravenous hyperalimentation   Nutritional supplementation by peripheral intravenous or central venous line infusion; also known as Total Parenteral Nutrition.

Hyperplasia   Any abnormal increase in the number (quantity) of cells in a tissue or part of a tissue, resulting in increased tissue mass. May be benign or malignant.

Hyperthermia   Greatly increased body temperature.

Ileostomy   Surgical procedure creating an opening into the ileum.

Immunotherapy   An investigational antineoplastic medical treatment modality in which the individual with cancer is administered certain antigens in the attempt to stimulate the client's own immune system to recognize the malignant cells as "not self" and destroy them.

Induction therapy   Specific and intensive chemotherapeutic drug administration in an attempt to put the client's malignancy into remission.

Inflammatory response   A tissue response to injury or destruction of cells with three sequential physiological events: vascular dilitation, leukocytosis, and fluid exudation. The inflammatory response has four classic symptoms: heat, swelling, redness, and localized pain. Occasionally, loss of function at the site of injury occurs.

In situ (carcinoma in situ)   A lesion with all the histological characteristics of malignancy except invasion.

Internal environment   The holistic physiological, personal, and social components within the individual's self.

Intra-arterial injection   Fluids or drugs injected into an artery.

Intracavity injection   Fluids or drugs injected into a body cavity.

Intrapleural injection   Fluids or drugs injected into the lung(s).

Intrathecal injection   Fluids or drugs injected into the cerebrospinal fluid, thus bypassing the blood-brain barrier.

Intravenous injection   Fluids or drugs injected into a vein.

Karnowsky scale   An assessment tool used to evaluate the overall condition and performance ability of a client.

Lectin   Also known as *Agglutinin*. Multivalent carbohydrate-binding proteins that attach to certain cell-surface receptor sites; thought to control the adhesion of one cell to another.

Leukemia   A diffuse malignant tumor characterized by abnormal proliferation and release of leukocyte precursors. Classification is based upon (1) predominant cell type and (2) whether the disease is acute or chronic.
  Acute leukemia   Characterized by the proliferation and release of blast (immature) leukocytes. More virulent than chronic leukemia.
  Chronic leukemia   Characterized by the presence of more mature leukocytes. Less virulent than acute leukemia.

Leukocyte   White blood cell; a colorless blood corpuscle whose chief function is to defend the body against pathogenic microorganisms causing disease. There are five types of leukocytes: lymphocytes, monocytes, neutrophils, eosinophils, and basophils, the last three often referred to collectively as granulocytes.

Leukocytosis   An abnormally high quantity of leukocytes in the circulating blood.

Leukopenia   An abnormally low quantity of mature leukocytes in the circulating blood.

"Liver flap"   See *Asterixis.*

Locus of control   An individual's perception of who or what controls his/her life events.
  External locus of control   The perception that luck, chance, fate, or powerful others control one's life events.
  Internal locus of control   The perception that one controls one's own life events.

Lumpectomy   A surgical procedure for breast tumors in which only the tumor and a small amount of surrounding tissue are removed.

Lymphedema   A postoperative pathological condition associated with mastectomy in which there is dysfunction of the lymph system in the arm on the side of the mastectomy; results in swelling, pain, inflammation, and possibly infection.

Lymph node   One of the accumulations of lymphoid tissue organized as lymphatic organs along the course of the lymphatic vessels. Their purpose is to filter and destroy invasive bacteria. Lymph nodes are the site or production of lymphocytes and certain antibodies.

Lymph node metastasis or "involvement"   Establishment of new tumor growth in a lymph node after a tumor cell has broken off from the primary tumor, gained access to the lymphatic system, has been carried as emboli directly to a lymph node, and arrested in the subcapsular sinus of the lymph node.

Lymphocyte   A leukocyte that arises in the reticular tissue of lymph nodes, generally described as non-granular.

Lymphocytosis   An abnormally high quantity of mature lymphocytes in the circulating blood.

Lymphoid tissue   Connective tissue with meshes that lodge lymphoid cells.

Lymphoma   A nodular or diffuse malignancy arising from lymphoid tissue and classified according to (1) cell type, (2) degree of differentiation, (3) type of reaction elicited by the tumor cells, and (4) pattern of growth.

Malignant   Cancerous; having the characteristics of anaplasia and disorderly, uncontrolled, chaotic pro-liferation.

Mammography   Roentgenography (X-ray) of the breast with or without injection of an opaque sub-stance into its ducts; used in early diagnosis of breast cancer.

Mastectomy   Surgical removal of a breast containing a malignant tumor.

Melanoma   Virulent malignant disease of the skin divided into three distinct groups: (1) lentigo malig-nant melanoma, (2) superficial melanoma, and (3) nodular melanoma.

Metaplasia   A reversible, benign change in which an adult cell changes from one type into another.

Metastasis   Secondary malignant lesions originating from the primary tumor but located in anatomically distant places.

Monocyte   The largest in size of the leukocytes, normally constituting 5%–10% of the leukocytes in the circulating blood.

Moribund   In a near-death condition.

Mucositis   Inflammation of mucous membranes, usually due to antineoplastic chemotherapy or head/neck irradiation, and which may include open lesions, infection, and necrosis in the gastrointestinal (and especially oral) mucous membranes.

Multiple myeloma   A diffuse malignancy characterized by abnormal proliferation of plasma cells, which are normally responsible for synthesis of immunoglobulins.

Myeloid tissue   Red bone marrow tissue.

Myeloma   See *Multiple Myeloma.*

Myelosuppression   A reduction in bone marrow function, resulting in a reduced release of erythrocytes, leukocytes, and platelets into the peripheral circulation and/or the release of immature (and therefore less-functional) cells into the circulating blood.

Nadir   The period of time when an antineoplastic drug has its most profound effects on the bone marrow.

Natural killer (NK) immunity   One of the three forms of immunological activity, but not mediated by either B- or T-cells. NK cells are probably a type of lymphocyte and seem to be stimulated by viral infections, possibly through production of interferon.

"Natural morphine"   Endogenous opiate-like hormones found in the central nervous system, the gas-trointestinal system, and plasma. They include enkephalins, endorphins, and serotonin; they mimic the action of morphine, including being nullified by naloxone (Narcan), a narcotic antagonist. Located in synapses between nerve fibers, they inhibit the release of Substance P, a peptide that transmits painful stimuli. The natural opiate-like hormones are found in reduced quantities in persons with chronic pain.

Neoplasia   "New growth." May be benign (e.g., common wart) or malignant (cancer).

Nerve block   Neurosurgery at the first level (peripheral) neurons for analgesia. Local anesthetics or neurolytic agents (e.g., alcohol, phenol, saline solution) are injected into a peripheral or sympathetic nerve in order to reduce or eradicate the nerve's capacity for transmission of pain messages. May also be used in spinal nerves. Analgesia is temporary.

Neurectomy   Neurosurgery at the first level (peripheral) neurons for analgesia, where a peripheral nerve is surgically cut. May cause loss of motor function as well as analgesia. Analgesia is temporary.

Neurosurgery at the third level (thalamic) neurons   Rarely performed resection of nerve roots in the thalamus and frontal lobe of the cortex for intractable pain. Analgesia is permanent.

Neutrophil   A medium-sized, mature form of leukocyte with small granules (therefore, part of the group of leukocytes collectively termed granulocytes), normally constituting 60%–70% of the leukocytes in the circulating blood.

Nitrogen balance   The state of the body in regard to the ingestion and excretion of protein.
 Positive nitrogen balance   The amount of nitrogen excreted is less than the quantity ingested; indicates adequate protein intake.
 Negative nitrogen balance   The amount of nitrogen excreted is greater than the quantity ingested; indicates protein depletion and malnutrition.

Nucleolus (pl. Nucleoli)   A round body rich in RNA within the nucleus of a cell.

Oat-cell carcinoma   An extremely virulent type of lung cancer associated with smoking; five-year survival rate approaches zero.

Oncogenic   Causing tumor formation.

Oncologist   A physician especially trained and educated in cancer treatment and certified to administer antineoplastic treatments, both FDA-approved and investigational.

Oncology   The scientific study of tumors.

Oncology nurse   A professional Registered Nurse especially trained and educated in oncology and the administration of antineoplastic treatments.

Opsonin   An antibody.

Opsonization   A specific antigen-antibody reaction in which the antibody prepares the foreign antigen so that it may be more easily destroyed by phagocytes.

Osteosarcoma   A malignant tumor arising from undifferentiated fibrous tissue of bone.

Pain trajectory   Pain pattern.

Pancreatic oncofetal antigen (POA)   A fetal protein thought to be a tumor marker strongly associated with pancreatic malignancies.

"Pap" smear   Papanicolaou Smear Test; a simple, painless test used to detect early cancer of the uterus and cervix, based on the phenomenon that malignant cells do not adhere well to one another and slough off easily into surrounding vaginal fluid or onto a swab.

Percutaneous cordotomy   Neurosurgery at the second level (spinal cord) neurons in which the spinothalamic tract within the spinal cord is cut. Results in temporary analgesia below the surgical site with preservation of sensory and motor control.

Phagocyte   Any cell, such as a polymorphonuclear leukocyte, that engulfs and destroys pathogenic microorganisms or harmful cells.

Phagocytosis   The engulfment and destruction of pathogenic or harmful cells by normal body cells.

Platelet   Also called a *thrombocyte*. The smallest of the formed elements in circulating blood, principally concerned with coagulation of blood and clot formation. Formed in the red bone marrow, they average 150,000 to 300,000 per cubic millimeter of blood.

Pleomorphic   Occurring in various distinct forms.

Prostate-specific antigen (PSA)   A highly specific tumor marker for prostate cancer.

Prostatic acid phosphatase (PAP)   An enzyme tumor marker classically associated with prostate cancer.

Proteolytic enzymes   Enzymes that break down proteins into simpler compounds.

Quadrantectomy   A partial mastectomy in which approximately one-fourth of the breast tissue, including the malignant lesion, is surgically removed.

Radiotherapy   The use of X-rays, radiation from radioactive substances, and other similar forms of radiant energy in the cytostatic treatment of cancer.
   External beam radiotherapy   Radiotherapy delivered by a machine external to the client's body, delivering a definite amount of radiation to a specific lesion in a dosage large enough to treat the lesion but not enough to permanently damage surrounding tissue.
   Internal beam radiotherapy   The use of radioactive needles, seeds, or other such implants to deliver radiation to a prescribed area of tissue.

Reed-Sternberg cells   A type of malignant cell characteristic of Hodgkin's disease.

Relapse   The return of signs, symptoms, and indications of proliferation and/or spread of a malignancy after remission has been achieved.

Remission   The abatement of signs and symptoms of a malignancy without indications of active spread or proliferation of malignant cells."Remission" is not synonymous with "cure."

Rhabdosarcoma   A sarcoma containing striated muscle fibers.

Rhizotomy   Neurosurgery at the first level (peripheral) neurons for analgesia, in which a spinal nerve root is cut at its entrance into the spinal cord. Produces analgesia in the body area innervated by the nerve root.

Sarcoma   A malignant solid tumor composed of tissues of mesodermal origin.

Sepsis   A morbid, serious pathological condition resulting from the presence of pathogenic bacteria and/or their toxic by-products.

Septicemia   The presence of bacteria and/or their toxins in the circulating blood.

Sequela(e)   A pathological condition following or occurring as a consequence of another condition or event.

Serotonin   A hormone that inhibits the activity of pain-transmitting neurons, among other functions.

Stage, staging   A method of classifying malignancies on the basis of the presence and extent of the tumor within the body; usually based on the TNM (tumor-nodes-metastases) system and is often not used for large-bowel tumors (see Dukes' Criteria).
   Stage I   Tumor mass limited to organ of origin. 70%–90% chance of survival.
   Stage II   Tumor shows evidence of local spread into surrounding tissue and first-station lymph nodes. 45%–55% chance of survival.
   Stage III   Tumor shows an extensive primary lesion with fixation to deeper structures. Lymph nodes positive for malignant invasion. 15%–25% chance of survival.
   Stage IV   Evidence of distant metastases beyond the primary lesion. Less than 5% chance of survival.

Stomatitis   Inflammation of the mucosa of the mouth and occasionally the rest of the gastrointestinal tract, usually because of antineoplastic chemotherapy and/or head/neck irradiation. The inflammation may proceed to open lesions in the mucosa, infection, and necrosis. See *Mucositis.*

Stressor   Any event—biological, personal, social, internal, or external—that comes into contact with an individual and that demands adaptation either by change in the internal environment or in the external environment. Stressors may be positive or negative in the perception of the individual, but the bio-psycho-social response may be identical.

Stupor   Partial or nearly complete unconsciousness; a state of lethargy and immobility with diminished responsiveness to stimulation.

Substance p   A neurological peptide that transmits painful, noxious stimuli.

Suffering   A subjective, emotional, evaluative response to pain and to fear of the unknown.

Sympathectomy   Neurosurgery at the first level (peripheral) neurons in which sympathetic ganglia are cut at various points along the sympathetic nerve fiber chain.

T-cell immunity   See *Cellular immunity.*

Tennessee antigen (TennaGen)   A glycoprotein tumor marker associated with colorectal cancer.

Teratogenetic   Causing fetal deformities. For example, a teratogenic drug given to a pregnant woman may produce spontaneous abortion or a defective infant.

Thanatology   The study of death and the dying process.

Thrombocyte   Platelet.

Thrombocytopenia   An abnormally low quantity of platelets in the circulating blood.

Thrombocytosis   An abnormally high quantity of platelets in the circulating blood.

Total parenteral nutrition   A method of administering all necessary nutrients to an individual by intravenous infusion. See *Hyperalimentation.*

Tractotomy   Neurosurgery at the second level (spinal cord) neurons in which the spinothalamic tract is severed in the mesencephalon. Performed by occipital craniotomy and has a high mortality rate.

Transcutaneous electrical nerve stimulation (TENS)   A nonpharmaceutical analgesic method utilizing the stimulation of large-diameter nerve fibers by low-dosage electricity.

Treatment protocol   A specific method of treatment of a disease, usually including the pattern of drug administration, drug dosage, laboratory monitoring, clinical examination requirements, and so on.

Tumoricidal   Destructive to malignant cells.

Tumor burden   The ratio of the quantity of tumor cells to the quantity of normal cells in a person's body.

Tumor marker   Specific bodily substances that seem to indicate tumor progression or regression.

Undifferentiated cells   Cells that have lost the capacity for specialized functions.

Vesicant   An intravenous drug that causes severe irritation to surrounding tissues if it extravasates.

Vinca alkaloid antineoplastic drugs   Anticancer drugs derived from the periwinkle plant. They probably act by inhibiting the construction of the protein structure necessary for the segregation of DNA into two separate groupings.

Wilms' tumor   A virulent sarcoma of the kidney, comprised of embryonal tissue and occurring chiefly in children under the age of five.

Zinc glycinate marker (ZMG)   A tissue-associated antigen thought to be a tumor marker associated with gastrointestinal malignancies.

Index

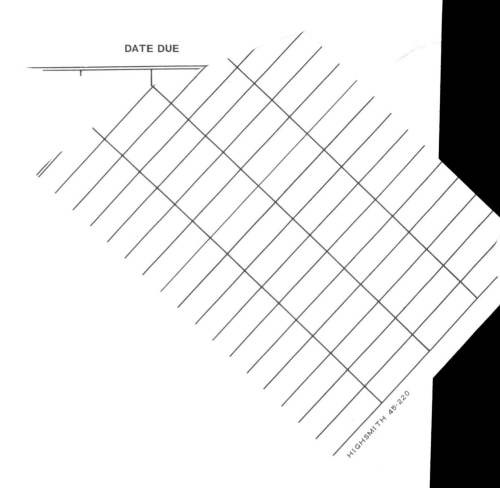